PHARMAC... FO

The first year's proceeds from sales of this text will be donated to The Bays' Project, Swansea and the money will go towards supporting their work with homeless mothers and babies.

Pharmacology for Midwives

The Evidence Base for Safe Practice

Sue Jordan MB, BCh, PhD, PGCE (FE)

Editorial Advisors

Kate Isherwood RGN, RM, ADM
Fiona Murphy RGN, BN, MSc, PGCE
Vicky Whittaker BA, PGCEA, ADM, H.V.Cert.,
R.M., RGN, PGDM

palgrave

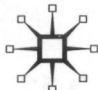
First published 2002 by
PALGRAVE
Houndmills, Basingstoke, Hampshire RG21 6XS and
175 Fifth Avenue, New York, N.Y. 10010
Companies and representatives throughout the world

PALGRAVE is the new global academic imprint of
St. Martin's Press LLC Scholarly and Reference Division and
Palgrave Publishers Ltd (formerly Macmillan Press Ltd).

ISBN 0–333–97138–8 hardback
ISBN 0–333–69396–5 paperback

This book is printed on paper suitable for recycling and made
from fully managed and sustained forest sources.

A catalogue record for this book is available
from the British Library.

10 9 8 7 6 5 4 3 2
11 10 09 08 07 06 05 04 03 02

Printed and bound in Great Britain by
Creative, Print and Design (Wales), Ebbw Vale

My family

Contents

List of Implications for Practice

List of Figures

List of Tables

List of Boxes

Preface

Midwives have an increasingly important role in the management of drugs during pregnancy, labour and the postnatal period. Their responsibilities include: drug administration; monitoring the woman, fetus and neonate for adverse effects; and prescribing specified drugs under locally agreed protocols. In addition, they are a primary source of client education, providing women with information and advice on drug use, for example pain relief in labour and management of the third stage of labour. It is essential, therefore, that midwives understand the actions, side effects, cautions and contra-indications of the drugs used in pregnancy and childbirth (UKCC, 1992).

Traditionally, midwifery practice has been primarily concerned with caring for healthy, 'low risk' women during normal childbirth. However, in recent years increasing numbers of women with pre-existing medical conditions and serious complications of pregnancy are achieving successful pregnancy outcomes under medical and midwifery care. This means that midwives will be involved in the administration of an increasing number of drugs to a client group whose conditions necessitate close monitoring.

Midwifery practice is dynamic, constantly evolving in response to internal and external pressures. Changing socio-economic conditions, government policy and developments in medical technology have all impacted on maternity service provision. In addition, tensions within the midwifery profession have produced complementary and co-existing paradigms. On the one hand, midwives working in consultant units are closely involved in the medical management of labour and may assume many of the functions previously undertaken by junior doctors. In contrast, government policy and consumer pressure support the establishment of team midwifery and caseload practice, with the midwife rather than the doctor undertaking the role of lead professional in the provision of maternity care. Across this continuum runs an acknowledgement of the increased responsibility and autonomy of midwifery practice which is pertinent to the administration of drugs.

The tragedy of thalidomide in the 1960s highlighted the potential for iatrogenic morbidity. The response of the pharmaceutical industry has been to recommend caution when administering drugs to pregnant or breastfeeding women. For both ethical and practical reasons, research, particularly randomized controlled trials, is very difficult, if not impossible, in women who are pregnant or breastfeeding. Therefore, much drug administration is based on custom and practice rather than research evidence. These uncertainties surrounding pharmacological research and knowledge, together with increased

public awareness and burgeoning professional concern, make drug administration a very difficult aspect of the midwife's role.

This book will review the available literature on drugs commonly prescribed
during pregnancy, labour and the puerperium, highlighting problems frequently experienced as well as indicating others that may be encountered only
occasionally. The aim of this text is to enable the midwife to discharge her
statutory responsibilities effectively in respect of drug administration and
monitoring.

Sue Jordan
Professor Dame June Clark
Professor Anne Williams
Vicky Whittaker
Kate Isherwood
Fiona Murphy

Acknowledgements

Sue Jordan wishes to thank: Chris Ruby, midwifery lecturer for help with the early stages of the book; Alison Schooler, midwfery lecturer, Sue Philpin, nurse lecturer, for help with final drafts; Stephen Storey, librarian, Helen Myfannwy McAteer, co-ordinator midwifery education, and Karen Davies, Diane Mort, programme managers for support with the project.

The authors and the publishers are also grateful to the following for their kind permission to use the copyright material listed beneath:

Oxford University Press for Figure 1.1, adapted from Grahame-Smith and Aronson: *The Oxford Textbook of Clinical Pharmacology and Drug Therapy* (1985).

The McGraw-Hill Companies for Figure 1.4, adapted from Hardman et al: *Goodman and Gilman: The Pharmacological Basis of Therapeutics,* 9th edition (1996).

Professor S. C. Hughes at the Department of Anesthesia, San Francisco General Hospital for Figure 4.3, adapted from Hughes: Analgesia methods during labour and delivery; *Canadian Journal of Anesthetics* 39:5 (1992).

Every effort has been made to trace all the copyright holders, but if any have been inadvertently overlooked the publishers will be pleased to make the necessary arrangements at the first opportunity.

List of Abbreviations

ACE	*Angiotensin converting enzyme*
ADH	*Anti-diuretic hormone*
BP	*Blood pressure*
	Britsh Pharmacopoeia
CESDI	*Confidential Enquiry into Stillbirths and Deaths in Infancy*
CNS	*Central nervous system*
CSE	*Combined spinal epidural*
CVS	*Cardiovascular system*
DoH	*Department of Health*
DVT	*Deep vein thrombosis*
ECG	*Electrocardiograph*
ECT	*Electro-convulsive therapy*
EEG	*Electro-encephalograph*
FEV_1	*Forced Expiratory Volume in 1 second*
FVC	*Forced Vital Capacity*
HELLP	*Haemolysis, Elevated Liver Enzymes, Low Platelets*
HR	*Heart rate*
IUGR	*Intrauterine growth retardation*
LFTs	*Liver function tests*
MAOI	*Monoamine-oxidasse inhibitors*
MCHRC	*Maternal and Child Health Research Consortium (CESDI authors)*
MI	*Myocardial infarction*
mOsm/kg	*milli-osmoles per kilogram*
NSAIDs	*Non-steroidal anti-inflammatory drugs*
OTC	*Over the counter (drugs sold by a pharmacist)*
PE	*Pulmonary embolus*
PEFR	*Peak Expiratory Flow Rate*
pO_2	*partial pressure of oxygen (effectively the concentration of oxygen)*
pCO_2	*partial pressure of carbon dioxide (effectively the concentration of carbon dioxide)*
SIADH	*syndrome inappropriate ADH (excessive secretion of ADH)*
TFTs	*Thyroid function tests*
UTI	*Urinary tract infection*
im	*intramuscular*
iv	*intravenous*
sc	*subcutaneous*

Notes on dosage abbreviations

1000 nanograms (ng) = 1 microgram (μg)
1000 micrograms   = 1 milligram (mg)
1000 milligrams   = 1 gram (g)

Micrograms and nanograms should not be abbreviated as confusion is likely to arise (BNF, 2000).

Quantities less than 1 gram should be written as milligrams.
Quantities less than 1 milligram should be written as micrograms.

> For example 500 mg is better than 0.5 g
> 500 micrograms is better than 0.5 mg
> This minimizes the use of the decimal point, which is easily misread.

List of Contributors

Maria Andrade School of Health Science, University of Wales, Swansea, Wales

Nick Clerk University Hospital of Wales, Heath Park, Cardiff, Wales

Cheryl Davies The Pharmacy, Singleton Hospital, Swansea, Wales

Simon Emery Singleton Hospital, Swansea, Wales

Richard Griffith School of Health Science, University of Wales, Swansea, Wales

Billy Hardy UKCP Registered Family Therapist with The Family Institute, Cardiff, Wales

Bronwen Hegarty Nursing and Midwifery Department, Otago Polytechnic, New Zealand

Kate Isherwood Community Midwife, Withybush Hospital, Haverfordwest, Wales

Sue Jordan School of Health Science, University of Wales, Swansea, Wales

Fiona Murphy School of Health Science, University of Wales, Swansea, Wales

Yamni Nigam School of Health Science, University of Wales, Swansea, Wales

Rena McOwat School of Health Science, University of Wales, Swansea, Wales

Scott Pegler The Pharmacy, Singleton Hospital, Swansea, Wales

Mike Tait School of Health Science, University of Wales, Swansea, Wales

Vicky Whittaker School of Health Science, University of Wales, Swansea, Wales

Using this Book

This book aims to provide midwives with an understanding of the principles of drug actions as well as useful references and some clinical guidelines.

In several chapters, in order to explain drug actions and side effects, we have been encouraged to offer readers an explanation of the underlying physiology and pathophysiology. We hope that readers will find these sections informative as few books for midwives discuss common disorders such as asthma, diabetes, epilepsy and mental illness, which all occur in at least 1 per cent of the UK population. Where our explanations are incomplete the comprehensive referencing of the text offers readers signposts to further reading.

For a variety of reasons, including practical considerations, this book has been limited to drugs commonly prescribed during pregnancy. We have therefore been unable to include: drugs used largely for recreational purposes such as alcohol and tobacco; drugs sold as 'herbal remedies'; drugs prescribed by specialists in unusual circumstances such as the management of cancer or arthritis in women who are pregnant.

In the UK, practitioners rely heavily on the *British National Formulary* (BNF) and this is reflected in the text. Implementation of an EEC directive (92/27) has involved name changes for several drugs; to accommodate these changes, some drugs have been dual named. A glossary of terms is appended to the book.

Features of this Book

Implications for practice

The tables summarize and highlight the links between pharmacology and clinical practice for the most commonly used drugs. As far as possible they have been adapted from published guidelines, which are referenced in the text. They aim to provide the busy practitioner with an easily accessed practice checklist or guideline.

Practice points

Over three hundred practice points are provided throughout the text. These sections are designed to provide an immediate link to practice so that the relevance of the text is not lost to the reader.

Case reports

The core sections of the book contain illustrative case reports, instances where pharmacology could have been applied to practice to influence the outcome for an individual woman.

Quick reference for major drugs

Appendix 1 provides a summary of: uses, side effects cautions and interactions for the most commonly used drugs. This is intended not only to highlight common problems but also to provide a reference point for those seeking information on rarer conditions and drug interactions.

PART I

INTRODUCTION TO PHARMACOLOGY

The administration of medicines is always undertaken with due regard for the relevant bioscience principles, evidence base and legal considerations. This first part of the book outlines these issues in relation to current midwifery practice.

CHAPTER 1

Principles of Pharmacology

SUE JORDAN

This chapter sets the scene by describing the state of the evidence base in midwifery pharmacology; it continues with an account of pharmacological principles, terms and definitions as they relate to midwifery practice.

Chapter Contents

▦ The evidence base for pharmacological interventions

▦ Drug therapy

▦ Conclusion

Pharmacology is the science dealing with the interactions between a living system and chemicals introduced from outside the system. *A drug may be defined* as any small molecule that, when introduced into the body, alters body function by interactions at molecular level.

The evidence base for pharmacological interventions

All treatments and their effects are multidimensional. When assessing the contribution made by drugs to health care, we could consider the available evidence under the headings:

- magical/placebo and nocebo effects [glossary]
- empirical evidence
- rational/scientific evidence

Magical

The *'power of the placebo'* should not be underestimated (Beecher & Boston, 1955; Turner et al, 1994). The non-specific effects of treatment (placebo/nocebo) interact, probably at a biological level, with disease, therapeutic interventions and psychosocial factors. It is important to separate the results of the placebo effect from other treatment effects and the natural course of the condition or disease.

Empirical

Many remedies or treatments are given on an *empirical* or 'trial and error' basis, as they have been for thousands of years. For example, salicylates, as willow bark or aspirin, have long been used to relieve the symptoms of headache. Many of the questions about why drugs work or do not work are still unanswered.

Monitoring for the side effects of drugs is based on empirical evidence. For example, on administering a drug known to lower blood pressure (BP), such as nifedipine or bupivacaine, it would seem sensible to monitor blood pressure at regular intervals. Using case study data, the author's research has demonstrated how this approach can contribute to care (Jordan & Torrance, 1995; Jordan, 1998). However, there are no randomized controlled trials demonstrating the advantages of monitoring orthostatic hypotension. Despite the absence of controlled trials indicating the value of monitoring patients for side effects, we believe this to be an important aspect of patient care.

Rational or scientific

The 'gold standard' in scientific research methods is the *randomized controlled trial* (RCT); all other research methods are compared to this. However, it is important that controlled trials have sufficient numbers of subjects to demonstrate an effect, that is they are not underpowered (Anthony, 1999). Practice based on the results of RCTs can claim to be evidence-based. Medicine's stated goal is for practice to be based on rational, scientific evidence, largely derived from meta-analyses of the findings of RCTs (EBM Working Group, 1992). In some areas, this has been achieved and research is ongoing.

Example
The value of metronidazole plus erythromycin mid-trimester has become clearer following the RCT conducted by Hauth et al (1995). From this study, it would appear that this antibiotic combination is effective in reducing the incidence of pre-term delivery only in women with bacterial vaginosis with a risk factor for pre-term delivery, and further studies are in progress.

Several initiatives are underway to assist the transfer of research findings to clinical practice: for example the Cochrane Centre's Pregnancy and Childbirth database in Oxford, the NHS Centre for Reviews and Dissemination at the University of York (Welsh Office, 1996; NHS Executive, 1998). The success of the clinical effectiveness initiative depends on keeping practitioners informed of research developments.

The use of many drugs is based on the evidence of RCTs, and practice evolves and beliefs change as the evidence emerges (Jones et al, 1998).

Example

Although we have been aware of the potential benefits of magnesium sulphate infusions in eclampsia, and have been teaching this for several years, until recently clinicians have been deterred from its use by the difficulties of measuring serum magnesium levels and the consequent dangers of respiratory arrest. While the experience with magnesium infusions in coronary care has reassured us of the safety of this procedure, the significant development which has led to the widespread adoption of magnesium sulphate in eclampsia has been the RCT involving 1687 women with eclampsia (Eclampsia Trial Collaborative Group, 1995). Significantly fewer convulsions occurred in women treated with magnesium sulphate than either diazepam or phenytoin; the use of phenytoin was associated with significantly more adverse outcomes in women and infants.

While the literature contains examples of clinicians ignoring the results of scientific research (for example Mather et al, 1976), in the current climate of research-based practice and clinical effectiveness, the RCT is likely to displace the case report as the currency of clinical communication (Hunter, 1991; Jordan, 1997).

The evidence base in practice

The library searches for this book have revealed the dearth of research evidence on which practice is based. For example: in midwifery, for the last four decades, we have faced an epidemic of bottle feeding. In a small study (n = 127), the onset of lactation was delayed by at least 13 hours if medication was administered during labour (Hildebrandt, 1999). However, the impact on breastfeeding of many commonly prescribed medications, such as prochlorperazine and ergometrine, is unknown. To address such issues, we shall require research funding and funding bodies sympathetic to the interests of women and children rather than pharmaceutical companies.

Unfortunately to date, women's issues in therapeutics have often been neglected by the medical and pharmaceutical research community (Jordan and Hughes, 1996). It is therefore unsurprising that the nascent disciplines of nursing and midwifery pharmacology have been unable to conduct large scale studies. The reluctance of funding bodies to support trials of medication

monitoring means that the guidelines suggested are often based on bioscience principles, empirical evidence and case data. Nevertheless, it is hoped that by supplying busy practitioners with this information they will be better placed to inform clients, thus empowering women in making what can be difficult decisions, both in normal childbirth and in situations where women's needs are rather more specialized.

Drug therapy

The interactions between the drug and the person receiving it can be divided into four stages:

- Getting the drug into the body – pharmaceuticals
- Getting the drug around, about and out of the body – pharmacokinetics
- Actions of the drug on the body – pharmacodynamics
- Effects of the drug on the person – therapeutics

Pharmaceuticals: getting the drug into the body

Two issues are considered here:

- compliance
- drug formulation

Compliance

Compliance or concordance with medication is the extent to which clients adhere to prescribed regimens and the associated professional advice. Although studies on compliance give conflicting results, it is estimated that up to 40 per cent of patients make major errors in compliance and only 1–5 per cent comply exactly. Interviews by professionals are generally unsuccessful at detecting non-compliance (Sackett et al, 1991).

Factors associated with non-compliance include:

Women in pregnancy who consider themselves to be healthy
Fear of harming the unborn child
Living alone
Taking more than three drugs
More than two drug administrations per day
Reduced oesophageal motility, for example dehydration

Drug formulation

The storage requirements of each preparation depend on the formulation. Therefore, the data sheet for each product and brand should be consulted for instructions on storage.

Packing chemicals

All tablets and medicines sold or administered contain specified active ingredients plus other 'packing' chemicals, which may be there to stabilize the active ingredient or modify its release into the body. The 'packing' chemicals for any drug may differ between brands. We cannot always assume that different brands of any one drug are bioequivalent [glossary]. Important examples include: antiepileptic drugs, lithium preparations, antipsychotic medications. Because different brands of these drugs are not bioequivalent, they cannot be interchanged without consulting the prescriber.

The 'packing' chemical in a tablet can have clinical effects. For example some preparations contain sodium or potassium ions. This is important if a patient is on a salt-restricted diet.

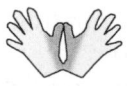 **Practice Point**

The sodium content of many antacid indigestion remedies may be enough to precipitate fluid retention and pulmonary oedema in pregnancy or in people with mild heart failure.

Liquids and solids

The formulation of a drug affects its *rate of absorption*.

Before being absorbed, all tablets must disintegrate and the active ingredients must dissolve. The rate at which this occurs depends on the drug formulation, particularly the size of the particles in the tablet or capsule. For example, the liquid form of a drug will be absorbed more rapidly and completely than a solid tablet. This can be of clinical importance: for example paracetamol given as a liquid acts more rapidly than when given as a tablet.

Pharmacokinetics: how the body handles the drug

This section addresses the questions:

- Is the drug getting to the desired site of action? (absorption and distribution)
- Is the drug getting out of the body? (elimination)
- Is there a risk of accumulation and toxicity?

The actions and side effects of any drug depend on the concentration of the drug in the tissues.

Therapeutic range

Every drug has a *therapeutic range* or a desirable range for the concentration of drug in plasma. Above the therapeutic range, toxic effects may appear. Below the therapeutic range, the drug does not have the desired effect. (see Fig. 1.1) For some drugs this range is very narrow, and the therapeutic concentration is very close to the concentration at which adverse effects appear, for example lithium, digoxin, anti-epileptics, warfarin, insulin. Therefore, people receiving these drugs must be monitored closely. For some drugs, such as phenytoin and gentamicin, the plasma concentrations are measured regularly. However for most drugs the therapeutic effects are assessed more directly by patient observation: for example insulin regimens are monitored by measurement of blood glucose concentrations. For other drugs, the therapeutic range is wide in most individuals, and there is a larger 'safety margin' between therapeutic dose and toxic dose. For example in people not suffering from epilepsy, penicillins and folic acid are relatively safe, even in overdose.

The concentration of any drug in the plasma and tissues depends on the way the drug is treated by the body. The body handles all drugs in three stages (see Fig. 1.2):

- Absorption
- Distribution
- Elimination

These process are affected to some extent by pregnancy. The clinical significance of these changes is greatest for women taking regular anti-epileptic therapy (see Chapter 19).

Absorption

Absorption is the process by which a drug is made available to the body fluids for distribution. The absorption of a drug will depend on: the route of administration (see Box 1.1), formulation (see above) and the way the drug molecules move across cell membranes throughout the body.

In this example, the drug is scheduled to be administered four times per day or every six hours. If this is done strictly, for example at 6.00 am, 12 noon, 6.00 pm and midnight, although the concentrations fluctuate, they remain within the therapeutic range. This is illustrated:

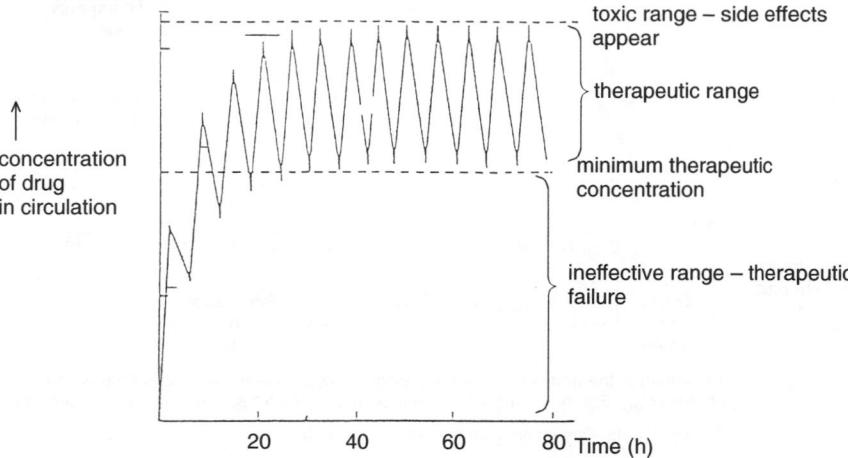

However, if the ward is busy, the dosing may be rescheduled to accommodate other tasks, with the result that the drug is administered at 10.00 am, 2.00 pm, 6.00 pm and 10.00 pm. Therefore, the concentrations fluctuate wildly. At times the drug is below the minimum therapeutic concentration and ineffective, but at other times it causes toxicity, as illustrated:

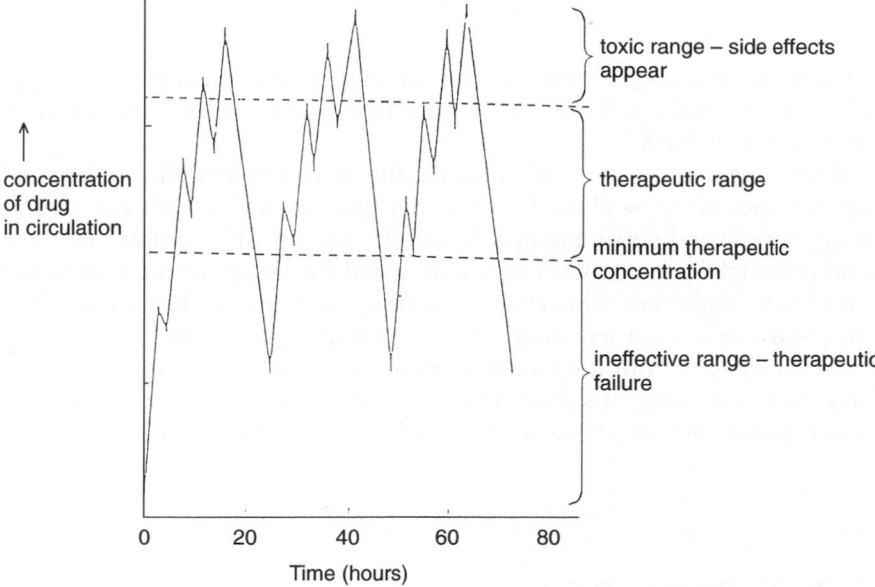

Figure 1.1 'Peaks and troughs' of Bolus Dose administration
Source: Adapted from Grahame-Smith, P. & Aronson, J.K. (1985)
The Oxford Textbook of Clinical Pharmacology and
Drug Therapy, Oxford University Press.

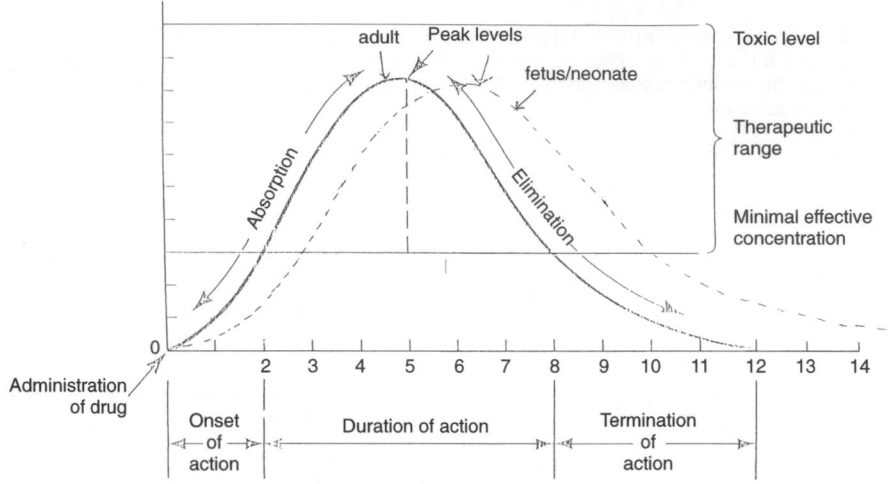

Absorption of the drug into the fetus may be delayed unless the drug is administered intravenously. For most drugs, the elimination from the fetus or neonate will be delayed.

----- represents elimination from the fetus or neonate

Figure 1.2   Changes in plasma concentration of a drug following a single dose
Source: Adapted from McKenry & Salerno (1995).

Important barriers to drug absorption and distribution include: the gut wall, capillary walls, cell membranes, the blood/brain barrier, the placenta, the blood/milk barrier.

Most drugs are given orally because this is convenient. All tablets and capsules should be swallowed with a full glass of water, with the patient sitting upright and remaining upright for 30 minutes. This ensures that there is no prolonged contact between the drug and the linings of the mouth and oesophagus, which are vulnerable to corrosive substances such as aspirin, iron and potassium salts. A few drugs, including aspirin and alcohol, are partially absorbed straight from the stomach; most others are passed into the small intestine before being absorbed. Pain, particularly migraine and labour pain, reduce gastric motility, delaying the absorption of oral medications.

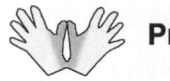 **Practice Point**

It is important that migraine sufferers take analgesia at the first warning of an attack. During a migraine attack, analgesics such as paracetamol and anti-emetics such as metoclopramide can not be absorbed efficiently because they are not passed into the small intestine. Under these circumstances, liquid paracetamol can be useful.

Box 1.1   Routes of drug administration

Oral administration. Several factors need to be considered:

STATE OF THE STOMACH:
   presence of food
   motility of the stomach, for example altered by pain, pregnancy, labour
   pH of the stomach for a few drugs, for example aspirin, iron

MALABSORPTION

METABOLISM BY THE LIVER

Sublingual (under the tongue) administration is sometimes used for a rapid action. Venous blood from this area enters the systemic circulation, not the hepatic portal vein, and therefore bypasses the liver.

Rectal administration partly bypasses the liver, for example diclofenac suppositaries (Voltarol ®).

Intramuscular injection causes pain and gives erratic absorption.
   Only low volumes of drugs of neutral pH can be administered this way.
   Absorption depends upon site and the state of the circulation, and the temperature of the muscle (see Rodger & King, 2000).
   Long term depot injections are administered this way, for example medroxyprogesterone acetate (Depo-Provera), anti-psychotic agents.

Subcutaneous administration is affected by blood flow, exercise and site of injection but is less painful than intramuscular injection (Chapter 17 insulin). Absorption is usually slower than intramuscular administration.

Intravenous injection or infusion brings the drug straight into the circulation, for example magnesium sulphate (Chapter 9).
   The drug's action is rapid and not disturbed by other factors such as circulatory shock. Intravenous injections are given slowly to minimize side effects.

Spinal or *epidural* administration (Chapter 4).

Inhalation is used to treat asthma and for administration of anaesthetics.

Eye drops. These are absorbed into the nose and swallowed, causing side effects.

Other topical applications, for example prostaglandins per vaginam.

   Systemic side effects may result from all routes of application.

The presence of food in the stomach influences the absorption of many drugs, such as iron (Chapter 11), antimicrobial agents (Chapter 14) and nifedipine (Chapter 7). The presence of food in the stomach may reduce the nausea associated with some drugs such as iron and aspirin. The absorption of some drugs is increased by gastric acidity.

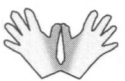 **Practice Point**

Iron is best absorbed in its ferrous form. However, this is converted to the less soluble ferric form if the gastro-intestinal contents are not sufficiently acid. To prevent this, pregnant women are advised to take any iron tablets with vitamin C, for example with orange or tomato juice. Any iron taken with antacid preparations will not be absorbed.

The decline in gastro-intestinal motility associated with pregnancy (due to increased progesterone and decreased motilin) delays the absorption of certain drugs from the gastro-intestinal tract. This may reduce the efficacy of anti-epileptics (see Chapter 19). During pregnancy, the peripheral circulation is dilated which may enhance the absorption of drugs given by subcutaneous or intramuscular injections. Women with diabetes should be alerted to the added risks of hypoglycaemia in early pregnancy (Carlson & Byington, 1998) (see Chapter 17).

Distribution

Distribution is the movement of the drug around the body. It is affected by:

1. plasma protein binding;
2. the lipid solubility of the drug (that is whether it dissolves in fatty tissues);
3. the binding properties of the drug;
4. blood flow to the organs and the state of the circulation;
5. stage of life cycle, for example pregnancy, infancy;
6. disease state, for example pre-eclampsia or heart failure.

Plasma proteins

Drugs are bound to the plasma proteins to a varying extent. Some drugs (for example warfarin, nifedipine, tricyclic antidepressants), some hormones and bilirubin circulate largely bound to plasma proteins, particularly albumins. Normally the free and bound forms are in equilibrium or a state of balance. Only the free drug is biologically active. The bound drug acts as a storage reservoir. The availability of protein for binding is reduced in pregnancy, neonates, malnutrition and extensive burns. This increases the effects, and side effects, of some drugs such as anti-epileptics. Protein binding is a source of drug interactions. Some drugs, for example aspirin, displace bilirubin from its binding sites on plasma albumins.

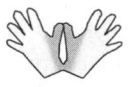 **Practice Point**

Aspirin should not be administered to neonates or nursing mothers because the displaced bilirubin may cause jaundice and kernicterus in the infant.

Lipid solubility

This is the extent to which the drug dissolves in the body's fatty tissues. It is possible to visualize the body as chemically composed of fluid compartments plus fatty tissues. Most drugs arc spread throughout the body's fluid compartments and pass into the fatty tissues to a greater or lesser extent. Because of its high myelin content the brain can be regarded as a fatty tissue. The extent to which the drug spreads throughout the body is referred to as the *volume of distribution*.

Examples

The benzodiazepines (for example diazepam, temazepam) have a high volume of distribution and pass into all fatty tissue. When these drugs are discontinued, the effects of withdrawal are prolonged for many people. This is attributed to the drugs dissolving extensively in the fat and passing out into the circulation gradually over time.

When an anaesthetic gas such as nitrous oxide is administered, it will dissolve to some extent in fatty tissues. In women with generous deposits of adipose tissues, more of the gas will enter the body fat, leaving less in the circulation. Therefore, such women will require a larger dose to achieve the desired analgesic effect. Also, when the inhalation is discontinued, they will take longer to recover since the drug, which has passed into the body fat, will take time to clear (see Chapter 4).

Binding characteristics

A few drugs have unusual binding characteristics. For example, tetracyclines bind to growing bones and teeth and can not be given to anyone who is growing, pregnant or breastfeeding. The antimalarial chloroquine can bind to the retina of an adult or fetus. A high dose can cause retinal damage. Pregnant women should seek specialist advice regarding travel to countries where malaria is endemic.

Blood flow to the tissues

Some tissues receive a better blood supply than others; for example the blood flow to the brain is much higher than that to bone. The local and general state of the circulation determines the distribution of drugs. In shock [glossary], the distribution of the circulation and any drugs administered is impaired. Drugs administered orally, subcutaneously or intramuscularly may not be absorbed adequately. The circulation is preferentially redistributed to the heart, brain and lungs. Therefore any drug administered will be circulated into these organs, bypassing others. Because the volume of the circulation is restricted, the drugs will be at a high concentration in the tissues they do reach. This can be critical when administering drugs with a narrow safety margin such as magnesium sulphate (Chapter 9).

Neonates

The body of the neonate contains a relatively high proportion of water and a low proportion of fat. Any fat soluble drugs are therefore distributed into a small volume. For example vitamin K is administered to neonates in its fat soluble form. The relatively low body fat content of neonates limits its distribution. Any water soluble drugs will be diluted over a relatively larger body volume. This means that neonates, particularly premature babies, receive different drug doses from adults, even when body weight is taken into consideration.

Example
Naloxone (Narcan ®) is given to neonates in a dose of 10 micrograms/kg, (subcutaneous, intramuscular or intravenous injection) repeated every two–three minutes as necessary, whereas the corresponding adult dose is 1.5–3 micrograms/kg (BNF, 2000).

The blood/brain barrier is not fully developed in the neonate. Therefore drugs taken in with breast milk may enter the brain with relative ease while remaining undetectable in the blood. This is particularly relevant for mothers taking drugs for mental illness who wish to breastfeed (see Chapter 16, mental health drugs).

Pregnancy and lactation

With the exception of anti-epileptics, the main practical considerations are the introduction of extra body compartments: the developing fetus and breast milk. The placenta is not an effective barrier to the passage of drugs. Most drugs are lipid soluble and therefore cross the placenta. However not all drugs are harmful to the developing fetus in all cases. Estimates vary as to the incidence of teratogenesis: 2–26 per cent with phenytoin, 10–33 per cent with warfarin, 1–10 per cent with sodium valproate (Rubin, 1995). It should be remembered that 2–4 per cent of all neonates have some congenital abnormalities. As the placenta thins towards the end of pregnancy, the amount of drug reaching the fetus increases. The infant may be born experiencing drug side effects and withdrawal syndromes, most of which are potentially dangerous. Where the midwife has been able to obtain a history of drug use or misuse, she should advise hospital delivery and alert the neonatalogists (see Table 1.1). Most drugs pass into breast milk, but the concentrations are sometimes too small to be harmful (see Table 1.2). The content and composition of breast milk can also be affected by the mother's diet and any exposure to environmental toxins such as weed killers.

Disease state of the patient

Renal or hepatic failure will impair the body's ability to eliminate most drugs (for example eclampsia or severe pre-eclampsia). Drugs will also accumulate in the body if the woman or neonate is dehydrated. If the drug accumulates, side effects will intensify. Other conditions affecting drug distribution include: heart failure, shock, thyroid disease, gastro-intestinal disease.

Elimination or clearance

The route of elimination varies with individual drugs. Some drugs are eliminated unchanged whereas others are extensively metabolized. Most drugs are excreted via the kidneys, although the bile is also an important route of excretion. Many drugs are passed into breast milk. Alcohol is unusual in that 5–10 per cent is eliminated unchanged via the lungs, sweat and urine. For most drugs, elimination involves metabolism in the liver plus excretion by the kidneys.

Drug metabolism

Most metabolism takes place in the liver, but the gastro-intestinal tract and the central nervous system (CNS) contain enzymes responsible for the metabolism of some drugs. These metabolic processes allow the body to deal with and detoxify foreign substances. All drugs given orally must pass through the liver to reach the circulation. Drugs administered by other routes reach the liver after passing round the general circulation. Metabolism in the liver occurs in two stages: (1) The products of digestion are transformed by metabolism or detoxification; (2) The metabolites are then rendered soluble in water (by conjugation, [glossary]) so that they can be excreted via the kidneys. Both

Table 1.1   Some drugs known to be potentially harmful to the fetus
For a more complete list, the midwife should refer to the current BNF, and consult the manufacturers if uncertainty persists. Further examples are given in the relevant chapters

Drug	Potential problem
ACE inhibitors, e.g. enalapril, captopril	Renal damage, skull defects, olighydramnios.
Alcohol (including some cough remedies)	Fetal alcohol syndrome, poor growth and learning disabilities. Withdrawal syndrome in neonates.
Amitriptyline	Neonatal irritability.
Amphetamines ('Ecstasy' is an amphetamine)	Irritability and poor feeding. Tachycardia. Cardiovascular and musculoskeletal malformations.
Anabolic steroids	Masculinization of female fetus. Adrenal suppression (see Chapter 15).
Antihistamines	Manufacturers advise to avoid on the basis of animal studies.
Antimalarials SPECIALIST ADVICE MANDATORY	Some risks of congenital abnormalities. Extra folate supplements may be recommended.
*Antipsychotics (see Chapter 16)	Central nervous system may be affected.
Aspirin, non-steroidal anti-inflammatory drugs	Possible intrauterine growth retardation, bleeding complications. Delayed labour.
Barbiturates	Risk of congenital abnormalities. Vitamin K deficiency and bleeding. Dangerous withdrawal syndrome in neonates.
Benzodiazepines	Possibility of facial clefts, cardiac anomalies, microcephaly. Respiratory depression or withdrawal syndrome in neonate.
Beta blockers	Intrauterine growth retardation, neonatal hypoglycaemia.
Buspirone (for anxiety)	Teratogenic in animals. Manufacturer advises to avoid.
*Cancer chemotherapy and radiotherapy	Risk of miscarriage, growth delay.
Carbenoxolone, in mouthwashes and gels (Bioplex mouthwash®, Bioral gel®) and liquorice	Fluid retention and oedema. Avoid.
Chloral hydrate	This acts like alcohol.
Chlorpromazine	Possible ocular damage. Hypotension during labour.
Cimetidine, ranitidine, misoprostol	Theoretical risk of miscarriage, manufacturers advise to avoid. Congenital facial paralysis and vascular disruption with misoprostol.
Cocaine	Intrauterine growth retardation, congenital malformations of bones, eyes or heart. Abrupt withdrawal causes premature labour.
Danazol	Masculinization of the neonate
Diuretics furosemide (frusemide) thiazides	Hypoperfusion of placenta and sudden death. Thrombocytopenia, electrolyte disturbances.
Ephedrine, in 'cold cures' OTC[+]	Possible link to club foot. Fetal tachycardia.

Table 1.1 (Cont'd)

Drug	Potential problem
General anaesthetics, mainly staff exposure	Small increase in miscarriage and anomalies.
*Gold salts, for rheumatoid arthritis	Teratogenic in animal studies.
Ibuprofen, indometacin	Possible *in utero* constriction of ductus arteriosus, and lung damage. Delayed labour.
Imipramine, other tricyclic antidepressants	Irritability and muscle spasms in neonate.
Iodine, topical povidone iodine, anti-thyroid agents (amiodarone is an important source of iodine)	Neonatal goitre and hypothyroidism.
*Lithium	Possibility of cardiac abnormalities. Detailed ultrasound investigations recommended. Risks of toxicity in neonates.
Live vaccines MMR smallpox vaccine	Fetal infections. Fetal death.
Mineral oils (as laxatives)	Vitamin deficiencies, particularly K.
Nicotine	Intrauterine growth retardation.
Opioids	Possibility of respiratory or gastro-intestinal defects. Withdrawal syndrome in neonates after regular use.
Oral contraceptives	Risk of cardiovascular abnormalities, In first trimester, not supported by epidemiological studies.
Oral hypoglycaemics	Poor glycaemic control.
Paracetamol	Possible association with hip dislocation, club foot. Considered safe at usual doses.
Quinine (in tonic water, for cramps)	High doses are teratogenic.
*Retinoids, for acne, including topical preparations	Teratogen. Microcephaly, cardiac and ear defects reported. Avoid. Requires effective contraception for one month before treatment and two years after discontinuation.
Selective serotonin re-uptake inhibitor anti-depressants (see Chapter 16)	Some studies have found increased congenital malformations. Sertraline manufacturer advises to avoid.
Statins to lower cholesterol	Congenital abnormalities. Avoid.
Sumatriptan, related drugs for migraine and lysergic acid diethylamide (LSD)	Manufacturer advises to avoid (see ergometrine, Chapter 6). Risk of uterine cotnractions.
Theophylline, in some 'cold cures' such as Franol®.	Irritability or apnoea in neonate. Possible link to cardiac abnormalities.
Vitamins, large doses (see Chapter 11) A	Kidney damage, congenital abnormalities including central nervous system and craniofacial defects. Vitamin A may take two years to be eliminated.
C	Scurvy in neonate.
D	Learning disabilities.

+ OTC over-the-counter products sold to the public in retail outlets.
* Specialists will always be involved in the prescription of these drugs.

Table 1.2   Breastfeeding: some drugs to avoid

Drug	Potential problem
Alcohol (including some cough remedies)	Sedation.
Anabolic steroids	Maculinizes infant.
Antihistamines, particulalry clemastine	Sedation.
Anti-microbials	May affect gut flora, causing diarrhoea.
Antipsychotics	Possible sedation. Central nervous sytem damage reported in animal studies.
Aspirin, ibuprofen	Risks of bleeding and Reye's syndrome. Some manufacturers advise to avoid, including topical use.
Caffeine (large doses), theophylline (e.g. OTC medication, Franol®)	Large doses cause jitteriness, inattentive feeding and poor sleeping.
Cimetidine, ranitidine	Further decrease in gastric acidity. Cimetidine may affect male infants (see Chapter 12).
Combined oral contraceptives	Diminish milk supply. Progesterone only pill considered safe.
Cytotoxic drugs	Damage to white blood cells and infection.
Diuretics	May impair milk production.
Ergometrine, ergotamine	Impairs milk production (see Chapter 6)
Fluoride in high concentrations	Mottling of teeth
Fluoxetine (Prozac®)	Irritability, gastro-intestinal upsets. Risk of hypersensitivity responses.
Iodine, including topical preparations	Hypothyroidism in neonate.
Lithium compounds	Gastro-intestinal upset. Risk of damage to central nervous system and kidneys.
Nicotine, including patches	Irritability. Gastro-intestinal upset.
Pyridoxine (vitamin B6) in large doses, bromocriptine	Inhibit milk production
Retinoids for acne	Risk of damage to sight, hearing, bones or liver. Increased skin fragility. Risk of convulsions. Avoid, including topical preparations.
Sedatives: benzodiazepines, antipsychotics, prochlorperazine, some tricyclic antidepressants (doxepin), anti-histamines, alcohol, opioids	Difficulty establishing feeding. Neonate becomes too drowsy, and muscle tone is too weak. May fail to gain weight and length appropriately.
Stimulant laxatives, e.g. senna	Diarrhoea in infant
Stimulants: ephedrine (cold cures), amphetamines	Neonate becomes irritable and sleeps poorly.
Sumatriptan and related preparations for migraine	Withold breastfeeding for 24 hours after administration (see ergometrine, Chapter 6). Risk of vasoconstriction.
Vitamins A & D, high doses	Risk of damage to liver and bones.

For a more complete list, the midwife should refer to the current BNF, and consult the manufacturers if uncertainty persists. Further examples are given in the relevant chapters on antimicrobials and anticonvulsants: 14, 19.

these processes depend on liver enzymes. The activity of the liver enzymes is affected by:

- genetic make-up/familial tendencies
- the liver's environment, that is what reaches the liver from the gut and the circulation
- liver impairment. This is likely to occur in women with malnutrition, cirrhosis of the liver, hepatitis, HELLP syndrome or in malnourished babies.

Neonates (particularly premature babies) metabolize and eliminate drugs more slowly than adults.

Examples
Following administration during labour, it can take a neonate two to three days to clear the metabolites of meperidine (pethidine), during which time the neonate may be irritable (see Chapter 4).

Breastfed infants are less able to metabolize the caffeine that their mothers ingest. If a mother takes several cups of filtered, boiled or strong coffee, she may feel no ill effects, but the caffeine can accumulate in the baby, making him/her unduly irritable and unable to concentrate on feeding. Women should be aware that some over-the-counter analgesics contain appreciable amounts of caffeine.

Rate of metabolism   This is affected by the liver enzymes. Depending on what has been ingested, the liver enzymes can be speeded-up (induced) or slowed down (inhibited).

Enzyme induction   The liver enzymes adapt to their environment, that is they become accustomed to whatever is ingested – diet or drugs. Regular ingestion of some drugs accelerates the liver enzymes with the result that the drug, and sometimes other substances, are eliminated more efficiently and more rapidly. The induction of enzymes takes days or weeks. Many drugs, including rifampicin, barbiturates, phenytoin, carbamazepine, alcohol, caffeine and tobacco and a high protein diet, all speed up the actions of the liver enzymes. This means that any drugs or hormones eliminated by these enzymes are metabolized away more rapidly and become less effective. For example rifampicin and some anti-epileptics (phenytoin, carbamazepine) render the standard dose oral contraceptive pill ineffective. Therefore, for effective contraception, women taking phenytoin or carbamazepine must take a higher daily dose of oestrogen (50 μg rather than 30 μg). In women taking anti-epileptic medication, 25 per cent of unplanned pregnancies can be attributed to 'pill failure' (Fairgrieve et al, 2000).

Enzyme inhibition   The liver enzymes can be stopped suddenly (inhibited) by enzyme inhibitors, including alcohol in high doses, grapefruit juice, erythromycin, cimetidine (Tagamet), some antifungal preparations such as ketoconazole (Chapter 14). For example concurrent administration of cimetidine with meperidine (pethidine) impairs the metabolism and elimination of the opioid, which may then accumulate and cause severe side effects such as respiratory depression. This drug interaction is not shared by ranitidine.

Drug excretion

Most drugs are dependent on the kidneys for excretion, but some drugs are excreted via the bile, for example corticosteroids and oestrogens. The functioning of the kidneys can be considered as two distinct processes: glomerular filtration rate (GFR) [glossary] and tubular secretion and reabsorption. Excretion of drugs from the kidneys may rely on either or both of these processes, depending on the drug involved. Some drugs, for example lithium and magnesium, are eliminated entirely by filtration, and their clearance is thus directly dependent on the GFR. Therefore GFR is assessed before these drugs are administered. If GFR falls, the elimination of most drugs is impaired, causing accumulation and even toxicity. If the GFR is below normal, most drugs are administered in reduced doses or at prolonged intervals. Therefore, those administering medications, particularly magnesium sulphate, should be aware of the circumstances likely to be associated with a low GFR and impaired renal elimination.

Causes of a low GFR

- dehydration (including the use of diuretics)
- renal disorders (for example urinary tract infection (UTI) and pre-eclampsia)
- shock and/or heart failure
- administration of non-steroidal anti-inflammatory drugs (NSAIDs) (including ibuprofen)

GFR is often estimated from serum creatinine concentrations. In normal pregnancy, the concentration of serum creatinine falls, and any value over 70 micromoles/litre is indicative of renal compromise. In contrast, for non-pregnant adults, values above 120–133 micromoles/litre are indicative of renal problems. This is particularly important in the interpretation of results of laboratory investigations for women with pre-eclampsia or urinary tract infections (Chapter 9).

The GFR of the neonate is only 30–40 per cent of adult values (Suri et al, 1998). Therefore, there is a danger that certain drugs, such as magnesium, may accumulate following maternal administration. These neonates should be observed for signs of muscle weakness, including respiratory depression for 48 hours after delivery. Pregnancy increases GFR 30–50 per cent. This increases the elimination of certain drugs (Loebstein et al, 1997).

Examples

The elimination of ampicillin is increased, and therefore higher doses (at least 500 mg every eight hours) are administered to combat infections.

In women with epilepsy, seizure frequency may worsen during pregnancy. Therefore, careful monitoring of anti-epileptic therapy is required. This should include venous blood samples to assess the plasma concentrations of anti-epileptic drugs.

Elimination half-life

The elimination half-life for each drug is the time taken for the concentration of the drug in blood or plasma to fall to half its maximum value (see Fig. 1.3).

A knowledge of a drug's half-life is essential for planning dose regimens. Drugs are administered approximately every half-life. Should drug administration deviate too much from this, the fluctuations in the concentration of the drug in the plasma will lead to therapeutic failure and/or toxicity.

Example (see Fig. 1.1)

Erythromycin may be prescribed for intravenous or oral administration every six hours. If administration is irregular, the plasma concentration of the drugs

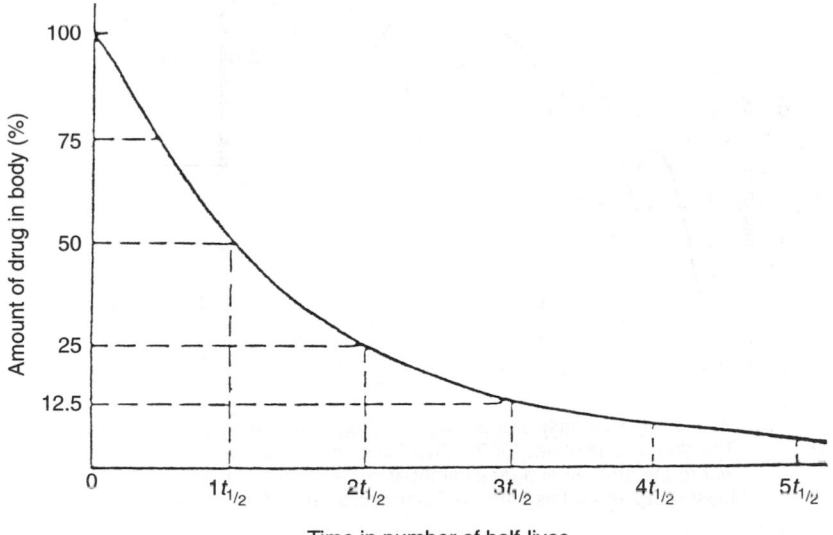

Time in number of half-lives

Most drugs follow this pattern of elimination.
During the first half-life, 50% of the drug is eliminated from the body.
After 3 half-lives, 87.5% or $\frac{7}{8}$ of the drug has been removed.
After 4–5 half-lives, this dose of the drug has effectively disappeared.

Figure 1.3 Graph to illustrate elimination half-life following a single intravenous dose

may at times fall so low as to be ineffective, allowing regrowth of micro-organisms; at other times, plasma concentrations may become so high that toxicity ensues.

Administration every six hours presents practical problems. For example, oral erythromycin, four times per day is sometimes prescribed for UTI ante-natally. It is also advisable to administer oral erythromycin one hour before or after meals. Therefore, it is not easy to calculate the timing of erythromycin administration to provide maximum clinical effect.

With repeated dosing, many drugs will accumulate in the body (see Fig. 1.4). The time taken for this to happen depends on the drug's elimination half-life. For most drugs in normal doses, repeated administration at regular intervals will result in a relatively constant plasma concentration or a steady state. At this concentration, the rate of drug elimination is equal to the rate of administration: what goes in, goes out. The time taken to achieve steady state is between three to five half-lives. Side effects often do not appear until the steady state is reached. If the midwife knows the half-life of a drug, she will therefore know when side effects are most likely to appear for the first time. In emergency situations, it is not possible to wait for three to five half-lives for a drug to reach a constant plasma concentration. Therefore a high

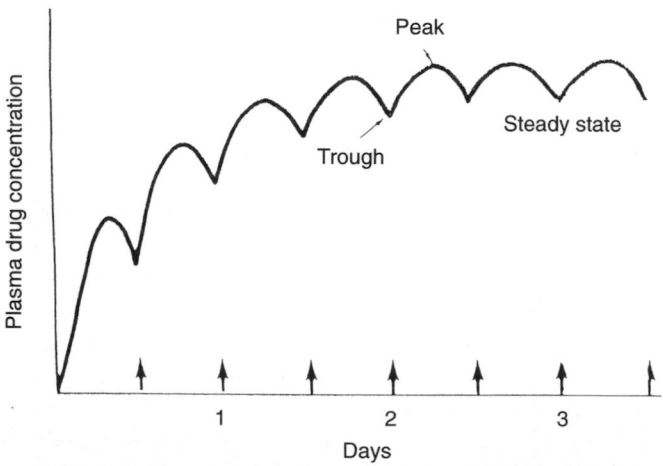

Repeated twice daily oral dosing of a drug with a half-life of 12 hours.
The drug accumulates for 3–5 half-lives, then it reaches a steady state,
where the amount of drug eliminated equals that taken in.
Most drugs show this pattern of elimination at normal doses.

Figure 1.4   Diagram to illustrate the accumulation of a drug with
repeated dosing

Source: Adapted from L. Benet (1996) General principles. In: Hardman,
J., Limbard, L., Molinoff, P., Ruddon, R., & Goodman Gilman, A. (eds)
Goodman & Gilman's: The Pharmacological Basis of Therapeutics,
9th edition, New York, McGraw-Hill.

dose will be administered to achieve a therapeutic concentration rapidly. This is known as a *loading dose*.

Pharmacodynamics: actions of the drug on the body

This section addresses the question: what are the effects of the drug on the tissues? Drugs work as a result of the physiochemical interactions between drug molecules and the patient's/recipient's molecules. These chemical reactions may alter the way the cells are functioning which in turn may lead to changes in the behaviour of tissues, organs and systems. Drugs modify the existing functions of the body; they cannot introduce new functions.

Most drugs act on more than one type of cell and therefore have multiple effects on the body. An example of this would be nicotine, which acts on the CNS to 'calm the nerves', on the blood vessels to raise blood pressure and on the respiratory epithelium to cause irritation. Similarly, opioids act on the pain pathways, the respiratory cilia and the gastro-intestinal tract. Other drugs are relatively specific, for example penicillins act almost exclusively on bacterial cell walls.

Most drug molecules work via:

- protein receptors in cell membranes or within cells
- ion channels in cell membranes
- enzymes in cells or extracellular fluid
- non-specific actions.

Drug–receptor interaction – the Lock and Key Hypothesis

Many drugs work by acting on specific receptor proteins. These are components of the cell membrane which normally respond to the body's hormones and neurotransmitters – the endogenous ligands [glossary]. Examples include: insulin receptors, opioid receptors, dopamine receptors, histamine receptors. Many drugs imitate the actions of the body's own ligands. Some drugs are direct replacements, for example insulin and epinephrine (adrenaline). Others provide an artificial boost to certain receptors, for example opioids.

Each receptor shows a high degree of specificity for its own ligand, so that histamine receptors are bound only by histamine, and not by insulin and vice versa. This idea of specificity, based on the three-dimensional shape or structure of ligand and receptor, is referred to as the 'Lock and Key Hypothesis' (Clark, 1933) (see Fig. 1.5; Ross, 1996).

Drugs with the same, or similar, three-dimensional structures as endogenous ligands (hormones, neurotransmitters) can bind to their receptors in their place and modify the actions of the system controlled by the receptor. When drugs (or endogenous ligands) and receptors interact, changes in the

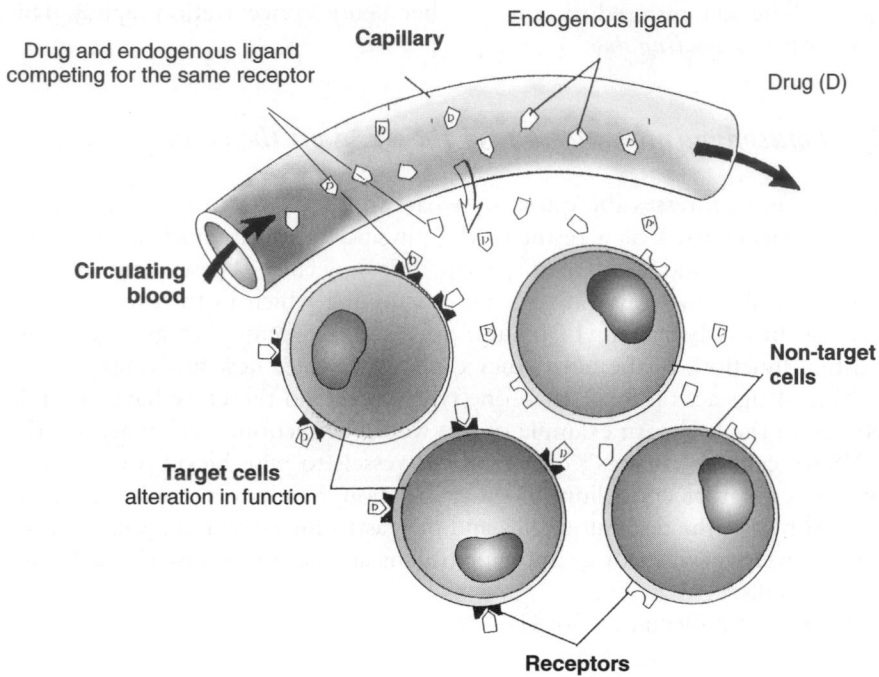

Figure 1.5   Dragram to illustrate the 3D fit between receptors and endogenous ligands or drugs

cell's metabolism are initiated. This alters the functioning of the cells which in turn affects organs and body systems. These changes in functioning show wide individual variation. However there is usually a relationship between dose and response, that is the higher the dose, the greater the effect on the body.

Drugs which 'fit into' binding sites on receptors may either activate them (agonists) or inactivate them (antagonists).

An agonist [glossary] will bind to a receptor and alter its functioning. For example salbutamol, prescribed for asthma or tocolysis, is a beta$_2$ agonist, meperidine (pethidine) is an opioid agonist, dopamine is a dopamine agonist. Agonists usually augment the normal function of the receptors to which they bind. For example meperidine stimulates the opioid receptors, increasing analgesia, sedation and constipation. Likewise, beta agonists mimic some of the actions of the sympathetic nervous system, increasing heart rate, dilating bronchioles and relaxing the uterus (Chapter 7).

An antagonist [glossary] will bind to a receptor and block the receptor and prevent the agonist working. For example naloxone (Narcan ®) blocks the opioid receptors and reverses the actions of meperidine/pethidine, reducing analgesia and sedation. Similarly, the beta blockers (propranolol, atenolol) block the actions of the sympathetic nervous system, slow and stabilize the heart rate and induce bronchoconstriction. Some drugs have intermediate actions, and are 'partial agonists' (see Galbraith et al, 1999).

Some drugs are specific for one receptor type (for example ranitidine), whereas others block more than one type of receptor (for example prochlorperazine (Stemetil ®)). Drugs which act on several types of receptors have diverse side effect profiles, affecting many systems of the body. This is well illustrated by prochlorperazine (Chapter 5).

Tolerance

The cells' receptors are continually being renewed by the protein-synthesizing machinery of the cells. When a drug is administered over a period of time, the cells or their receptors may adapt to the drugs. The number of receptors available on the cell surface may change in response to the presence of drugs. The continued presence of a drug may reduce the number of receptors available for it to act. This *down regulation* of receptors is believed to be responsible for the tolerance seen with continued use of opiates or beta$_2$ agonists.

Drugs which act on ion channels

Ion channels are similar to receptors in the way they bind to certain drugs. Examples include: calcium antagonists (nifedipine) and local anaesthetics such as lignocaine. However, because ion channels are present in a wide variety of cells and tissues, the side effects of these drugs can affect several body systems. For example, local anaesthetics affect both nerves and muscles (see Chapter 4).

Drugs which act on enzymes

Enzymes are present in all cells, catalysing their vital biochemical reactions. Some drugs bind to enzymes and inhibit their actions. Examples include, NSAIDs (non-steroidal anti-inflammatory drugs, such as aspirin, ibuprofen), MAOIs (mono amino oxidase inhibitors for depressive illness). It is likely that these drugs are able to interact with certain enzymes by virtue of their shape and structure in a similar manner to the drug–receptor interaction.

Most reactions between drugs and receptors, ion channels or enzymes are reversible, and eventually wear off when the drug is discontinued. One exception to this is aspirin. One of the actions of aspirin is to bind to and inhibit platelet enzymes responsible for synthesizing chemicals which promote clotting. This binding is irreversible. The effect of aspirin on the coagulation process takes several days to wear off, and clotting is only returned to normal when new platelets have been synthesized in the bone marrow which takes up to a week. Therefore, if aspirin is administered within a week of delivery, the risk of post-partum haemorrhage is markedly increased.

Drugs with non-specific actions

Some drugs are presumed to act by virtue of their physiochemical properties, rather than as a result of the specific shape of their molecules. For example antacids such as sodium bicarbonate or aluminium hydroxide neutralize gastric secretions without acting on the cells of the body.

Therapeutics: the effects of the drug on the person

This section addresses the questions: has the drug produced any effect on the recipient? If so, is the result therapeutic or toxic?

Changes in physiology of cells, tissues and organs

Even if a drug is working on the body's cells, there may be no noticeable response. For example, due to individual differences, an oxytocic or a tocolytic [glossary] may be ineffective.

Clinical effects

Clinical response shows considerable individual variation. This is not always entirely predictable, and idiosyncratic reactions can occur. For example, some women are unduly sensitive to oxytocin, and therefore infusions are commenced using a very low dose (BNF, 2000). Clinical effects also depend upon age, gender, pregnancy, disease state, drug interactions, weight, height, and genetic make-up. For example, women generally require lower doses of drugs than men, even when body weight is taken into consideration.

Side effects

Side effects are adverse drug reactions that occur within the normal range of therapeutic doses. Most drugs have potential side effects. These can be grouped under the headings:

- RELATED TO THE DRUG'S MAIN ACTIONS
- UNRELATED TO THE DRUG'S MAIN ACTIONS:

- Related to subsidiary actions
- Hypersensitivity responses
- Cell damage

These effects may be experienced by mother, fetus or neonate (see Tables 1.1 and 1.2).

Side effects related to the drug's main actions

These are often the drug's main side effects. Severity is usually related to the dose administered. Since such side effects are often highly significant and entirely predictable, appropriate monitoring systems must be in place. For example unless adequate checks are undertaken anti-coagulants can cause bleeding, and insulin can cause hypoglycaemia. With other drugs, the link between drug actions and side effects is less obvious and requires rather more understanding of physiology. For example metoclopramide and prochlorperazine (Stemetil ®) are dopamine antagonists. They are useful anti-emetics because they block the excitatory action of dopamine on the vomiting centre. However, they also block the actions of dopamine that can cause side effects in the areas of the brain which control posture and movement (the basal ganglia). For many drugs, such as metoclopramide, this type of predictable side effect limits the dose which can be administered (see Chapter 5).

Side effects related to subsidiary actions

Many drugs act on more than one type of cell receptor; this consequence gives the potential for diverse side effects. Again, these side effects are predictable, and the midwife should monitor or caution the woman appropriately. For example, oxytocin acts on the oxytocic receptors of the uterus, but it also acts on the anti-diuretic (ADH) receptors in the nephrons. This property gives it the potential to trigger water retention and fluid overload. Therefore, the midwife must monitor fluid balance (see Chapter 6). Similarly, prochlorperazine acts on muscarinic receptors in addition to dopamine receptors. By blocking the action of muscarinic receptors, prochlorperazine is responsible for drying the body's secretions such as saliva. Therefore, the midwife should advise the woman of the likely side effect and offer her frequent sips of water.

In pregnancy, the subsidiary actions of drugs on the uterus assume great importance. Any drugs which stimulate uterine contractility should be avoided, including stimulant laxatives (Chapter 13), misoprostol (Chapter 6) and all drugs chemically related to ergotamine (Chapter 6). This last group includes most drugs prescribed for migraine, such as sumatriptan, which are therefore contra-indicated in pregnancy and lactation (Pfaffenrath & Rehm, 1998). These medicines are often prescribed on an 'as needed' basis, to be stored and administered only during an attack of migraine; the woman must be careful not to continue use of such medicines during pregnancy.

Hypersensitivity responses (allergies)

A hypersensitivity [glossary] response is possible with almost all drugs, although antimicrobials are particular offenders. Individuals with a history of atopic [glossary] disorders, such as asthma or eczema, are particularly vulnerable. The Confidential Enquiry into Stillbirths and Deaths in Infancy (MCHRC, 2000) reports two cases where infant death followed maternal anaphylaxis following administration of a general anaesthetic for Caesarean section. Occasionally, the excipients (packing chemicals) used in tablets or injections may be responsible for hypersensitivity responses. Serious hypersensitivity responses, such as anaphylaxis, bone marrow depression and haemolysis, are rare but can be fatal (Rang et al, 1999). Most drugs or their metabolites can combine with carrier proteins in the circulation to form *immunogens*, substances which produce an immune response. This may affect any one of several organs such as skin, liver or bone marrow. The severity of the hypersensitivity response is also variable, ranging from a temporary skin rash to life-threatening aplastic anaemia. A mild drug reaction usually takes the form of an erythematous rash or an urticarial ('nettle') rash. In all cases, it is important that the offending drug is discontinued. Once someone has experienced even a mild allergic skin reaction to a drug they are likely to be sensitized and more likely to have an anaphylactic reaction at the next exposure (see Box 1.2: anaphylaxis and angioedema).

Box 1.2   Anaphylaxis and angioedema

The most immediate type of hypersensitivity response is anaphylaxis. This can also arise from allergens in food or bee stings. Anaphylaxis is characterized by the sudden onset of urticarial rash, tissue swelling (particularly around the mouth), obstruction of the respiratory tract, bronchoconstriction and hypotension. Bronchospasm may be the first indication of a problem. The patient may visibly swell and lose consciousness as blood pressure plummets. Death is most likely to occur from oedema of the airways (angioedema).

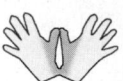   **Practice Point**

A hypersensitivity response may occur within seconds or up to one hour after injection. Therefore, observation for at least 15 minutes when the first dose of a new intravenous drug is given is vital.

Box 1.2 *(Continued)*

Almost any medication can cause a hypersensitivity response; common offenders include antimicrobials, hormone preparations, dextrans, heparin, vaccines, blood products, iron injections, local anaesthetics and streptokinase. Where drugs have similar chemical structures, *some cross allergies exist*: for example some people who are allergic to penicillins will also be allergic to cephalosporins.

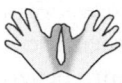 **Practice Point**

A history of previous drug responses is vital, as most severe reactions occur on a second or subsequent exposure to the drug.

Management of anaphylaxis involves stopping the drug, maintaining the airway, elevating the feet, calling help, administering oxygen and epinephrine (adrenaline).

Adrenaline/epinephrine is usually given intramuscularly as 500 micrograms or 0.5 ml of 1 in 1000 solution, repeated, if necessary, five minutes later. In extreme emergencies, if the circulation is inadequate, adrenaline/epinephrine may be given by slow intravenous injection; the dose is then 500 micrograms or 5 ml of 1 in 10000 solution injected over five minutes. Vital signs are monitored concurrently. Adrenaline/epinephrine may not be effective in patients taking beta blockers (such as atenolol or labetolol) and intravenous salbutamol may be needed. In anaphylactic shock, cardiac output is so low that adrenaline can only enhance the blood supply to the placenta, therefore concerns regarding vasoconstriction by adrenaline/epinephrine are misplaced (MCHRC, 2000).

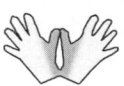 **Practice Point**

Two different strengths of adrenaline/epinephrine solution are available. This could lead to confusion in an emergency: should 5 ml of the stronger (1 in 1000) solution be administered intravenously, fatalities could occur.

Intravenous antihistamine (chlorphenamine/chlorpheniramine) is also administered intravenously (10–20 mg over one minute) and continued for 24–48 hours to prevent relapse (BNF, 2000).

Cell damage

Some drugs can cause direct damage to cells. For example, in large doses, paracetamol (acetaminophen) can damage the liver and kidneys. Other drugs, such as components of tobacco, damage cells by altering the DNA regulating oncogenes which control cell division.

Drug-induced teratogenesis [glossary] is a result of cell damage. This is relevant to a wide variety of drugs, from alcohol to thalidomide. The cells of the developing fetus are most vulnerable during the first trimester; however the inner ear remains vulnerable during the fourth month of pregnancy. Drugs impairing cell division (such as cytotoxic drugs) should be avoided during the first 14–17 days of gestation when they are most likely to cause abortion. Drugs impairing organ differentiation should be avoided between the 18th and 55th days of pregnancy, for example tetracyclines, lithium, benzodiazepines (Rubin, 1996). However other drugs influence fetal development at later stages of pregnancy, for example insulin, furosemide (frusemide) and antithyroid agents.

The risks of fetal damage depend on several factors as well as the chemical composition of the drug (Lipkin, 1993):

- The stage of pregnancy
- The amount of drug ingested
- The number of doses – a single dose may be less damaging than repeated exposure
- Other agents to which mother and fetus are exposed
- The mother's nutritional status
- The genetic makeup of mother and fetus.

The picture is complicated by epidemiological work which indicates that some congential malformations, particularly cleft lip, cleft palate and congenital heart malformations, are associated with severe maternal stress during the first trimester (Hansen et al, 2000). Some fetal abnormalities, including cardiac anomalies and neural tube defects, can be detected *in utero* by screening with high resolution ultrasound.

Table 1.1 lists some common medications which may adversely affect the fetus. A further list is included in Chapter 14, antimicrobial agents. For many drugs and herbal remedies, the manufacturers advise against use in pregnancy on the grounds that there are insufficient human data to demonstrate safety. No drugs have been subjected to randomized controlled clinical trials in human pregnancy. Therefore, no drug has been demonstrated as 'safe'. Evidence is gradually being accumulated from case series and retrospective analysis (see for example, Yoshida et al, 1999; McElhatton et al, 1999). Retrospective reporting of drug-induced fetal damage may lead to a bias towards over-reporting, but this is often the only available data. However, years of experience with some drugs, such as paracetamol and penicillins, indicate that use at usual dosage is not manifestly harmful to the fetus.

Conclusion

It is hoped that the framework for the bioscience principles outlined here will offer a useful guide to the practitioner. More detailed accounts are available in medical textbooks.

Further Reading

Rang, H. et al (1999) *Pharmacology*, 4th edition Edinburgh, Churchill Livingstone.

Mycek, M. et al (1997) *Pharmacology* Philadelphia, Lippincott-Raven.

Saeb-Parsy, K. et al (1999) *Instant Pharmacology*, Chichester, Wiley.

CHAPTER 2

Pharmacological Considerations for Intravenous Therapy

SUE JORDAN

This chapter outlines the extra considerations involved when intravenous (iv) drug administration is undertaken outside specialist intensive care facilities.

Chapter Contents

- Getting the drug into the person
- How the body handles IV drugs
- Actions and side effects of the drugs
- Conclusion

The intravenous (iv) route, using either central or peripheral lines, is used for the infusion of fluids and electrolytes, drug administration and parenteral nutrition. An indwelling iv line is extremely useful in medical emergencies such as anaphylaxis. Drugs commonly given intravenously include: antimicrobials, oxytocin, tocolytics, anticonvulsants, heparin and anaesthetics.

Getting the drug into the person

Administration

Intravenous administration may be by continuous infusion, intermittent infusion or as bolus doses. The formulations are not interchangeable: a patient died when a 60-minute intravenous infusion (ivi) of vancomycin was mistakenly administered as a bolus dose (Cousins, 1995).

Case Report

This case illustrates the importance of careful supervision of all intravenous infusions.

A 39-year-old woman had given birth and had developed a fever, for which an antibiotic was prescribed, to be administered diluted in 0.9 per cent saline or water for injection. Unfortunately, strong potassium chloride solution was mistakenly substituted and administered intravenously. An immediate cardiac arrest occurred. Despite instant attempts at resuscitation, the woman sustained massive brain damage. The Health Authority settled the claim for £845 000.

It is recommended that potassium chloride is kept securely away from the general drug stock, and extensive checks are carried out before it is ever infused (Cousins, 1994).

Continuous intravenous infusions

Continuous ivi aims to establish and maintain a steady concentration of drug in the circulation, for example oxytocin (Syntocinon ®). The drug is administered as a dilute solution to reduce irritation of the vein. However it is important to ensure that the drug is compatible with the infusate. For example, frusemide (furosemide) is incompatible with glucose/dextrose solutions.

Intermittent infusion

Intermittent infusion may cause the concentration of the drug in plasma to 'peak and trough', and fall above and/or below the therapeutic range (see Chapter 1). This can cause both toxicity and therapeutic failure. This could occur, for example, in a woman treated with intravenous antibiotics or heparin.

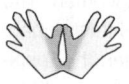 **Practice Point**

Because of the rapid absorption of iv drugs, it is very important that they are administered strictly 'on time'. Delays and subsequent 'bunching' of administration cause exaggerated 'peaks and troughs' in drug concentrations. This is illustrated in Figure 1.1.

Bolus doses

An injection can be given directly into a vein or into an existing intravenous line. Direct injection into a vein is usually avoided because:

- Using a steel needle for repeated intravenous injections risks extravasation and tissue damage.
- Without continuous venous access, any adverse reactions will be difficult to manage.

Bolus doses must be given slowly enough to allow the flow of infusate to continue and dilute the drug. The rate of administration will depend on the drug. Generally, unless the patient has suffered a cardiac arrest, or a severe haemorrhage, no dose should be administered in less than one minute (Loeb et al, 1993; McKenry & Salerno, 1995). Most drugs can be administered over one to three minutes, with several important exceptions such as epinephrine (adrenaline), ephedrine and aminophylline (Swonger & Matejski, 1991).

Rapid administration of drugs is likely to cause:

- trauma to the veins
- a severe hypersensitivity response
- serious side effects
- pulmonary oedema or embolization if large volumes of fluid are administered.

Mixing

Any drug added to an infusion must be *mixed thoroughly*. This involves detaching the container from the giving set. Without thorough mixing, delivery will be uneven. If potassium or magnesium are allowed to 'layer' at the bottom of an infusion bag, a high concentration will be delivered, risking a cardiopulmonary arrest. The use of ready-prepared solutions is safer (BNF, 2000).

Case Report

Magnesium sulphate was administered for tocolysis in a healthy 20-year-old woman. The solution was prepared by injecting magnesium sulphate into the intravenous infusion bag. The woman complained of feeling slightly hot. The infusion was stopped when the respiratory rate was five/minute and BP was 135/45 mmHg. Venous blood sampling revealed a high concentration of magnesium (6.95 mmol/l). Oxygen and calcium gluconate were administered, and the situation was 'rescued' with no long term consequences. Investigations revealed that the magnesium had not been thoroughly mixed prior to administration (Cao et al, 1999).

This case illustrates the importance of thorough mixing when magnesium sulphate is added to an infusion bag.

Storage

Some drugs are inactivated by light, for example ephedrine, adrenaline (epinephrine), amphotericin, sodium nitroprusside. Since these drugs are retained for emergency use, it is important that storage conditions are checked regularly.

Incompatibilities

Drugs may be added to infusion containers when constant plasma infusions are needed or when the administration of a concentrated solution would be harmful. When this is done, problems with delivery rate and incompatibilities can occur. The longer drugs or chemicals remain in contact with each other, the greater the chance of incompatibilities arising. Penicillins and cephalosporins are not sufficiently chemically stable for continuous infusion.

Many drugs interact with the infusate or other drugs, resulting in loss of effect, toxicity or other actions. Therefore, whenever possible, *only one drug should be added to any infusion container* and never to *blood products, mannitol, amino acids or sodium bicarbonate* (BNF, 2000). For example: glucose causes red cells to clump together; oxytocin is inactivated in blood.

When infusates are incompatible, chemical reactions occur which can cause solid particles to form in the giving set. For example furosemide (frusemide) and dopamine interact and may form a visible precipitate, causing solid white particles to appear in the infusion line. Unfortunately, this may not become apparent immediately. Precipitates can cause thrombophlebitis or, if the infusion leaks, skin sloughing. Infusates of different pHs [glossary] are likely to be incompatible. For example frusemide (furosemide) is incompatible with infusates of a low pH such as glucose.

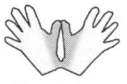 **Practice Points**

- Infusions should be checked regularly for signs of incompatibility: cloudiness, colour change or crystallization. However, **the absence of visual changes does not exclude the possibility of incompatibility**. For example, the combination of heparin and gentamicin is incompatible, but there may be no visible changes to the infusion. This mistake may only be recognized when the infection fails to respond to the antimicrobial or a thromboembolic event occurs.
- To reduce the risk of chemical reactions causing drug incompatibilities, the giving set should be changed every 24 hours if it is used to administer a drug (BNF, 2000).

Cannulation

For ease of venous access, it is important that the site to be cannulated should be vasodilated. It is therefore important to ensure that the area is warm.

Pain

Venepuncture or venous cannulation may be painful. This can be reduced by application of local anaesthetic cream. Amethocaine (tetracaine) gel may be faster acting and more effective than other local anaesthetic creams (see p. 107). Amethocaine causes vasodilation unlike lignocaine, which can cause vasoconstriction. This is clearly important when obtaining venous access (Russell & Doyle, 1997). However as with all applications, there is a small risk of side effects, mainly from systemic absorption.

Selection of venous access

Peripheral veins may collapse and provide inadequate venous access in shock, such as post partum haemorrhage. Veins may also become scarred and inaccessible from frequent access, for example in women who have received lithium therapy, with the associated regular blood sampling. In general a peripheral vein can only be expected to remain patent for 48 hours.

A central line is used for long term therapy, administration of concentrated or irritant solutions, or if the peripheral veins are inaccessible. However, air embolism and pneumothorax are greater risks with central venous lines. The subclavian vein provides suitable central access.

Electronic pumps and controllers are useful for very low or very precise infusion rates and for central venous lines. They are widely used in neonatal care. However, they are a potential source of infection (see Pickstone et al, 1994).

Maintaining venous access

The intravenous infusion site must be checked for patency at every use. An injection port must be 'flushed' with 2 ml of fluid (see Box 2.1) before and immediately after every use to ensure complete delivery, and at least every 24 hours to prevent clot formation (Ben-Arush & Berant, 1996). If the venous access is failing, resistance to the injection will be felt at this time.

Extravasation

Direct injection may exert too much pressure on fragile veins, causing thromboembolism or extravasation. Leakage (or extravasation) of isotonic fluid in

---

Box 2.1 Maintaining patency of a vein

Either saline (0.9 per cent physiological saline) or heparin (for example Hepsal ® or Hep-flush ®) may be used to maintain venous patency. If heparin (10–200 units every four hours) is used, the woman may experience the side effects of heparin (Chapter 8; *American Journal of Hospital Pharmacy*, 1994). Saline flushes have been shown to be as effective as heparin in maintaining venous patency for up to 48 hours. Heparin flushes are only recommended for infusions destined to continue for longer than this or for infusion sites where blood is aspirated (*American Journal of Hospital Pharmacy*, 1994).

In some situations, it may be necessary to maintain venous patency, although it is not currently required for infusion. In these circumstances, an infusion of physiological saline (0.9 per cent) is administered at a rate of 42–50 ml per hour or 1 litre over 24 hours (Huffman, 1994). This should be taken into consideration when calculating fluid balance.

---

small amounts is not damaging, but fluid containing drugs may be extremely irritant. Severe tissue necrosis and skin breakdown, requiring skin grafting (or even amputation in neonates) may follow the extravasation of noradrenaline (norepinephrine) or adrenaline (epinephrine). Fluids containing potassium or glucose are also highly irritant.

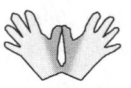 **Practice Point**

Extravasation or leakage is more likely if:
- steel needles are used in preference to plastic catheters
- the intravenous infusion is sited near a joint
- a vein has been punctured for more than two days
- the needle is not inserted deeply enough.

The extent of any extravasation can be limited by frequent checks and transparent dressings. An extravasated drug is an emergency. The infusion should be stopped, the amount in the tissues estimated, the limb elevated and medical help called. Any inflammation can be treated by ice packs. However, warming the site will increase fluid reabsorption from the surrounding tissues.

Antidotes, or dispersion agents, given in small amounts subcutaneously around the damage are available for some extravasated drugs. For example, **hyaluronidase** (Hyalase ®) is used when aminophylline, calcium, potassium, dextrose, total parenteral nutrition or contrast media leak, or when excess fluids need to be absorbed. Hyaluronidase acts by breaking down the ground substance [glossary] of the dermis, thereby allowing the fluid to disperse. 1500 units in 1 ml water for injection or 0.9 per cent sodium chloride are infiltrated into the affected area as soon as possible. Hyaluronidase is not indicated for infants in unexplained premature labour or in sites where infection or malignancy are present (BNF, 2000).

Phlebitis

Phlebitis is inflammation of a vein, usually due to damage to the wall, which causes release of inflammatory mediators and clot formation. Redness, pain and oedema usually occur two to three days after insertion of the needle. If the venous catheter is not removed, infection will result. Phenytoin, erythromycin and diazepam are particularly irritant, as are high concentrations of potassium, multivitamins, dextrose and amino acids. Phlebitis is more likely when the infusion is acid or alkaline or is very concentrated.

Precautions taken to reduce extravasation and phlebitis include:

● *ensuring the iv line is patent;*
● *avoiding the back of the hand, where tendons and nerves are easily damaged;*
● *avoiding compromised circulations, for example veins which have been traumatized by venepuncture;*
● *avoiding wrists and digits which are hard to immobilize;*
● *selecting a site which allows proximal access;*
● *checking for leaks before giving the drug. A tourniquet above the vein should stop the flow of infusate if it isn't leaking;*
● *observing the infusion site for swelling or redness;*
● *asking the patient to report any burning or itching or pain;*
● *using a dressing which allows inspection;*
● *flushing the drug through with a few millilitres of saline.*

Infections

Intravenous lines are notorious sources of infection; common micro-organisms include *Candida sp., Enterobacter sp., Staphylococcus epidermis, Staphylococcus aureus and Klebsiella sp.* Strict asepsis is always necessary when handling intravenous giving sets (Perry & Leaper, 1994). The use of ready-prepared infusions is much less likely to introduce infection than ad hoc/extemporaneous additions to infusions on the ward. Similarly, ready-prepared infusions for administration over 30–60 minutes are preferable to manual intravenous injections.

The incidence of infection can be reduced by:

● *replacing intravenous cannulae every 48 hours;*
● *hand disinfection with soap and water before handling intravenous cannulae;*
● *use of gloves;*
● *disinfection of the patient's skin;*
● *leaving only sterile tape in contact with the entry site;*
● *firmly anchoring the intravenous catheter;*
● *transparent dressings to allow site inspection;*
● *change of dressing if moisture visibly collects under the dressing;*
● *assessing the site at least daily for signs of redness;*
● *asking the patient to examine the site for signs of redness;*
● *assessing the patient for signs of fever.*
                    (Keenlyside, 1992; Loeb et al, 1993; Wilson, 1994)

Infection is more dangerous with a central line (see Loeb et al, 1993).

How the body handles IV drugs

Intravenous infusion is the fastest and most certain route of drug administration. A single bolus injection will produce a very high concentration of the drug in the plasma. The drug rapidly reaches the therapeutic range which is useful in emergencies. If the drug is administered too rapidly, the concentration is likely to overshoot the therapeutic range and enter the toxic range. If the drug is administered slowly, the concentration rises less rapidly. With care, the rate of infusion can be adjusted to optimize the therapeutic effects and minimize the side effects.

Intravenous administration means that all the drug administered is absorbed. There is no need to take account of any uncertainties in dose or timing due to individual differences involving the gut or the liver enzymes. Doses can be calculated and adjusted to the patient's needs more precisely than with other routes of administration.

Although the intravenous route minimizes potential problems with drug absorption, consideration must be given to potential problems with drug distribution and elimination (see Chapter 1). When giving any drug, distribution will be reduced and the chances of toxicity increased in renal failure, heart failure and shock; patients with severe pre-eclampsia or eclampsia are particularly at risk.

Circulatory overload

If the amount of fluid in the blood vessels is increased beyond the heart's capacity to pump it, the circulation becomes overloaded and blood backlogs into the pulmonary veins. This causes pulmonary oedema and breathlessness, which may progress to adult respiratory distress syndrome (ARDS), followed by systemic oedema and heart failure. Women with pre-eclampsia/eclampsia or diminished renal or cardiac reserve are at particular risk of circulatory overload. This is a particular danger with the administration of isotonic solutions (for example 0.9 per cent sodium chloride, Ringer's lactate @ 275 mOsm/kg) or hypertonic solutions (for example dextrose 5 per cent in 0.45 per cent saline @ 406 mOsm/kg) [glossary].

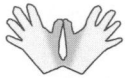 **Practice Points**

- The flow rate is checked at regular intervals, when the patient changes position and if the height of the infusion stand is altered. If an infusion is falling behind schedule, only minor adjustments to rate may be made, that is within 30 per cent, without consulting a doctor (Loeb et al, 1993). Too rapid an infusion may cause circulatory overload.
- A record of all fluids administered must be kept. Even small imbalances can cause overload in vulnerable patients such as neonates or those with severe pre-eclampsia. Many problems could be avoided by checking vital signs and state of hydration before and during administration of infusions (Clayton & Stock, 1993: 111). The frequency with which ARDS appears as a cause of maternal death has forced the DoH assessors to issue a terse warning regarding the risks of circulatory overload in pre-eclamptic women (DoH, 1998: 45).

Case Report

In the triennium 1994–6 three deaths occurred due to ARDS in eclamptic/pre-eclamptic women.

At 27 weeks gestation, a woman developed HELLP syndrome. During transfer between hospitals, the fetus died *in utero*. While labour was being induced, excessive amounts of fluid were transfused. This caused pulmonary oedema, and positive pressure ventilation was needed to maintain oxygenation prior to Caesarean section. The lung damage was so severe that ARDS followed (DoH, 1998: 42).

This case illustrates the dangers of fluid retention associated with oxytocin (see Chapter 6). In pre-eclampsia, the vessels are so damaged, and the vascular space is so reduced, that excess fluid readily passes into the tissue spaces, causing pulmonary oedema and further damage leading to ARDS.

Raised intra-cranial pressure

If hypotonic solutions are administered, in effect excess pure water is infused which will pass into cells, causing them to swell. This can damage the cells of the brain or the cardiac conduction system. Hypotonic solutions (for example 0.45 per cent saline @ 154 mOsm/l) are not given to patients at risk of raised intra-cranial pressure: for example eclampsia, severe pre-eclampsia, head injury, cerebrovascular accident.

Protein deficiency

The osmotic activity of the plasma proteins is important in maintaining the distribution of body water. When reduced concentrations of plasma proteins are present, for example due to liver disease, malnutrition, burns, they are unable to hold water in the blood vessels. The water is then likely to enter body cavities, tissue spaces and cells. Therefore, such patients should not receive hypotonic infusions.

Lactate infusions

Lactate (as in Ringer's lactate) is metabolized into bicarbonate ions by the liver. Therefore administration of lactate is avoided in:

- alkalosis (for example hyperventilating women);
- liver disease (for example HELLP syndrome).

Hypersensitivity responses

Most hypersensitivity responses are harmless skin eruptions, presenting as an itchy 'nettle' rash and swelling around the infusion site. However, bronchospasm and anaphylaxis can occur. Not only the drug but the preservative of the infusion can trigger a hypersensitivity response: for example sulphites can precipitate an asthma attack (see Box 1.2).

Actions and side effects of the drugs

In general, the actions and side effects of drugs are not affected by the route of administration. However, the onset of adverse effects may be much more rapid when drugs are administered intravenously, and extra precautions are needed. Ampicillin and diazepam are taken as illustrative examples.

Ampicillin

Intravenous administration poses several potential problems, not normally encountered with oral administration (Gahart, 1992):

- In an infusion, ampicillin is incompatible with many other drugs, for example gentamicin.

- Ampicillin is inactivated by contact with tetracyclines or erythromycin.
- Heparin may be potentiated by contact with ampicillin.
- Fits can occur if injections are too rapid, especially in neonates and patients with renal impairment.
- Hypersensitivity responses are likely to be very severe. Patients receiving beta blockers (for example labetolol) are particularly at risk.

Diazepam

Intravenous diazepam is very important in seizure control. However, it can cause several problems not usually seen with oral administration:

- Respiratory depression can occur in susceptible individuals. Therefore, respiratory support should be available for emergency use.
- Diazepam can not be diluted or mixed with other drugs or infusions.
- Diazepam tends to precipitate onto plastic tubing, and is therefore given directly into a vein if possible.
- Diazepam is an irritant, so small veins are avoided, and leakage is hazardous. There is a high risk of thrombophlebitis.
- Other sedatives (for example pethidine) are potentiated; therefore respiratory support should be available. Bed rest should be maintained for three hours after injection.
- After a large dose, withdrawal symptoms, (such as anxiety, insomnia, photophobia, tinnitus, nausea) can last for several weeks.

Conclusion

The site of infusion is an important source of potential discomfort, which can disturb much needed sleep in the puerperium. This can be minimized by regular observations of the site and resiting as needed.

When administering intravenous infusions, the midwife must be aware not only of the side effects of the drugs but also of the particular hazards of infusions. Compatibilities between drug and infusate and any co-administered drugs must be checked before administration. Unfortunately, neither the BNF nor the ABPI Data Sheet Compendium are always adequate sources for this information, and information must be sought from pharmacy (Dean, 1996).

Further Reading

Loeb, S., Holmes, N.H., Charnow, J., Fandek, N., Johnson, P. & Sloan, G. (1993) *Clinical Skillbuilders: Medication Administration and IV Therapy Manual*, 2nd edition. Springhouse, Pennsylvania, Springhouse Corporation.

CHAPTER 3

Law, Medicines and the Midwife

RICHARD GRIFFITH

This chapter describes the statutory framework for the control of medicines and discusses the implications for midwives.

Chapter Contents

- Introduction

- Accountability

- The legal regulation of medicines

- Administration of prescription only medicines

- Patients group directions (group protocols)

- Professional requirements

- Civil liability

- Conclusion

Introduction

Medicines are mainly recognized for their therapeutic benefits but they also have great potential to harm those who take them. Drugs such as Thalidomide (*J v. Distillers Co (Biochemicals)* (1969)) and Opren (*Nash v. Eli Lilly & Co* (1993)) demonstrate the tragic consequences that may follow medication administration. Therefore, the law regulates the arrangements for the supply of medicines to patients. Traditionally, the law has divided the supply process by allowing doctors to prescribe a drug, a pharmacist to dispense the drug and the midwife or nurse to administer it. However, the Cumberlege report (DHSS, 1986) recommended that suitably qualified nurses and midwives working in the community should be able to prescribe from a limited list of items and adjust the timing and dosage of medicines within set protocols. However this is still under discussion. With this authority comes increased accountability and midwives must be aware of the legal framework for the prescription, supply and administration of medicines.

Accountability

As registered practitioners, midwives are accountable or answerable for their actions to four main legal sources. A range of sanctions may be applied for failing to adequately meet the required standard in each case.

The profession

A midwife who is found guilty of professional misconduct is liable to removal from the professional register. The UKCC has the authority to hold midwives to account through the Nurses, Midwives and Health Visitors Act 1997. The professional standard required of a midwife by the governing body is given in the UKCC's Code of Professional Conduct (1992) and is further elaborated by the Midwives Rules and Code of Practice (UKCC, 1998). However, there may be change in the future, as the UKCC may be replaced with a Council of Nursing.

The employer

Midwives have legal binding contracts of employment with their employers that require, among other duties, that they obey the reasonable requests of the employer and work with due care and skill. The contract further requires that midwives are duty bound to account for their actions and to disclose any misdeeds. An employer may therefore hold an employee to account through reasonable disciplinary policies and procedures that ultimately may lead to dismissal.

   As a result of the control employers exercise over their employees, the law holds them vicariously liable for any tort [glossary] committed by an employee during the course of their employment that has the effect of indemnifying the employee against damages for harm caused to another in the course of their employment. Independent midwives are self-employed and do not have this protection. They therefore require insurance indemnity against claims for compensation.

The client

A mother or child who feels they have been harmed by the carelessness of a midwife can seek redress though the civil court system. This remains a lengthy and costly process and is still a relatively rare occurrence. The great majority of clients will usually complain to the midwife's employer or the UKCC rather than go to law. However, when a case is successfully brought the award of damages can run to millions of pounds. In *T (A Minor) v Luton & Dunstable Hospital NHS Trust* (1998), T suffered cerebral palsy as a result of a prolonged delivery during which placental abruption and type II (late) heart decelerations went unnoticed. The NHS Trust accepted that it was vicariously liable and agreed damages amounting to £1 736 347.

Society

We are all accountable to society through the criminal law. A midwife who breaks the law is as liable to prosecution as any other person. The tatutes concerned with the regulation of medicines, such as the Medicines Act 1968 and the Misuse of Drugs Act 1971, carry criminal penalties if breached. It is vital therefore that midwives are within the law when working with medicines.

Summary

The four spheres of accountability regulating the practice of the midwife are not mutually exclusive. It is entirely possible that a midwife might be removed from the professional register, dismissed from her post, sued by a patient and receive a fine, community penalty or imprisonment. It is essential therefore that the midwife understands that the notion of accountability is always considered as a whole through all four spheres. This will ensure safe and effective practice that will benefit the patient and avoid being called to justify one's actions.

The legal regulation of medicines

Medicines Act 1968

The principle statute regulating the use of medicines is the Medicines Act 1968. This provides an administrative and licensing system to control the sale and supply of medicines to the public. Before a drug can be marketed for sale to the public it must have a Marketing Authorization issued by the Secretary of State for Health. A Marketing Authorization cannot be issued unless the committee on the safety of medicines has been consulted (section 2, Medicines Act 1968). This body is charged by the 1968 act with looking at matters such as the quality of the drug and its usefulness for the purpose for which it is marketed. The Committee on the Safety of Medicines is further charged with the promotion of the collection of data on adverse reactions to drugs (section 4, Medicines Act 1968).

Drugs that have a manufacturer's authority are categorized into three types for the purpose of supply to the general public.

General sales list drugs

This type of drug may be sold through a variety of outlets without need for a registered pharmacist. Examples include paracetamol and aspirin.

Pharmacy only

This category of medicine can only be purchased under the supervision of a registered pharmacist in a retail pharmacy. Examples include ranitidine, cimetidine and piriton.

Prescription only

This category of medicine can only be obtained from a registered pharmacist by prescription from a registered doctor, dentist or eligible nurse, midwife or health visitor. They cannot normally be supplied unless a prescription has been issued from an appropriate practitioner. The criteria for determining which products should be available on prescription only are regulated by European Directive 92/26/EEC. These medicines are listed in article 3 of the Prescription Only Medicines (Human Use) Order 1997. Under the Medicines (Products Other Than Veterinary Drugs) (Prescription Only) Order 1983 in exceptional circumstances pharmacists may supply five days' emergency treatment of a prescription only product.

Appropriate practitioners

The Medicines Act 1968 bestows prescribing authority to registered medical practitioners, dentists and vets who are able to issue prescriptions from their relevant formularies. The Medicinal Products: Prescribing by Nurses etc. Act 1992 extended the range of appropriate practitioners to include registered nurses, midwives and health visitors who are of such a description and comply with such conditions as may be specified by order. As of this writing, this currently excludes midwives.

Definitions

Administration

This is not generally defined but accepted as involving the drug being given by a practitioner or a practitioner supervising the patient taking the dose. The

Prescription Only Medicines (Human Use) Order 1997 defines parenteral administration as administration by breach of the skin or mucous membrane.

Supply

Section 131 of the Medicine Act 1968 defines supply as supplying a drug in circumstances corresponding to retail sale. However if a midwife were providing any prescription only medicine for patients to take away and administer themselves, then that would amount to supply.

Prescription

Means a prescription issued by an appropriate practitioner under or by virtue of the NHS Act 1977. That is, it is written on the proscribed form and is signed and dated by the practitioner, for example FP10.

The form of a prescription

Article 15 of the Prescription Only Medicines (Human Use) Order 1997 requires that a prescription must be completed in ink, or be otherwise indelible, on the statutory form and must contain the following information:

- The name and address of the patient;
- The drug described clearly;
- The signature of the prescriber and;
- The date of signing.

Administration of Prescription Only Medicines

A drug categorized as a prescription only medicine can normally only be administered by or under the direction of an appropriate practitioner. Section 58(2)(b) Medicines Act 1968 states that:

> *No person shall administer otherwise than to himself any such medicinal product unless he is an appropriate practitioner or a person acting in accordance with the directions of an appropriate practitioner.*

However article 9 of the Prescription Only Medicines (Human Use) Order 1997 limits the restriction on the administration of prescription only medicines to those that are for parenteral administration.

The restriction imposed by s 58(2)(b) shall not apply to the administration to human beings of a prescription only medicine which is not for parenteral administration.

Furthermore, the Prescription Only Medicines (Human Use) Order 1997 allows registered midwives to be exempted from the regulations relating to supply and administration of named prescription only drugs under certain conditions. Such medicines that are normally only available on a prescription issued by a medical practitioner may be supplied to midwives who have notified their intention to practise for use in their practice under Part III Medicines Act 1968.

Summary of Relevant Aspects of the Prescription Only Medicines (Human Use) Order 1997. SCHEDULE 5

Article 11(1)(a)

EXEMPTION FOR CERTAIN PERSONS FROM SECTION 58(2) OF THE ACT

PART I

EXEMPTION FROM RESTRICTIONS ON SALE OR SUPPLY

Persons exempted	Prescription only medicines to which the exemption applies	Conditions
4. Registered midwives.	**4.** Prescription only medicines containing any of the following substances: Chloral hydrate Ergometrine maleate Pentazocine hydrochloride Triclofos sodium.	**4.** The sale or supply shall be only in the course of their professional practice and in the case of ergometrine maleate only when contained in a medicinal product that is not for parenteral administration.

Article 11(2)

PART III

EXEMPTIONS FROM RESTRICTION ON ADMINISTRATION

Persons exempted	*Prescription only medicines to which the exemption applies*	*Conditions*
2. Registered midwives.	**2.** Prescription only medicines for parenteral administration containing any of the following substances but no other substance specified in column 1 of Schedule 1 to this Order:	**2.** The administration shall be only in the course of their professional practice and in the case of promazine hydrochloride, lignocaine and lignocaine hydrochloride shall be only while attending on a woman in childbirth.
	Ergometrine maleate Lignocaine Lignocaine hydrochloride Naloxone hydrochloride Oxytocins, natural and synthetic Pentazocine lactate Pethidine hydrochloride Phytomenadione Promazine hydrochloride.	

Exemption for the administration of a prescription only medicine in an emergency

In addition to the specific exemptions for midwives in schedule 5 of the 1997 order, a general exemption on restriction from administration is allowed for the following medicinal products for the purpose of saving life in an emergency:

- Adrenaline/epinephrine injection 1 in 1000 (1 mg in 1 ml)
- Atropine sulphate injection
- Chlorpheniramine injection
- Dextrose injection strong BPC
- Dicobalt edetate injection
- Diphenhydramine injection
- Glucagon injection
- Hydrocortisone injection

- Mepyramine injection
- Promethazine hydrochloride injection
- Snake venom antiserum
- Sodium nitrite injection
- Sodium thiosulphate injection
- Sterile pralidoxime

Similar arrangements exist for the supply of prescription only medicines in an emergency.

Patient group directions (group protocols)

While most medicines are provided by using individual, named patient prescriptions, one way of giving increased flexibility to midwifery practice is through the use of group protocols. The Department of Health's *Review of Prescribing, Supply and Administration of Medicines* (1998) described a Group Protocol as:

> *a specific written instruction for the supply or administration of named medicines in an identified clinical situation. It is drawn up locally by doctors, pharmacists and other appropriate professionals, and approved by the employer, advised by the relevant professional advisory committees. It applies to groups of patients or other service users who may not be individually identified before presentation for treatment.*

Since individual patients are not named, group protocols appeared to contravene the restrictions on the sale, supply and administration of prescription only medicines under section 58 (2) of the Medicines Act 1968. The legal uncertainty was removed by the Prescription Only Medicines (Human Use) Amendment Order 2000 that provides for the use of Patient Group Directions (Group Protocols) in NHS-related work. This order exempts midwives, and other named classes of health professionals, from the restriction on supply and administration of prescription only medicines where this is done as part of a Patient Group Direction, signed by a senior doctor and senior pharmacist and authorized by the relevant health service body such as a health authority, local health group or NHS Trust.

Developing a Patient Group Direction

The Department of Health and National Assembly of Wales (2000) recommend Patient Group Directions should be drawn up on a multi-disciplinary basis involving a doctor, a pharmacist and a representative of any professional group expected to supply or administer medicines under their direction. Since each practitioner involved in the direction would be individually named and accountable, it should clearly specify the role of practitioners, who must sign their agreement.

In addition a Patient Group Direction must by law contain the following information:

(a) The period during which the direction shall have effect;
(b) The description or class of prescription only medicine to which the direction relates;
(c) Whether there are any restrictions on the quantity of medicine which may be supplied on any one occasion and, if so, what restrictions;
(d) The clinical situations which prescription only medicines of that description or class may be used to treat;
(e) The clinical criteria under which a person shall be eligible for treatment;
(f) Whether any class of person is excluded from treatment under the direction and, if so, what class of person;
(g) Whether there are circumstances in which further advice should be sought from a doctor or dentist and if so, what circumstances;
(h) The pharmaceutical form or forms in which prescription only medicines of that description or class are to be administered;
(i) The strength, or maximum strength, at which prescription only medicines of that description or class are to be administered;
(j) The applicable dosage or maximum dosage;
(k) The route of administration;
(l) The frequency of administration;
(m) Any minimum or maximum period of administration applicable to prescription only medicines of that description or class;
(n) Whether there are any relevant warnings to note and, if so, what warnings;
(o) Whether there is any follow up action to be taken in any circumstances and, if so, what action and in what circumstances;
(p) Arrangements for referral for medical advice;
(q) Details of the records to be kept of the supply, or the administration, of medicines under the direction.

Failure to comply with the requirements of the order would be a criminal offence under the Medicines Act 1968. The use of Patient Group Directions by independent midwives or those working for private or voluntary organizations will be restricted to NHS-related work. If medicines are supplied by a midwife under a Patient Group Direction for self-administration by the patient, care must be taken that the labelling and product information associated with the drug meets EC Labelling and Leaflet Directive 92/27.

Midwives are already exempt from the restriction on supply and administration of certain medicines used in their practice and this exemption is unaffected by the provisions relating to Patient Group Directions. Controlled drugs continue to be regulated by the Misuse of Drugs Act 1971 and its regulations, and are therefore currently excluded from inclusion in a Patient Group Directive.

Misuse of Drugs Act 1971

Controlled drugs are prescription only medicines that are further regulated by the Misuse of Drugs Act 1971. In health contexts, Misuse of Drugs Regulations 1985 categorizes controlled drugs into five numbered schedules:

1. No health purpose (for example lysergic acid);
2. Opiates (for example pethidine, diamorphine) and major stimulants (cocaine, amphetamines);
3. Barbiturates and minor stimulants (for example temazepam);
4. Benzodiazapine tranquillisers, anabolic steroids;
5. Preparations with minimal risk of abuse.

Drugs from schedules 2 and 3 can only be dispensed on prescription. A valid prescription must be written indelibly, be dated and signed by the prescriber. The dose and name and address of patient must be stated. For schedules 1 to 3 the dose of the drug must be in words and figures.

Special record keeping requirements apply for controlled drugs. Drugs in schedules 1 and 2 of the 1985 regulations must have a record, kept in a bound register, each time the drug is obtained or supplied. Midwives may possess and use specified controlled drugs under a midwives' supply order signed by a doctor or supervisor of midwives. Currently, the Prescription Only Medicines (Human Use) Order 1997 allows a midwife to possess and administer pethidine hydrochloride under these arrangements for use in their professional practice.

Professional requirements

Although the general legal requirements for the supply and administration of prescription only medicines have exemptions for registered midwives, a midwife must have regard to her professional accountability and obligations when supplying or administering medicines.

Midwives Rules and Code of Practice

The UKCC (1998), through the Nurses, Midwives and Health Visitors (Midwives Amendment) Rules, as in the *Midwives Rules and Code of Practice* (1998), regulates a midwife's professional practice with regard to the supply and administration of medicines. While the midwife's code of practice (1998) acknowledges that midwives may be supplied certain medicines listed in schedule 5 of the Prescription Only Medicines (Human Use) Order 1997, the UKCC stresses that the actual drugs used by the midwife in practice are agreed in a local policy in collaboration with a senior midwife, medical and pharmacy staff.

Midwives are also required to limit the administration of medicines and dosages to those that they have been trained to use and administer. Furthermore, a midwife shall administer medication by means of apparatus only if it meets the requirements for use by a midwife (Paragraph 41, *Midwives Rules 1998*; Paragraphs 20 and 21, *Midwives Code of Practice 1998*).

Requirements relating to controlled drugs

When administering a controlled drug in the NHS, a midwife is required to comply with locally agreed health authority policies and procedures. The UKCC acknowledges that this might include a standing order signed by a consultant and senior midwife authorizing the administration of controlled drugs and medicines for the midwife's use in her practice in an institution (Paragraphs 16 and 24, *Midwives Code of Practice 1998*).

The UKCC requires the midwife to comply with the procedure for the destruction and surrender of controlled drugs laid out in the Misuse of Drugs Regulations 1985. This allows for the destruction of the drugs by the midwife in the presence of a person authorized by regulation 26 of the 1985 regulations. Alternatively the midwife may surrender stocks of controlled drugs to the pharmacist from whom they were obtained or to an appropriate medical officer but not to a supervisor of midwives (Paragraphs 17 and 18, *Midwives Code of Practice 1998*).

A prescription for controlled drugs that has been issued directly to the expectant mother is regarded in law as her property. As such, the midwife cannot lawfully possess such drugs and cannot return unused drugs to the pharmacist. It is the responsibility of the mother to destroy unused controlled drugs, and the midwife should encourage the mother to do this in her presence. A record must be kept of any advice the midwife gives, any action taken and the quantities of controlled drugs (Paragraph 19, *Midwives Code of Practice 1998*).

Civil liability

Negligence

It can be seen that considerable flexibility is afforded midwives in the supply and administration of medicines during the course of their practice. The standard required of the midwife is that of the 'ordinary [person] professing to have and exercise that particular skill or art' (J. McNair in *Bolam v. Friern*

HMC (1957)). The House of Lords in *Whitehouse v. Jordan* (1981) confirmed that this standard applied to errors in the course of treatment, including childbirth and surgery. In common law [glossary], there are several cases where a health professional has been found liable in negligence for falling below the required standard.

Parenteral administration of medicines usually involves the use of an injection. The breaking of a needle during an injection is a matter that would require an explanation but has not to date given rise to liability in negligence, but failure to deal with the aftermath of a broken needle has done so. In *Gerber v. Pines* (1934) a GP was held to be negligent for failing to inform a woman that a piece of needle remained in her after it broke during an injection. In *Henderson v. Henderson* (1955) a surgeon was found negligent after causing scarring when he persisted in trying to remove a needle that broke during suturing. Negligence can also occur where a practitioner injects into the wrong site. In *Daly v. Wolverhampton Health Authority* (1986) liability was conceded where an injection caused a permanent neuroma. Similarly a midwife was found liable when she injected pethidine into the inside of the woman's leg damaging a superficial nerve. (*Walker v. South Surrey District Health Authority* (1982)). A further cause of action in negligent injection giving might arise from giving the injection at a time when a skilful practitioner would wait.

Failure in communication in relation to drug administration has also been shown to be negligent. In *Collins v. Hertfordshire County Council* (1947) the mishearing of a prescription resulted in a lethal dose being administered. Allowing the administration of four extra injections of streptomycin above the 30 prescribed, resulting in permanent loss of balance, rendered a ward sister liable in negligence. (*Smith v. Brighton & Lewes Hospital Management Committee* (1958))

In *Dwyer v. Rodrick* (1983) a doctor was found liable in negligence when an incorrectly written prescription resulted in an overdose of the drug. Similarly in *Prendergast v. Sam & Dee Ltd* (1989) both the doctor and pharmacist were found liable in negligence when an illegibly written prescription resulted in the wrong drug being supplied to the patient.

A further failure in communication that can render a midwife liable in negligence is a failure to inform a patient of the side effects of a drug (*Goorkani v. Tayside Health Board* (1991)) It is hoped that this book will assist the midwife here. It is essential therefore that a midwife adheres to the standards of prescribing required by law and the profession in order to avoid liability in negligence or a charge of professional misconduct.

Congenital Disability (Civil Liability) Act 1976

As well as the common law [glossary] duty of care owed towards the mother, a midwife also owes a duty to the unborn child. The 1976 act allows a child born alive to sue a person for negligence for damage caused to it in the womb. This would include a midwife who through carelessness harmed the child before or during birth. On the grounds of public policy, section 1(1) of the Congenital Disabilities (Civil Liability) Act 1976 excludes the child's mother from liability under the act even if the child was born disabled as a result of her misuse of drugs, alcohol or tobacco.

Conclusion

The legal regulation of medicines and the professional and contractual regulation of midwifery practice seek to protect the public from harm. Nevertheless, midwives are afforded considerable discretion and flexibility within these frameworks to exercise professional judgement when supplying and administering medicines. When informing their decision making, midwives would do well to heed the requirements of the statutory framework on medicines, professional guidance on the use of medicines and court decisions on negligent care. In this way midwives will ensure that their practice meets the standards required by the accountability bestowed upon them by the law, their profession, their employers and their moral obligation to the women in their care.

Further Reading

Montgomery, J. (1998) *Health Care Law*. Oxford, Oxford University Press.

Mason, J.K. & McCall Smith, R.A. (1999) *Law & Medical Ethics*, fifth edition. London, Butterworths.

PART II

DRUGS IN LABOUR

For myriad reasons, very few deliveries take place without some form of pharmacological intervention. Ideally, all labours would require no more than inhalational analgesia, but in practice such labours are the minority, and even Entonox® is not without its hazards. Administration of analgesia would appear to be linked with use of anti-emetics and possibly oxytocics. This core section of the book describes the drugs regularly administered to healthy women in labour. We aim here to present the evidence base for these interventions which, in some centres, have become routine practice.

CHAPTER 4

Pain Relief in Labour

SUE JORDAN

This chapter describes the analgesics commonly administered to labouring women, starting with the least invasive and progressing to the most technically compli-cated. This ordering has entailed dividing the discussion of the opioids in accor-dance with their routes of administration.

Many women request pain relief during labour and a wide range of pharma-cological and non-pharmacological options exist. These options should be carefully discussed with the woman during ante-natal visits so that she is able to choose a method of pain relief appropriate to her individual needs. This decision should then be documented in the case notes. Nevertheless, it is rec-ognized that women's requirements for pain relief are not always predictable and may change during labour and therefore the midwife should be able to discuss with the woman the specific advantages and disadvantages of all the pharmacological options available (Dickersin, 1989; Simpkin, 1989).

Pathophysiology of pain

Most authorities define pain as: '*an unpleasant sensory and emotional experi-ence associated with actual or potential tissue damage, or described in terms of such damage*' (IASP, 1986: S217). The experience of pain is individual and contextualized; there is not always a clear relationship between tissue damage and pain experience. Pain scores offer a useful communication tool to assist in assessing the need for analgesia (Fairlie et al, 1999).

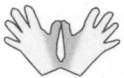 **Practice Point**

Analgesia should be monitored using a 'pain scale' such as a visual analogue scale.

The individual's learnt experience is an important determinant of pain perception and the development of pain syndromes (see Loeser & Melzack, 1999). Therefore, experience in previous deliveries will influence each woman's analgesic requirements.

The **anatomy** of the pain (or nociceptive) pathways is outlined in Figure 4.1. Aspects most relevant to pharmacology include:

- The passage of pain impulses depends on action potentials in the neurones of the pain pathways. These are blocked by local anaesthetics.
- The integration of pain fibres, touch fibres and descending analgesic tracts occurs in the dorsal horn of the spinal cord, the 'pain gate' (see Melzack and Wall, 1996). This is one site of opioid action.
- The pain pathways synapse in the reticular formation in the brain stem. Here they activate the sympathetic nervous system and increase:

  - level of arousal and consciousness;
  - respiration;
  - heart rate;
  - blood pressure;
  - emesis;
  - sweating/perspiration.

  Anaesthetic gases (for example nitrous oxide) and opioids act in the brain stem.
- The pain pathways can overwhelm the cerebral cortex, to the exclusion of other considerations. The cerebral cortex is one site of opioid action.

Severe, unrelieved pain may not only provide the woman with a very negative experience of childbirth, but can also have **adverse physiological consequences**.

Increased rate and depth of respirations (see nitrous oxide)

Hyperventilation rapidly reduces the carbon dioxide in the body, leading to vasoconstriction of the maternal and placental circulations, jeopardizing the

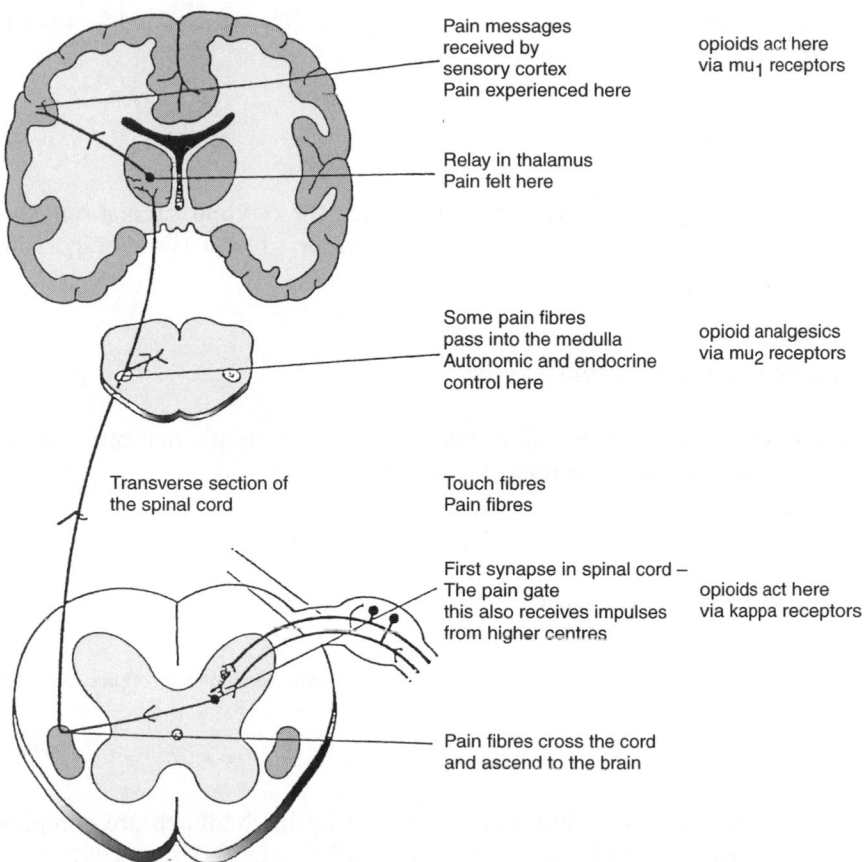

Pain messages
received by
sensory cortex
Pain experienced here

opioids act here
via mu$_1$ receptors

Relay in thalamus
Pain felt here

Some pain fibres
pass into the medulla
Autonomic and endocrine
control here

opioid analgesics
via mu$_2$ receptors

Transverse section of
the spinal cord

Touch fibres
Pain fibres

First synapse in spinal cord –
The pain gate
this also receives impulses
from higher centres

opioids act here
via kappa receptors

Pain fibres cross the cord
and ascend to the brain

During the first stage of labour, the pain fibres stimulated enter the spinal cord from T$_{10}$ to L$_1$.
During the second stage of labour, the pain fibres from the perineum are stimulated and
enter the spinal cord from S$_2$ to S$_4$.

Figure 4.1   Diagram to illustrate the pain pathways
Source: Adapted from Jordan, 1992.

fetus. Between contractions, the lack of carbon dioxide reduces the respiratory drive and decreases respirations. This can lead to hypoxia of mother and fetus.

Tachycardia

The increase in heart rate increases the work and oxygen needs of the heart while simultaneously reducing coronary blood flow. Ischaemic changes in the ECG are not uncommon in labour. Tachycardia can reduce cardiac output. In labour, cardiac output must increase to meet the work requirements of the muscles. If cardiac output declines, insufficient oxygen will be delivered to the muscles for aerobic respiration to take place. Therefore, lactic acid will accumulate, making the woman acidotic.

Hypertension

Any sudden rise in blood pressure can threaten the cerebral circulation. The physiological changes of pregnancy render cerebral blood vessels especially vulnerable to hypertensive episodes.

Gastric stasis and emesis

Pain causes gastric stasis and disturbances of the autonomic nervous system. Intense pain may lead to nausea and vomiting.

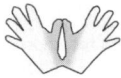 **Practice Point**

Even if a woman has received no analgesia, close observations of vital signs must be maintained.

The anatomy, physiology and psychology of pain in childbirth are complex issues (see Groer & Shekleton, 1989; Moore, 1993; Mas & Lamy, 1998; Carr & Goudas, 1999; Yerby & Page, 2000).

Inhalation analgesia

Introduction

Inhalation analgesia is achieved by the use of anaesthetic gases in sub-anaesthetic concentrations. The widespread use of inhalation analgesia in childbirth for over a hundred years has established its relative safety. Nevertheless, the administration of inhalation agents requires close supervision (Clyburn & Rosen, 1993). (See Implications for Practice). In the UK, only nitrous oxide is in regular use for inhalation analgesia in childbirth, although other anaesthetic agents may be employed for Caesarean section and surgical procedures. Therefore, the principles of inhalation anaesthetics, relevant to all gaseous agents, will be outlined in this chapter, with a more detailed review of nitrous oxide analgesia such as Entonox® (a mixture of 50 per cent nitrous oxide and 50 per cent oxygen).

Uses of inhalation agents

Nitrous oxide, as Entonox®, is normally available to women in all delivery settings and provides intermittent analgesia during uterine contractions (Clyburn & Rosen, 1993). Reynolds (1993a) suggests that it is most effective when reserved for use during transition, the second stage of labour, perineal suturing and while awaiting epidural analgesia. Studies have shown that women have found it to be a more effective analgesic than meperidine (pethidine) or TENS machines, but less effective than epidural analgesia (Reynolds, 1993a). The pharmacology of nitrous oxide described here is directly applicable to Entonox®, used in the UK.

Actions of inhalation agents

The precise mechanism of action of the anaesthetic gases remains uncertain. Although the chemistry of these agents is diverse, they share the properties of lipid solubility and the ability to bind to cell membranes at certain sites. This interaction with cell membranes affects the release of neurotransmitters at synapses and the transmission of nerve impulses in the central nervous system. Anaesthetics potentiate the actions of inhibitory neurotransmitters (Kennedy & Longnecker, 1996). The reticular activating system in the brain stem is an important site of action for inhalational agents. This is a network of neurones which transmits sensory input to the cerebral cortex, in a nonspecific manner, to control states of arousal and consciousness. Gradual suppression of the reticular activating system results in the four stages, or depths, of anaesthesia: analgesia, delirium, surgical anaesthesia and finally depression of the vital centres of the medulla.

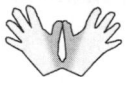 **Practice Point**

It is important to realize that an incorrect dose of an inhalation agent may produce a stage of anaesthesia which is not clinically desirable.

How the body handles inhalation agents

The effect of an inhalation agent depends on not only how much is absorbed but also on the concentration of gas reaching the brain. This is determined by:

- the concentration of the inspired gaseous mixture;
- the pulmonary ventilation delivering the gas to the lungs;
- the transfer across the respiratory (alveolar) membrane into the bloodstream;
- the solubility of the gas in blood;
- the loss of the gas into other body tissues;
- the cardiac output [glossary] and the blood supply to the brain.

Concentration of inspired gas

Nitrous oxide is not sufficiently powerful to produce surgical anaesthesia when used alone. Concentrations of 50 per cent nitrous oxide are needed for effective analgesia. If this is administered with air, rather than oxygen, hypoxia will ensue. Should high concentrations be administered (for example following improper storage; see below), hypoxia is an urgent consideration. When nitrous oxide was inhaled with air from the pre-1965 standard obstetric analgesic machine, oxygen concentrations as low as 1.8 per cent were inhaled and the women were so hypoxic they became cyanosed (Cole, 1975). Nitrous oxide is now administered as Entonox®, using pre-mixed cylinders of 50 per cent nitrous oxide in 50 per cent oxygen as a homogenous gas (BOC, 1996).

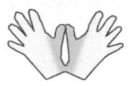 **Practice Point**

Improper storage of cylinders could allow administration of concentrations of nitrous oxide greater than 50 per cent, reducing the percentage of oxygen available. If this is suspected, oxygen saturation should be assessed.

Pulmonary ventilation

Increases in ventilation [glossary] will increase the delivery of gas to the blood and hasten the effects of gaseous analgesia and anaesthesia. Women given nitrous oxide tend to over-ventilate in order to maximize pain relief. The inherent danger is that they will exhale too much carbon dioxide, lowering the CO_2 concentration in the blood, which causes:

- vasoconstriction of the placental bed and hypoxia in the fetus;
- maternal hypoventilation between contractions, leading to fetal hypoxia;

- cerebral vasoconstriction, making the woman dizzy;
- alkalosis [glossary], which may induce tetany.

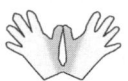 **Practice Points**

- It is important that the respirations of all women are supervised during the administration of inhalation agents and instructions are given to breathe slowly and fairly deeply (Clyburn & Rosen, 1993: 180).
- Tetany usually begins as painful involuntary spasms of the muscles of the hands and feet. If the early signs go unnoticed, it may develop into spasm of the larynx and obstruction of the airway.
- Any reports of dizziness, tingling or twitching in the woman's hands or feet should be an indication to monitor breathing patterns very closely for signs of over-breathing.
- The prolonged use of nitrous oxide from early labour should be avoided (Reynolds, 1993a).
- Women with diseases of nerves or muscles (such as disseminated sclerosis) may be unable to benefit fully from nitrous oxide inhalation.

Transfer across the respiratory membrane

This will be compromised in women with lung disease (such as severe asthma or cystic fibrosis), resulting in delays in both the absorption and elimination of the gas (Kennedy & Longnecker, 1996).

Solubility of the gas in blood

This determines the rate at which the gas is absorbed and eliminated from the body. Gases such as nitrous oxide, which dissolve in blood to a minimal extent, act on the brain very quickly, giving rapid analgesia (within 20–60 seconds) and are excreted rapidly. Due to its relatively low solubility in lipids (fats), nitrous oxide is rapidly eliminated from the blood and tissues with high blood flow, including the brain.

Transfer into tissues

The amount of gas transferred into different tissues depends on the flow of blood, the concentration of the gas and the nature of the tissue, since gases dissolve more readily in some tissues than in others. Anaesthetics have a tendency to accumulate in fat.

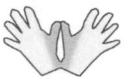 **Practice Points**

- Women with generous deposits of adipose tissue will require more anaesthetic agent than thin women.
- Recovery from all anaesthetics is delayed in obese people (Rang et al, 1999).

The blood/brain barrier [glossary] is freely permeable to anaesthetics and the brain is well perfused, therefore the concentration of gas in the brain is approximately equal to that in the blood. The analgesic effects of nitrous oxide are experienced some 25–35 seconds after administration.

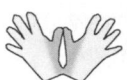 **Practice Point**

Ideally, nitrous oxide should be inhaled some 20 seconds before a contraction. There is a 15-second interval between a contraction becoming palpable to the midwife and the onset of pain. Therefore, palpation assists in the timing of administration of nitrous oxide (Beischer et al, 1997).

Cardiac output is important in determining blood flow to lungs and tissues; the distribution of inhalation agents may be impaired in women with pre-eclampsia or a compromised cardiovascular system (Nagelhout, 1992).

Elimination of inhalation agents

Being lipid soluble, inhalation agents cross the placenta, and accumulate in the fetus. They are eliminated via the lungs after delivery. This is an advantage over other analgesics, which depend on the immature liver and kidneys for removal (Clyburn & Rosen, 1993). In both mother and neonate it is estimated that the effects of Entonox® have worn off after two to three minutes (BOC, 1996), although removal from tissues with low blood flow, such as fat, takes longer (Kennedy & Longnecker, 1996).

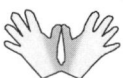 **Practice Point**

Opioids depress ventilation in mothers and neonates and therefore may retard the recovery from inhalational agents if co-administered (Rang et al, 1999).

When high concentrations of nitrous oxide have been administered for some time, 'diffusion hypoxia' may occur on abrupt discontinuation and resumption of breathing air. This is due to large volumes of nitrous oxide entering the alveoli and diluting the available oxygen. Therefore, for a brief period, the woman and neonate are inhaling a concentration of oxygen below 20 per cent.

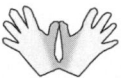 **Practice Point**

The resulting hypoxia can be prevented by administration of supplementary oxygen when nitrous oxide is discontinued to both the neonate at birth and the woman in the early recovery period (Clyburn & Rosen, 1993; Kennedy & Longnecker, 1996; Marshall & Longnecker, 1996).

Nitrous oxide

Nitrous oxide is colourless, odourless, heavier than air and non-explosive. It strongly supports combustion, and should not be allowed to contact lighted cigarettes, oils, greases, tars or many plastics. Should a fire occur, normal fire extinguishers are effective (BOC, 1995). It is available at concentrations of 50 per cent or 70 per cent in oxygen.

Side effects of nitrous oxide

The side effects of nitrous oxide impact in two areas (See Implications for Practice):

- the cental nervous systems of the woman and fetus/neonate;
- the bone marrow and reproductive systems of staff.

Nitrous oxide is not a muscle relaxant and, unlike other anaesthetic gases, it has no effect on smooth muscle, including the uterus (Marshall & Longnecker, 1996). All anaesthetic gases depress the nervous system. This involves both the higher functions and the vital centres of the medulla and brain stem.

Central nervous system depression (obtunding)

Nitrous oxide produces some maternal sedation. Self-administration provides some safeguard against overdosage: as the woman becomes drowsy, the mask or mouthpiece falls away. The manufacturers suggest that administration will cease before the laryngeal (gag) reflex is lost (BOC, 1996). However, overuse of inhalation agents can result in depression of the central nervous system, including the laryngeal reflex. If the laryngeal reflex is suppressed, and unable to protect the airway, there is a danger of aspiration of stomach contents, should any vomiting occur (Zelcer et al, 1989 Clyburn & Rosen, 1993).

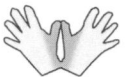 **Practice Point**

Close observation of the woman for any signs of sedation is extremely important.

Central nervous system depression, dizziness and confusion are usually mild, although it is recommended that no one should drive a motor vehicle or use machinery for at least 12 hours following the use of Entonox® analgesia (BOC, 1995). Only in very high concentrations does medullary paralysis (stage 4 of anaesthesia) occur, depressing respiratory and cardiovascular systems (Rang et al, 1999; Malseed et al, 1995).

Neonatal CNS depression is a potential hazard with all inhalational agents, including prolonged administration of nitrous oxide (Capogna & Celleno, 1993). In normal doses, nitrous oxide is eliminated so rapidly that neonates do not suffer adverse effects (Brownridge, 1991).

Hallucinations

Vivid dreams and hallucinations represent the delirium stage (stage 2) of anaesthesia and women should be warned that these may occur transiently, since the feelings of dissociation produced may be very unpleasant (Bushnell & Justins, 1993). Some of the analgesic properties of nitrous oxide are attributed to its effect on the affective and cognitive dimensions of pain (Carstoniu et al, 1994). Some people may find inhalation pleasurable and over-use Entonox® in early labour.

Nausea

Nausea is a common side effect of nitrous oxide and vomiting may occur (Reynolds, 1993a).

Hypoxia

Hypoxia is a particular danger if nitrous oxide is used without adequate supervision. All anaesthetics tend to depress the vital centres, but the effects of nitrous oxide are subtle and may be easily overlooked (Marshall & Longnecker, 1996). The use of nitrous oxide may worsen any existing fetal hypoxia and exacerbate any placental insufficiency. Zelcher et al (1989) suggest that if the fetal heart rate is abnormal, the use of nitrous oxide is ill-advised. In one study (n = 40), inhalation of Entonox® throughout the first and second stages of labour resulted in a higher incidence of maternal hypoxia than did epidural anaesthesia (Arfeen et al, 1994). Pulse oximeters were used to detect hypoxia in this study.

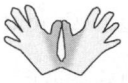 **Practice Points**

- A pulse oximeter assists in assessing the situation, since it provides continuous measurement of maternal haemoglobin saturation without causing discomfort. However, it **cannot detect changes in carbon dioxide** concentrations.
- Use of a pulse oximeter is advised if administration of nitrous oxide has been prolonged, the woman has dark skin, opioids are co-administered or any uncertainty exists (DoH, 1996; Marshall and Longnecker, 1996).

Side effects related to prolonged exposure (mainly staff)

Nitrous oxide inactivates vitamin B_{12}. The effect persists for several days. After brief exposure, this is rarely clinically significant. However, nitrous oxide should be avoided if pre-existing vitamin B_{12} deficiency exists, for example in pernicious anaemia (Rang et al, 1999). BOC (1995) recommend that the administration of Entonox® for longer than 24 hours (which is unlikely to occur in labour) should be accompanied by routine examination of the red and white blood cells for evidence of B_{12} deficiency.

Effect on reproduction

There is a possibility that prolonged occupational exposure to nitrous oxide may impair male or female fertility and increase the incidence of spontaneous abortions and preterm delivery (BOC, 1995; Reynolds et al, 1996; Rang et al, 1999). Nitrous oxide in low analgesic doses is teratogenic in rodents, but these findings have not been confirmed in humans (Rice, 1993). Use of, or exposure to, nitrous oxide during the first trimester may be harmful to the fetus, but is not absolutely contra-indicated, for example following trauma (BOC, 1995).

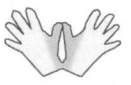 **Practice Point**

Because of the possible effects on staff, the concentration of nitrous oxide in the atmosphere should be maintained below a specified level.

The literature offers conflicting advice on the precise concentration considered safe.

- BOC (1995) recommend that the concentration of nitrous oxide should not exceed one hundred parts per million (ppm).
- Marshall and Longnecker (1996) state that the atmosphere of the delivery/operating room should not contain more than 50 ppm.
- Exposure limits given by the US National Institute of Occupational Safety and Health indicate that the maximum permissible dose for nitrous oxide is 25 ppm time-weighted average (West, 1993).

These concentrations may be achieved by effective ventilation and the scavenging of waste gases.

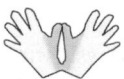 **Practice Point**

Health care workers should protect themselves by ensuring all gas cylinders are functioning correctly (not leaking) and avoiding the area within one foot of the client's face while the client is exhaling or administering nitrous oxide (McKenry & Salerno, 1998).

Storage

Entonox® may separate into nitrous oxide and oxygen if the temperature falls below −6°C (for example if it is stored outside). It is unsafe to administer in this condition. To ensure homogenization, cylinders should be stored horizontally above 10°C for 24 hours before use; if this is not possible, the manufacturers should be contacted to suggest alternatives (BOC, 1995). Incorrectly stored cylinders may administer insufficient oxygen (see below).

Drug interactions

The respiratory depressant action of opioids may be compounded by nitrous oxide, causing transient maternal hypoxia (Clyburn & Rosen, 1993). Most gaseous anaesthetics sensitize the heart to the action of adrenaline/epinephrine, risking cardiac dysrhythmias, but nitrous oxide is free from this effect.

Cautions

Nitrous oxide has the capacity to enter any pockets of gas trapped within the body and expand them. Therefore, it is contra-indicated in any situation where abnormal quantities of gas are trapped within the body, due to the risk of gas retention, for example in women with middle ear occlusion (BOC, 1995; Marshall & Longnecker, 1996; Twycross, 1994). Nitrous oxide may also diffuse into air bubbles formed by intra-spinal analgesia, hindering the spread of local anaesthetic (Reynolds et al, 1996). Nitrous oxide may impair levels of consciousness. It should not be administered to women whose level of consciousness is already impaired.

Conclusion

Although it is not always effective, nitrous oxide combined with oxygen has relatively few side effects and these can be minimized if administration is supervised and monitored by the midwife. Rapid elimination from maternal and neonatal circulations is an added advantage (Olofsson & Irestedt, 1998). In view of this, nitrous oxide remains a flexible and useful method of pain relief during labour.

Implications for practice: entonox®

Although the use of nitrous oxide is generally safe, careful supervision of the woman and her breathing pattern is important.

Potential problem	Management and care
Sedation	Supervise closely. Self administration. Be alert for vomiting.
Maternal and fetal hypoxia	Use premixed oxygen with nitrous oxide. Ensure the cylinder is correctly stored and fully mixed. Supervise – ensure slow, even inspirations. Use a pulse oximeter, for example if opioids are co-administered. Avoid prolonged use. Monitor fetal heart rate intermittently. Be prepared to administer oxygen to the neonate.
Dizziness, tetany	Prevent hyper-ventilation. Discontinue should tingling in hands and feet occur. Specifically question the woman about this.
Nausea	Supervise closely. Position to avoid aspiration.

> **Implications for practice: entonox® (*continued*)**
>
> | Potential problem | Management and Care |
> |---|---|
> | Hallucinations, dissociation | Warn recipients. Avoid over-use. |
> | Vitamin B$_{12}$ deficiency | Limit maternal administration to 24 hours. |
> | Affects on reproduction | Monitor the concentration in the environment. Avoid excessively close staff contact with gas. |
> | Risk of fire | Avoid contact with cigarettes, greases and oils. |

Opioids

Opioid drugs, such as meperidine (pethidine), are used extensively in labour. The term 'opioid' is used to describe any preparation acting on the body's opioid receptors, which normally respond to endorphins and enkephalins. Thus morphine, diamorphine, meperidine, meptazinol, codeine, buprenorphine (Temgesic®), pentazocine (Fortral) and the 'morphine antagonists' such as naloxone (Narcan®) are all opioids. In the absence of evidence favouring any particular opioid (Fairlie et al, 1999), the opioid offered is often based on institutional preference (Brownridge, 1991). This section considers the pharmacology of opioids. The distinctive features of meperidine, meptazinol and diamorphine are described below.

Uses of opioids

Opioids are used in labour, pre-operatively, intra-operatively, post-operatively and in intensive care for analgesia, sedation and reduction of anxiety. Opioids are able to reduce the hyperventilation induced by pain and maintain carbon dioxide at near normal concentrations (Clyburn & Rosen, 1993). Various low-dose opioid preparations are sold as over-the-counter preparations for controlling symptoms of cough or diarrhoea in all age groups.

Analgesia

Opioids provide greater pain relief in labour than either no treatment or injection of sterile water (Howell, 1994). Nevertheless, mothers frequently report that pain relief in labour from meperidine (pethidine) is inadequate (Ranta et al, 1995). However when opioids are discontinued, there is frequently a rebound increase in pain sensitivity. Opioids such as pethidine, morphine and the more powerful synthetic drugs, fentanyl and alfentanil, may also be administered epidurally or intrathecally and give rapid and effective analgesia

(Herpolsheimer & Schretenthaler, 1994). Although 6–30 hours of analgesia is provided by this route, the side effects may be troublesome, particularly urinary retention, sedation, nausea, itching, hypotension and respiratory arrest (Chrubasik et al, 1992). Intraspinal opioids are discussed at the end of this chapter. [The term 'intraspinal injection' is used to refer to administration within the spinal column, that is to encompass epidural, intrathecal (spinal) and combined spinal epidural administration (Wildsmith, 1996).]

Anaesthesia and reduction of anxiety

The benefits of opioids can be attributed to both their analgesic and anxiolytic actions. The release of adrenaline/epinephrine and noradrenaline/norepinephrine due to pain and anxiety decrease uterine blood flow. This is reversed by opioids, to the benefit of the fetus (Hollmen, 1993).

How the body handles opioids

Opioids are not given orally during labour, due to delays in absorption and metabolism. Intramuscular injection is the most convenient alternative. Opioids are metabolized in the liver and excreted via urine and bile. The metabolic pathways for each opioid differ.

Opioids are rapidly transferred across the placenta: changes are detected by fetal scalp electrodes within seven minutes of intramuscular administration of meperidine (pethidine). The fetus and neonate excrete opioids more slowly than adults, due to the immaturity of their liver enzymes (Chapter 1). In addition, due to the lower pH in the fetus, basic drugs, such as meperidine, are more likely to be ionized [glossary] in the fetus. Therefore, they may become 'trapped', unable to return to the maternal circulation. [Drugs are only transferred across the placenta in their non-ionized state.] At steady state, their concentration will always be higher in the fetal circulation than in the mother.

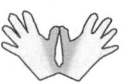 **Practice Points**

- If the fetus becomes acidotic due to lack of oxygen, the side effects of opioids are magnified (Clyburn & Rosen, 1993). Therefore, blood flow to the placenta and maternal oxygen saturation must be maintained at all times.
- The blood supply to the placenta is considerably reduced during uterine contractions. Therefore transfer of drug to the fetus may be minimized by intramuscluar administration immediately before a contraction (Carson, 1996).

Following a single intramuscular dose of meperidine (pethidine) to the mother, the fetus receives maximum exposure two to three hours later; therefore respiratory depression in the neonate is most likely in babies born at this time. If delivery occurs within one hour of meperidine administration, very little drug is transferred to the fetus. Should delivery occur more than six hours after administration, much of the meperidine will have been transferred back to the mother, although the active metabolite normeperidine will remain in the neonatal tissues. This is gradually excreted over several days. During this time the neonate's behaviour will be suboptimal (irritable and difficult to feed) (Crowell et al, 1994). The amount of normeperidine transferred to the baby is greater the longer the time between delivery and pethidine administration (Crowell et al, 1994).

Meperidine (pethidine) is metabolized to normeperidine, which is toxic in high concentrations. The half-life [glossary] of meperidine is three hours in the mother and four to five hours in the neonate. The half-life of normeperidine is 20 hours in the mother and 60 hours in the neonate. Therefore, this metabolite takes several days to clear from the neonate, during which time side effects persist. With multiple doses, normeperidine may accumulate in the fetus/neonate and cause respiratory depression and fits that are resistant to, or even exacerbated by, naloxone (Narcan®) administration.

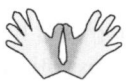 **Practice Points**

- Each institution imposes a maximum dose of meperidine/pethidine which is never exceeded. (The BNF (2000) gives 400 mg in 24 hours which will be excessive for some women.)
- Extra help will be needed to ensure the infant suckles correctly over the first three to five days of life. An irritable or jittery baby is unable to suckle the whole areola. Unless corrected, the resulting tissue damage will be painful and may lead to infection.

Meperidine/pethidine passes into breast milk which compounds early difficulties with feeding (Yerby, 2000). The dose of meperidine is subject to institutional preference and standing orders. Doses usually range from 50–100 mg by subcutaneous or intramuscular injection (BNF, 2000).

Actions of opioids

Opioids are chemically related to the body's endorphins and enkephalins, which are natural mood changers and analgesics, particularly in times of stress.

Opioids act at many sites in the central nervous system, including the spinal cord, the medulla, the midbrain and the cerebral cortex. (see Figure 4.1) Several classes of opioid receptors exist and different opiate drugs act selectively at different receptors to produce diverse responses. In some situations, the euphoriant or sedative effects of opioids predominate over their analgesic actions (Arner & Meyerson, 1988; Olofsson et al, 1996).

Opioids bind to the cell surface receptors for the endorphins and enkephalins, fitting in like keys into a lock (see Chapter 1). This binding triggers changes within the nerve or smooth muscle cells, usually inhibiting their activity and neurotransmitter release. In general, opioids (endogenous and pharmacological) depress the activity of target tissues and have a calming effect. They inhibit the hypothalamus and 'damp down' the level of activity in the autonomic nervous system, partly by reducing the stress response attributable to noradrenaline (norepinephrine).

There are several classes of opioid receptor, some are assigned a Greek letter. Several classes of opioid receptor are of pharmacological importance: μ_1,(mu1); μ_2,(mu2); δ,(delta); κ,(kappa) and peripheral opioid receptors. These are summarized in relation to common side effects in Table 4.1.

Table 4.1 Actions and side effects of opioids summarized

Actions of opioid receptors		
κ (kappa) receptors	analgesia, sedation and dysphoria	
μ_1 (mu 1) receptors	supraspinal analgesia, euphoria and addiction	
μ_2 (mu 2) receptors	depression of vital centres:	respiration
		heart rate
		orthostatic hypotension
		thermoregulation
		cough
	affect smooth muscle of:	
	uterus	prolonged labour
	urinary tract	retention of urine
	gut	constipation, ileus, gastric stasis
	blood vessels	hypotension
	eye	pupillary constriction
		(not seen in meperidine/pethidine overdose)
δ (delta) receptors	spinal and supraspinal analgesia	
Stimulation of		
Chemoreceptor trigger zone	nausea and vomiting	
Histamine release	pruritus	
	vasodilation and hypotension	
	bronchospasm in asthmatics	
Inhibition of		
Substance P release	spinal analgesia	
Neuroendocrine function		

Side effects of opioids *(see Implications for Practice)*

Central nervous system (CNS) – higher functions

Opioids act on more than one type of receptor in the cerbral cortex. While sedation is the usual result, central nervous system excitability, including hallucinations and convulsions, sometimes occurs.

Depression and obtunding of central nervous system

Opioids produce drowsiness, mental clouding and sometimes euphoria. These actions may be beneficial in some situations, for example in intensive care, but sedation is disadvantageous to both mother and baby in a normal labour. Opioids may provide sedation rather than analgesia (Olofsson et al, 1996): following administration of opioids, a woman may fall asleep, only to be woken by the pain of contractions (Fairlie et al, 1999). Central nervous system depression/obtunding [glossary] and sedation induced by opioids reduces the mother's ability to co-operate with labour. Sedation may be profound if any degree of thyroid imbalance is present. (see Chapter 18, thyroid disorders).

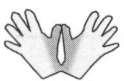 **Practice Point**

A woman who has received opioids may be sedated, and less able to 'push' in the second stage which will prolong labour.

For neonates, exposure to meperidine (pethidine) reduces the muscle tone and depresses the CNS (Wagner, 1993). This causes delay in the sucking and rooting responses (Nissen et al, 1995). The establishment of breastfeeding appears to be delayed by several hours if opioids are administered 1–5 hours before delivery (Crowell et al, 1994): several mothers in this study who had received meperidine discontinued breastfeeding because the infant was not feeding well. If delivery is delayed by more than eight hours after meperidine administration, there is less impact on feeding behaviour. In one study, infants who failed to suck had higher plasma concentrations of meperidine than those who started to feed, which suggests that failure to feed is a dose-dependent side effect (Nissen et al, 1997).

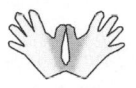 **Practice Point**

Problems with breastfeeding are more likely to arise if the dose of meperidine is 100 mg, rather than 50 mg (Nissen et al, 1997).

The fetal electroencephalogram is modified soon after the intramuscular administration of meperidine to the mother; this effect persists for the first four days of life, and corresponds to the neonate's decreased level of arousal and muscle tone (Clyburn & Rosen, 1993). Due to the long half-life (60 hours) of the metabolite (normeperidine), neonatal behaviour is depressed for approximately three days after the administration of meperidine (pethidine) during labour. During this time reflexes and thermoregulation are compromised and abnormal reflexes are more likely (Crowell et al, 1994).

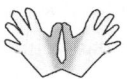 **Practice Point**

The poor muscle tone of affected infants means that they are less likely to suckle on the whole areola, thus traumatizing the nipple. It is better to supplement breastfeeding, preferably by expressed milk in a cup, over the first two to five days than to abandon it entirely.

Central nervous system excitability

Opioids may induce euphoria, dysphoria, tremulousness, restlessness or delirium. Visual disturbances, hallucinations and nightmares may accompany opioid use. Normeperidine (a metabolite of meperidine) may cause neurobehavioural abnormalities such as twitching and convulsions. Although respiratory depression produced by meperidine (pethidine) can be reversed by naloxone, any convulsions and respiratory depression caused by normeperidine are less likely to respond (Clyburn & Rosen, 1993).

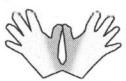 **Practice Point**

The midwife should be aware that not all respiratory depression will respond to naloxone, particularly in infants where normeperidine may have accumulated, for example following repeated doses and long delays between administration and delivery.

Central nervous system – brain stem

Opioids inhibit the activity of the vital centres in the brain stem. Therefore, midwives always pay close attention to the vital signs of the mother, fetus and neonate.

Respiratory depression

Opioids act directly on the respiratory centre in the medulla to depress respiration, and, also in rare instances, on the peripheral receptors to induce apnoea (Bowdle, 1998). Opioids reduce the sensitivity of the respiratory centre to carbon dioxide, thus reducing the normal drive to respiration (Reisine & Pasternak, 1996). Therefore, respiration fails to increase to meet the high metabolic demands of labour. Rate, depth and regularity of respirations are decreased, reducing alveolar ventilation and oxygenation. This effect is intensified if the woman becomes so sedated that she falls asleep. If the circulation is adequate, respiratory depression is maximal within 90 minutes of intramuscular administration. If the peripheral circulation is 'shut down' as in shock or haemorrhage, the absorption and side effects of intramuscular drugs can be delayed.

Depression of the carbon dioxide respiratory drive means that the patient's breathing depends on the hypoxic respiratory drive. Administration of a high concentration of oxygen to a patient (adult or neonate) whose respirations are depressed due to opioids can remove the remaining respiratory drive and precipitate a sudden respiratory arrest. This may be difficult to reverse, due to a sharp rise in carbon dioxide concentration (Reisine & Pasternak, 1996).

Respiratory depression of the woman during labour may lead to:
- retention of carbon dioxide and respiratory acidosis, in mother and fetus.
- hypoxia in mother and fetus which causes fetal heart rate decelerations.

Under these conditions, the fetus becomes acidotic, increasing his/her accumulation of meperidine and metabolites.

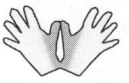 **Practice Points**

- Maternal respirations must be carefully monitored for rate, depth and rhythm.
- A pulse oximeter offers a useful guide as to the degree of oxygen saturation in the mother.
- Fetal monitoring for signs of acidosis is important in prolonged labours.

In the neonate, measurements with fetal scalp electrodes indicate that transcutaneous oxygen tensions (levels) fall to 37 per cent of baseline values seven minutes after the intramuscular administration of 50 mg meperidine (pethidine) but recover within 15 minutes (Clyburn & Rosen, 1993). Depression of the central nervous system (see above) reduces the neonate's reflexes, including the respiratory reflexes needed to cope with hypoxia and birth (Wagner, 1993).

The resultant respiratory depression in the neonate is potentially lethal; premature infants are particularly at risk (Karch, 1992). Rapid reversal with naloxone, an opioid antagonist [glossary] is mandatory. An overview of clinical trials found an association between opioid analgesia and low APGAR scores (Howell, 1994).

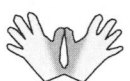 **Practice Point**

If opioids are administered, naloxone, oxygen and means of ventilation for the neonate must always be available.

Bradycardia

Opioids reduce the heart rate, by direct action on the cardiovascular centres in the medulla, by decreasing the activity of the sympathetic nervous system and by reducing anxiety. In labour, this may contribute to a fall in blood pressure and a reduction in placental perfusion. The subsequent depression of the fetal heart rate and loss of fetal heart baseline variability may be interpreted as fetal distress, triggering medical interventions.

Some fetal bradycardia on administration of analgesia is normal. This is attributed to the transient release of oxytocin (see below) which causes a brief tetanic contraction of the uterus (Eberle & Norris, 1996). However bradycardia lasting beyond five to eight minutes may be a sign of metabolic stress (Arkoosh, 1991).

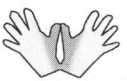 **Practice Point**

Fetal heart monitoring should be undertaken soon after administration of opioids and interpreted cautiously. Intermittent monitoring is often the preferred option.

Hypotension

Opioids act on the cardiovascular centres in the medulla, the blood vessels and the sympathetic nervous system to produce a fall in blood pressure. This is exaggerated on standing or sitting up, partly due to inhibition of the barore-ceptor reflex (Reisine & Pasternak, 1996). Sudden standing may result in dizziness, loss of balance or falls. Bed rest, fluid depletion, alcohol or phe-nothiazines such as prochlorperazine (Stemetil®) will exacerbate the effects of opioids on blood pressure. Hypotension can also impair placental and renal perfusion. Any hypotension is likely to be exaggerated by the fetal head com-pressing the maternal aorta and vena cava if the mother adopts the supine position.

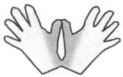 **Practice Points**

- The woman should not lie in a supine position.
- The woman will need assistance to get up slowly after administration of opioids.
- Opioids should be used with caution, if at all, in women with decreased blood volume, as the effects of hypovolaemic shock will be aggravated (Reisine & Pasternak, 1996).

Depression of thermoregulation

Opioids act on the hypothalamus to reduce the thermoregulatory set point. This has been recorded following meperidine (pethidine) administration during labour (Clyburn & Rosen, 1993). It is hazardous for the neonate, whose thermoregulatory mechanisms rely on the sympathetic nervous system. The vasoconstrictor and shivering responses are depressed in all neonates, and this is accentuated by opioids.

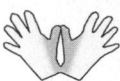 **Practice Point**

The neonate must be kept warm, preferably by the mother. However, the mother may be sedated following opioid administration, and she should be carefully observed to minimize any danger of 'over-lying'.

Cough

Opioids suppress the cough and sigh reflexes and depress the movement of respiratory cilia. This causes accumulation of the mucus secreted by the respiratory tract. Depression of the respiratory cilia is compounded by smoking. These factors increase the risks of pulmonary atelectasis [glossary] and chest infections (Govoni & Hayes, 1990).

Actions on smooth muscle

Generally, opioids cause relaxation of smooth muscle and contraction of sphincters.

Prolonged labour

Administration of intramuscular meperidine briefly stimulates the hypothalamus to release oxytocin, which causes a brief tetanic uterine contraction (Eberle & Norris, 1996). However, this effect is superceded by reduced contractility of uterine smooth muscle due to decreased release of oxytocin and the direct action on the mu_2/μ_2 opioid receptors. These actions are similar to those of endogenous opioids (Carson, 1996). Although the literature in this area suffers from absence of human randomized controlled trials, animal and *in vitro* studies suggest that meperidine and morphine reduce both the uterine response to oxytocin and the oxytocin release from the posterior pituitary gland (Thompson & Hillier, 1994). Uterine contractions may diminish following the administration of meperidine (pethidine) (Baxi et al, 1988), but this is disputed by some authorities (Reisine & Pasternak, 1996).

A literature review (Thompson & Hillier, 1994) indicated that the duration of both first and second stages of labour is directly related to the amount of meperidine (pethidine) administered during the first stage of labour.

Retention of urine and dysuria

Opioids reduce urine formation by increasing the secretion of antidiuretic hormone and reducing renal perfusion. They also inhibit the smooth muscle of the bladder. The voiding reflex is inhibited, while the tone of the internal urethral sphincter is increased. Combined with trauma to the urethra during labour, retention of urine is common following delivery.

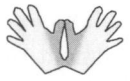 **Practice Points**

- Urine output should be monitored during and after labour.
- A full bladder may impede contraction of the uterus post partum, increasing blood loss.

Gastrointestinal tract

The motility of the stomach, small intestine and colon are decreased. Opioids inhibit the propulsive, peristaltic actions of the gut, while increasing seg-mental, non-propulsive contractions, particularly in the pyloric region of the stomach, the first part of the duodenum and the colon. Gastric stasis may cause oesophageal reflux (heart burn), nausea and vomiting. Opioids contribute to the constipation which commonly follows delivery. Opioids decrease gastro-intestinal secretions, causing a dry mouth. Spasm of the biliary tract, producing pain on the right side of the abdomen, is a rare side effect of opioids.

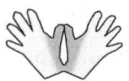 **Practice Points**

- Painful abdominal cramps may follow administration of opioids.
- The woman must be positioned so that gastric contents do not enter the airway.

Nausea and vomiting

Gastric stasis and stimulation of the chemoreceptor trigger zone (in the medulla) combine to cause nausea, which is experienced by 30–60 per cent of women receiving opioids. Ambulation and sudden movement stimulate the vestibular apparatus, and contribute to the nausea associated with opioids. Nausea and vomiting are less likely to occur if the patient remains resting. Pain, labour, fear and anxiety also induce gastric stasis, nausea and vomiting. When these physiological effects of labour are combined with the sedative actions of opioids, the dangers of gastric aspiration become very real.

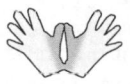 **Practice Points**

- A woman who has vomited following opioid administration should be warned that emesis is likely to recur on any subsequent administration of the same opioid.
- Vomiting can disrupt fluid and electrolyte balance, and increase the risk of thromboembolism (see Chapter 5, anti-emetics).

Histamine release

Opioids stimulate release of histamine. This may cause pruritus or bronchospasm and contribute to hypotension.

Pruritus

Histamine release may cause flushing, itching, 'nettle rash' and sweating, particularly in the upper part of the body. This is the most common side effect when opioids are given by the intrathecal route (Herpolsheimer & Schretenthaler, 1994).

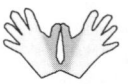 **Practice Points**

- Coolant gels may help relieve discomfort.
- Anti-histamine creams can be administered on medical advice, but they do not always abolish the itching.
- Naloxone may be effective in relieving symptoms (Reisine & Pasternak, 1996).

Bronchospasm

Histamine release causes bronchoconstriction and may occasionally precipitate an attack of asthma (Beischer et al, 1997). Opioids are not administered during an asthma attack since they may worsen symptoms.

Neuroendocrine actions

Opioids act on the hypothalamus to alter hormone secretion. With short term administration, problems may occasionally arise.

- In women whose adrenal or thyroid function are disturbed, opioids may suppress the release of these hormones.
- Opioids act on the hypothalamus to enhance the secretion of antidiuretic hormone. Occasionally, this can cause water retention and hyponatraemia [glossary] which is a *medical emergency*. This is described in Chapter 6.

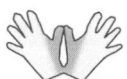 **Practice Point**

Women should be advised to drink only moderate quantities of plain water. Fluid balance must be checked following delivery.

Dependence

Some studies have linked the use of opioid analgesia in labour with an increased risk of opiate addiction in adult offspring in later life through a process of imprinting (Jacobson et al, 1990). However, Clyburn and Rosen (1993) suggest this work should be interpreted cautiously, since there were more males in the study group than the control group, and males have a greater risk of drug addiction.

Cautions

Opioids are used with caution, if at all, in the following circumstances:

- Reduced respiratory reserve: for example in asthma, obesity, kyphosis (excessive spinal curvature), disease of muscles or nerves (for example disseminated sclerosis). Opioids are contra-indicated if the partial pressure or concentration of carbon dioxide ($p\mathrm{CO_2}$) is raised, as in severe respiratory disease.
- With increasing age or debility or malnutrition, lower doses are needed since standard doses will produce excessive side effects. For example, a 40-year-old may need half the analgesic dose required by a 20-year-old (Twycross, 1994).
- Pre-existing hypotension may be dangerously worsened, for example, following haemorrhage.
- Excessive sedation and coma may result from administration of opioids to women with hypothyroidism or Addison's disease.
- Meperidine (pethidine) and propoxyphene are the opioids most likely to cause convulsions with repeated administration. This may be exacerbated by fluid retention following oxytocin administration.

- The CNS depressant effects of opioids will complicate any rise in intra-cranial pressure (for example following a CVA or an eclamptic seizure) by worsening respiratory depression and obscuring vital signs. Opioid-induced respiratory depression causes carbon dioxide retention, which will exacerbate any rise in intracranial pressure and increase cerebral ischaemia and seizures.
- Reduced doses of opioids are needed if liver or kidney function is impaired, for example in pre-eclampsia.
- Possibility of paralytic ileus.
- Known allergy to opioids.

Drug interactions

Opioids interact with many drugs, and this section offers only a guide.

Enhanced depression of CNS and vital centres

Administration of more than one depressant will intensify any opioid induced reduction in blood pressure, respiration and conscious levels. CNS depressants include: alcohol, anti-histamines, barbiturates, anaesthetics (nitrous oxide), benzodiazepines, metoclopramide, phenothiazines (for example prochlorperazine, Stemetil®), tricyclic antidepressants, and other non-opioid sedatives such as chloral hydrate. While phenothiazines have useful anti-emetic actions, they worsen postural hypotension, respiratory depression, sedation and bradycardia. Fentanyl plus diazepam or midazolam may cause hypotension and profound respiratory depression in adults and neonates (Stockley, 1999).

Case Report

This case illustrates the dangers of combining sedative drugs.

> A woman with severe pre-eclampsia was induced at 26 weeks' gestation. She received intravenous hydralazine and chlormethiazole, plus 100 mg meperidine (pethidine) intra-muscularly for analgesia. An hour later she was deeply sedated, and her airway was obstructed. The sedation was unrelieved and urine output was poor. She died later of adult respiratory distress syndrome, probably due to gastric aspiration while unconscious (DOH, 1991:79).

Two potent sedative drugs were administered. Together, these drugs inhibited the vital reflexes. Aspiration of stomach contents is a risk in unconscious or heavily sedated patients. The dose of meperidine (pethidine) seems high for a woman known to have a reduced circulatory volume due to pre-eclampsia.

Other interactions

- Selective serotonin uptake inhibitors (SSRIs) or monoamine oxidase inhibitors (MAOIs) (including moclobemide and fluoxetine (Prozac®)) and meperidine (pethidine), pentazocine, dextromethorphan or tramadol interact to produce hyperpyrexia, accompanied by either hypotension or hypertension, which can be fatal (Bowdle, 1998). (See the serotonin syndrome, Chapter 16.) *This drug combination must be avoided for two weeks after discontinuation of a MAOI.* This reaction is possible but less well documented with other opioids (*Drugs and Therapy Perspectives*, 1993b).
- **Gastric emptying**
  The gastric stasis induced by opioids is reversed by metoclopramide (Maxalon), cisapride and domperidone.
- **Drugs suppressing gastric acid secretion**
  Cimetidine inhibits liver enzymes, preventing the breakdown of other drugs. This may increase the concentration of meperidine (pethidine), methadone, fentanyl or morphine. Apnoea and confusion may result. Isolated reports exist of a similar reaction between morphine and ranitidine (Stockley, 1999).
- **Increased doses needed**
  Anticonvulsants (phenytoin, carbamazepine, phenobarbitone), rifampicin, oestrogens and tobacco all induce (speed up) liver enzymes. Therefore opioids (meperidine/pethidine and pentazocine) are more rapidly eliminated from the body, and more frequent dosing may be required to achieve pain relief (Stockley, 1999).
- Cyclizine co-administered with opioids can precipitate pulmonary oedema but only in seriously ill patients (BNF, 2000).

Implications for Practice: Opioids

Potential problem Maternal	Management
Respiratory depression, leading to hypoxia	Respirations should be assessed prior to, during and after administration of opioids, and if the respiration rate is below 12/min., or the breathing is unduly shallow or irregular, the opioid should be withheld until further assessment.
	A pulse oximeter should be used to check oxygenation (Bem et al, 1996). Administration of prochlorperazine will intensify these problems.
Respiratory arrest due to loss of carbon dioxide respiratory drive	Avoid administration of high dose oxygen to a patient whose respirations are depressed due to opioids.

Implications for Practice: Opioids (*continued*)

Potential problem Maternal	Management
Chest infection	The detrimental effects of reduced airway clearance can be mitigated by breathing exercises, positioning and turning. Avoid smoking until the opioid has been eliminated.
Hypotension	Women should be advised to mobilize slowly and to report any dizziness in order to reduce the likelihood of any falls. Monitor the lying and sitting BP and heart rate. This will also detect dehydration. Administration of prochlorperazine will intensify these problems. Fluid balance charts: intravenous fluid available to correct hypovolaemia and hypotension.
Prolonged labour	Monitor uterine contractions. Advise women of this prior to labour.
Nausea	Reduce anxiety, fear and pain. Avoid sudden movements. Resting decreases nausea.
Sedation	Monitor level of consciousness and drowsiness. Avoid other sedating drugs, for example prochlorperazine. Avoid administration to women with a history of thyroid or adrenal imbalance. Encourage the mother not to allow sedation to interfere with appropriate 'pushing'.
Aspiration of gastric contents	Prevent/minimize sedation and nausea. Adopt the recovery position should nausea and vomiting occur.
Reduced renal perfusion Retention of urine	Urine output should be monitored to exclude oliguria and retention of urine.
Pruritus	Coolant gels, calamine or anti-histamines should be available. For intraspinal administration, substitution of fentanyl may be helpful.
Scarring at injection site (meperidine)	Document site of injection. Do not reuse that site.

Potential problem Neonatal

Respiratory depression	Close observation. Availability of naloxone, oxygen and ventilatory support. If naloxone is required, a second dose will usually be necessary.

Implications for Practice: Opioids (*continued*)

Potential problem Neonatal

	If high doses of meperidine/pethidine have been administered, be aware that the infant may not respond to naloxone. Monitor to prevent fetal acidosis.
Fetal bradycardia	Monitor fetal heart rate regularly. Recognize a prolonged, abnormal fetal bradycardia and refer as appropriate.
Sedation and/or irritability	When an opioid analgesic has been administered during labour, babies should be left with their mothers and additional assistance given to establish breastfeeding.
Hypothermia	Ensure neonate is well wrapped and close to mother.

Features of individual opioids

Although opioids have many side effects in common, there are some important differences between individual agents. The main distinguishing features are listed below.

Meperidine (pethidine)

Meperidine given by subcutaneous or intramuscular injection causes local irritation and frequent repetition at one site may lead to severe fibrosis of muscle tissue. *It is recommended that no site is used twice during labour.* Meperidine is the opioid most likely to induce maternal tachycardia and myocardial depression; therefore it is contra-indicated in women with heart disease. Myoclonus and muscular rigidity, while potential side effects of all opioids, are most likely with meperidine (Cherny, 1996). This rigidity may be reversed with naloxone (Bowdle, 1998). Meperidine is more likely to cause nausea than either morphine or diamorphine (Olofsson et al, 1996) or tramadol (Elbourne & Wiseman, 2000). A woman who has experienced nausea with morphine may not feel sick with meperidine and *vice versa*. Meperidine has also been used as the sole agent for epidural analgesia since it has both local anaesthetic and opioid properties

Meptazinol

Meptazinol (Meptid®) produces less respiratory depression, but more nausea, than either meperidine or morphine. It is used intrapartum and post-operatively in some centres, but an anti-emetic is often necessary. Pain relief has been found to be indistinguishable from that of meperidine (Sheikh & Tunstall, 1986; Osler, 1987; Elbourne & Wiseman, 2000). Duration of action (two to seven hours) is shorter than morphine or meperidine. Unlike meperidine, meptazinol can be metabolized by the neonate (Bushnell and Justins, 1993).

Diamorphine (heroin)

Diamorphine is rapidly metabolized in the liver to 6-monacetylmorphine (6MAM) and then to morphine. Both diamorphine and 6MAM are highly lipid soluble (more so than morphine) and therefore readily cross the blood/brain barrier to achieve rapid symptom relief (Reisine & Pasternak, 1996). Due to its high lipid solubility, enough diamorphine for 24 hours can be placed in a small volume patient-controlled analgesia (PCA) device. Diamorphine is sometimes used in labour and post-operatively. It is reported to produce less nausea but more euphoria and CNS obtunding than equianalgesic doses of morphine. This may be useful if death *in utero* has occurred. One study found higher Apgar scores [glossary] in neonates whose mothers had received diamorphine rather than meperidine (Fairlie et al, 1999).

Naloxone

Naloxone (Narcan®) is an opioid antagonist: it reverses many of the actions of other opioids. It may be administered subcutaneously, intramuscularly or intravenously to reverse the respiratory depression of opioids in neonates following maternal intra-partum analgesia. The half-life of naloxone is 1.1 ± 0.6 hours; the duration of action is one to four hours (Reisine & Pasternak, 1996). These values are much shorter than (approximtely half) those of meperidine, meptazinol and morphine. Therefore, following administration of naloxone, close observation of the neonate is required to identify a recurrence of the initial respiratory depression, and *a second dose is usually required*. In adults, administration of naloxone is usually followed by a return of pain. Other side effects of naloxone include nausea, vomiting, tachycardia and ventricular fibrillation (BNF, 2000).

Conclusion

Although only 50 per cent of women feel that opioids offer adequate pain relief in labour, they are often preferable to no analgesia (Fairlie et al, 1999). Intramuscular opioids provide greater pain relief than a placebo. However, they may be providing sedation rather than analgesia (Olofsson et al, 1996; Reynolds & Crowhurst, 1997). Professionals are more likely than mothers to consider pain relief to be adequate and tend to underestimate the level of pain experienced (Rajan, 1993; Rajan, 1994).

The adverse affects of opioids on the mother, the fetus and the neonate are significant and therefore their use should continue to be approached with caution, as summarized in 'Implications for Practice'. Labour may be prolonged and breastfeeding more difficult to establish following the administration of intramuscular opioids. Meanwhile, intraspinal administration of opioids is becoming increasingly popular (see below).

Local anaesthetics

Introduction

Local anaesthetics have been developed from cocaine, which was first used in dentistry and ophthalmology in the 19th century. Cocaine has been superseded by lignocaine (lidocaine), bupivacaine (Marcain®), prilocaine and ropivacaine. Prilocaine is primarily used in topical preparations. This chapter focuses on bupivacaine and lignocaine/lidocaine. Ropivacaine is described on p. 104.

Uses of local anaesthetics

Local anaesthetics have an important role in providing short term pain relief. In midwifery, they may be administered by several routes:

● topical, for example for intravenous cannulation;
● subcutaneous/intradermal for suturing;
● infiltration around a single nerve, for example a pudendal block;
● epidural, on the surface of the dura for labour or Caesarean section;
● spinal (intrathecal), into the cerebrospinal fluid of the sub-arachnoid (intrathecal) space for labour and Caesarean section. (see Figure 4.2).

Local anaesthetics will be discussed first in relation to the drugs themselves, followed by a consideration of the routes of administration.

How the body handles local anaesthetics

Regardless of their route of administration, local anaesthetics pass into the blood stream, whence they are eliminated (Catterall & Mackie, 1996). Local anaesthetics pass from the woman to the fetus, where they may be responsible for side effects. As with meperidine (pethidine), placental transfer and 'trapping' is increased if the fetus becomes acidotic. Local anaesthetics are extensively bound to tissues and alpha 1-acid glycoprotein (a plasma protein) in the circulation of the woman and the fetus. Only the unbound (free)

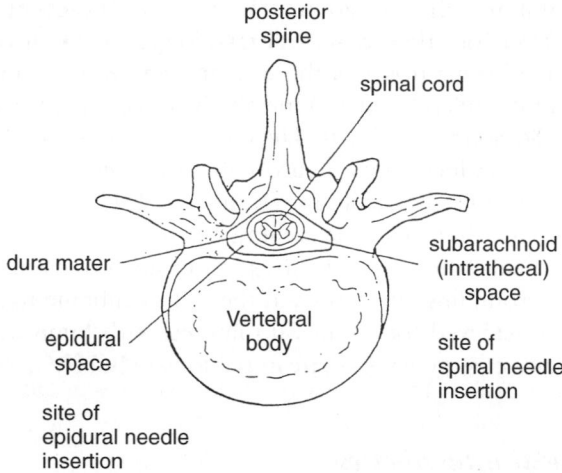

posterior
spine

spinal cord

dura mater

subarachnoid
(intrathecal)
space

epidural
space

Vertebral
body

site of
spinal needle
insertion

site of
epidural needle
insertion

Figure 4.2   Transverse section of the spine

fraction of the drug is responsible for actions and side effects. Since the fetus/neonate is relatively deficient in plasma proteins to bind these drugs, the proportion of free drug is higher and side effects are more likely

The elimination of local anaesthetics is important, because any failure to clear these drugs may result in toxicity. Local anaesthetics in the bloodstream are eliminated by metabolism in the liver of the woman, fetus or neonate and the metabolites are eventually excreted by the kidney. In view of this, local anaesthetics should be avoided in patients with liver problems as they may not be able to metabolize them effectively (BNF, 2000).

Lignocaine (lidocaine)

This has been used for over 50 years. It is metabolized in the liver of the woman, fetus and neonate into active metabolites. Although the duration of action and the half-life of lignocaine/lidocaine are relatively short (82 minutes in the woman and 95 minutes in the neonate), the metabolites continue to be excreted by the neonate for 36–48 hours after delivery, depending on the route of administration. These metabolites are responsible for some of the toxic effects of lignocaine (Kuhnert, 1993). With repeated administration, there is a danger of accumulation (Carson, 1996).

Bupivacaine (Marcain®)

This has a longer duration of action than lignocaine (two to three hours as epidural, or eight hours as nerve block) and because of this it is used extensively for epidural analgesia in labour. However, in the event of accidental overdose, the effects of bupivacaine will take longer to 'wear off'. The half-life of bupivacaine is nine hours in the woman and 18 hours in the neonate. Bupivacaine, and its (relatively inert) metabolites, continue to be excreted by the neonate for 36 hours after birth. The continued presence of the drug and its metabolites may induce subtle neuro-behavioural changes in the neonate which may not be clinically significant (Kuhnert, 1993).

To reach their site of action (the sodium channels in the axon membrane; see below), local anaesthetics must diffuse through surrounding tissues, the myelin sheath surrounding the axon and the cell membrane itself. Therefore, pain relief is not achieved for about 30 minutes, with bupivacaine, which is too slow for many emergency Caesarean sections (MCHRC, 2000).

Actions of local anaesthetics

Communication in the nervous system and mechanical activity in muscle depend on the electrical excitability of the cell membranes of those tissues. Nerve impulses depend on the generation of action potentials in the cell membranes of axons of neurones. The main action of local anaesthetics is to reduce the ability of nerves to conduct action potentials and impulses.

At rest, the cell membranes of nerve and muscle are polarized (or charged). When an action potential is triggered, the nerve is depolarized (or discharged) by a rapid influx of sodium ions, followed by repolarization (recharging), due to an efflux of potassium ions. The entire process takes about one millisecond. Local anaesthetics prevent the rapid influx of sodium ions by blocking the fast sodium channels in the nerve cell membranes. This inhibits the formation of action potentials, preventing the transmission of impulses and signals along the axons and therefore blocking normal nerve function. The action of local anaesthetics is reversed when the drug passes into the bloodstream and is excreted.

The effect of a local anaesthetic on any axon depends on both the size and myelination of the axon (Catterall & Mackie, 1996). Small diameter, unmyelinated axons which transmit pain sensation and impulses of the sympathetic nervous system are the most sensitive to local anaesthetics, while larger, myelinated axons responsible for movement and pressure/touch sensation are relatively resistant. The interruption of sensory functions in a nerve by the action of a local anaesthetic progresses in a definite order: the sensation of pain is the first to disappear, followed by cold, warmth, touch and pressure. This means that movement and coarse touch are often preserved during local anaesthesia. The interference with the functioning of the sympathetic nervous system (SNS) is responsible for many of the side effects of epidural anaesthesia such as hypotension.

Side effects of local anaesthetics

The potential side effects of local anaesthetics are the same, regardless of the route of administration. However, when normal doses are used topically and intradermally, problems are very rarely encountered. The midwife should be particularly alert for side effects when local anaesthetics are used via the epidural or spinal routes or if a local anaesthetic has been inadvertently injected into a vein (see 'Implications for Practice').

The side effects of local anaesthetics are related to their actions, in particular their ability to inhibit conduction of impulses in excitable tissues. Local anaesthetics block the fast sodium ion channels of *all* the body's conducting tissue, namely:

- central nervous system (CNS);
- heart and cardiovascular system;
- peripheral nervous system;
- sympathetic nervous system;
- smooth muscle – uterus, bladder, gut;
- skeletal muscle.

CNS excitation and inhibition

In the CNS, the sodium ion channels of the inhibitory neurones are blocked more readily than those of the excitatory neurones. Therefore, the CNS responses to local anaesthetics pass through several stages from excitation through to inhibition and depression:

- 'ringing in the ears'; 'funny taste in the mouth';
- confusion/agitation, blurred vision, shivering;
- restlessness, euphoria, chills;
- nausea;
- tremor;
- convulsions;
- respiratory depression;
- coma and death.

In the event of accidental intravenous administration, the initial response to local anaesthetics is usually excitation, restlessness, tremor and even convulsions (Hughes, 1992). This paradoxical excitation is followed by CNS depression, particularly respiratory depression. However, if the systemic administration of lignocaine/lidocaine or bupivacaine is rapid, the excitatory responses may not be seen. Instead, the woman may experience only CNS depression, and a sudden respiratory arrest.

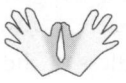 **Practice Points**

- It is important that the midwife is aware of these side effects. Failure to attribute the early signs of toxicity to excessive absorption of local anaesthetic could mean that:

  symptoms may be allowed to progress to more profound stages of CNS depression; further doses of local anaesthetic could be administered, intensifying the problem (Hughes, 1992).

- Nausea caused by local anaesthetics may be attributed to opioid administration or the physiological response to labour and treated with anti-emetics. However, nausea, disturbed mood, feelings of faintness or light-headedness may be due to hypotension, caused by local anaesthetics, and this possibility should be considered before further doses of local anaesthetic are administered (Brownridge, 1991).

Sympathetic blockade

Consequences of sympathetic blockade:

- reduced maternal blood pressure;
- maternal and neonatal thermoregulation failure;
- loss of neonatal asphyxia reflexes.

Local anaesthetics inhibit the functioning of the sympathetic nerves. These control the diameter of the blood vessels, and thus affect an important aspect of blood pressure regulation (the total peripheral resistance). With the activity of the sympathetic nerves impaired, blood vessels dilate, causing both a drop in blood pressure and an inability to vasoconstrict in response to a cold environment. The woman may complain of feeling cold, shiver uncontrollably or, conversely, may develop a pyrexia. Likewise, the neonate will be vulnerable to the cold (Howell, 1995a; Reynolds et al, 1996; El-Refaey et al, 2000).

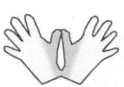 **Practice Point**

Blankets should be available to provide optimum comfort for the woman in labour. The neonate should be maintained in a warm environment, preferably by contact with the mother.

In association with the administration of epidural analgesia, pyrexia (>98°C or 100.4°F) was recorded in 16.6 per cent (120/724) of healthy parturients (n = 1218). Their infants were more likely to convulse or to be hypotonic and require resuscitation (Lieberman et al, 2000). These authors suggest that maternal intrapartum fever may induce an even higher temperature in the fetus (by 0.5–0.9°C); where the neonate is also suffering from an ischaemic insult, this degree of pyrexia may increase the extent of neurological damage.

At delivery, the neonate relies on his or her reflex response to asphyxia to take a first breath, and this reflex depends on the activity of the sympathetic nervous system. With the use of local anaesthetics, the neonate's reflex responses to delivery may be suppressed, requiring careful assessment and possibly prompt action by the midwife.

Hypotension

The fall in blood pressure that may accompany the intraspinal use of local anaesthetics is due to vasodilation plus simultaneous myocardial depression. However the relief of pain and distress afforded by effective analgesia may be a contributory factor.

Local anaesthetics inhibit the sympathetic nervous system, which is responsible for keeping the arterioles constricted and the blood pressure and heart rate within normal limits. Therefore they have the potential to compromise the cardiovascular system, causing hypotension, bradycardia and even cardiac arrest. Clinically significant maternal hypotension, defined as a fall of 20–30 per cent in pre-anaesthetic systolic blood pressure, or a systolic blood pressure below 100mmHg, occurs in 5–15 per cent of deliveries with epidural anaesthesia and 5–82 per cent of deliveries with spinal anaesthesia (Hollmen, 1993; Shennan et al, 1995).

The risk of hypotension is greater if the woman is dehydrated or hypovolaemic. Therefore prior to the intraspinal administration of local anaesthetics, intravenous fluids are infused, for example, 20–25 ml/kg crystalloid solution (Hollmen, 1993) or 1 litre of compound lactate solution (Sheenan et al, 1995). The infusion of fluids should maintain venous return and therefore cardiac output, thus countering any hypotension.

Case Report

A woman was given epidural analgesia 36 hours after a forceps delivery to control perineal pain, despite refusing an intravenous infusion. She was passing little urine, with evidence of dehydration; frusemide had no effect on the urine output. This indicates poor renal perfusion, due to hypotension. Her hands became numb, due to the effects of the local anaesthetics. There were no recordings of: blood pressure, respirations, level of block, pulse oximetry.

She received sedation when she became agitated. Restlessness may have been due either to hypoxia or the drugs administered. Hypoxia was diagnosed on the ECG. Only then was oxygen given. Hypotension developed, leading to cardiac arrest and death (DOH, 1996:93).

This woman died of hypoxia, due to hypotension and poor ventilation. Hypotension was caused by the combination of epidural opiates and local anaesthetics administered without intravenous fluids. With better monitoring and the appropriate use of intravenous fluids, this woman would have lived. However, rapid administration of crystalloid intravenous fluids (such as Ringer's, saline or glucose) may induce a diuresis and fail to prevent a drop in blood pressure (Richardson, 2000).

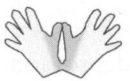 **Practice Point**

Cardiac output and circulating volume are assessed by careful monitoring of urine output, which can act as a 'early warning sign'. Oliguria (low urine output) indicates that renal autoregulation is occurring in an attempt to counteract impending or actual hypotension. It is essential that the midwife responds to any decline in maternal urine output.

Failure to monitor urine output in women receiving epidural anaesthesia is cited as a contributory factor in maternal deaths (DoH, 1998).

Case Report

Three hours after the administration of epidural analgesia, an emergency Caesarean section was performed for fetal distress. 0.5 per cent bupivacaine (2 × 10 ml) was administered prior to section. Recovery and initial observations taken by the midwife were normal. However, 40 minutes later, the woman was unrousable. Autopsy showed extensive haemorrhage into parametrial tissues (DOH, 1994:91).

The physiological signs of haemorrhage were modified by the blockade of the sensory and sympathetic nervous systems. The inadequacy of vital sign recordings indicated to the assessors that post-operative care was substandard.

Local anaesthetic induced vasodilation may reduce the ability of blood vessels to constrict in response to haemorrhage. Therefore even a moderate haemorrhage may cause hypotension and blood loss post-partum may be increased (Beischer et al, 1997). However, for Caesarean section, blood loss is less than with general anaesthesia (Lertakyamanee et al, 1999). It is important that any maternal hypotension is recognized immediately, because *the blood flow to the uterus, and hence fetal oxygenation, declines in direct relation to maternal blood pressure*. By jeopardizing the blood supply to the placenta, hypotension causes fetal acidosis, and depresses the neonate's central nervous system (Roberts et al, 1995).

Hypotension is compounded by aorto-caval compression by the baby's head, particularly if the woman is supine or obese, or if the uterus is enlarged due to multiple pregnancy, diabetes or polyhydramnios (Hollmen, 1993). To avoid compression of the vena cava, the uterus must be displaced laterally; a woman receiving local anaesthetics during labour should avoid the supine position, including reclining chairs, and the midwife should regularly ascertain the position of the uterus. A lateral position should be adopted, or alternatively, a 20-degree tilt achieved by using a 'wedge'. Aorto-caval compression may be less if the woman is upright and ambulant (Al-Mufti et al, 1997). If a woman (inadvertently) lies supine at term, the placental blood flow will decrease by 20–30 per cent, without any change in maternal vital signs. If position is not corrected, the *supine hypotension syndrome*, leading to maternal collapse, may follow. This suggests that practitioners should consider performing vaginal examinations with the woman in a lateral position (Yerby, 2000).

Case Report

A woman of 30 weeks' gestation was given a spinal anaesthetic. She was premedicated with 15 mg papaveretum and given 400 ml of Hartman's solution, followed by 1 ml of 0.5 per cent of heavy bupivacaine. She noticed her legs becoming weak, which was attributed to bupivacaine, and she was placed in a supine position with the table tilted laterally. Her blood pressure fell rapidly and she was treated with fluids and ephedrine (2 × 15 mg). Further measures taken were the administration of oxygen, atropine, epinephrine (adrenaline) and a further 1600 ml of fluids. Pulmonary oedema and subsequently death from adult respiratory distress syndrome followed. (DOH, 1994:83)

It is likely that the hypotension was due to aorto-caval compression, because a small degree of lateral tilt would not prevent this. The interventions which led to this catastrophe followed attempts to correct the hypotension. Pulmonary oedema was caused by the combination of fluids and two vasoconstrictors (that is epinephrine (adrenaline) + ephedrine).

Aldrich et al (1995) found that when 14 healthy labouring women, receiving effective epidural analgesia, 0.25–0.5 per cent bupivacaine, adopted the supine position for ten minutes, an 18 per cent fall in maternal lower limb

digital artery pressure and a, clinically significant, 8 per cent fall in fetal cerebral oxygen delivery occurred. The Hence measuring the maternal blood pressure in the arm could allow significant hypotension at the level of the uterus
to remain undetected. This suggests that the use of leg cuffs should be considered when intraspinal analgesia is used (Hollmen, 1993).

If placental blood flow is already compromised, for example by pregnancy
induced hypertension, the vulnerable fetus may not be able to withstand the
extra stress of low maternal blood pressure. Maternal deaths have occurred
when epidural analgesia has been used alone to control hypertension in
women with pre-eclampsia or eclampsia (DoH, 1994). Thus the use of
epidural analgesia in these women remains controversial (Hollmen, 1993).

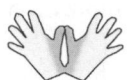 **Practice Point**

Particularly careful BP monitoring is needed on initial administration, during the first 30
minutes of spinal anaesthesia and when 'top-up' doses are administered into the epidural
space (Sheenan et al, 1995).

Hypotension is more likely with a spinal (intrathecal) than an epidural
anaesthetic. 'High risk' situations include:

- within the first 30 minutes of administration;
- when 'top-up' doses are administered;
- aorto-caval compression (exacerbated in the supine position);
- hypovolaemia;
- when anaesthesia reaches the level of the T_4 segment (nipple level);
- if there are pre-existing cardiac problems such as heart block;
- standing may induce postural hypotension.

Clinically significant maternal hypotension, jeopardizing the fetus, may not
be manifest as maternal symptoms. If hypotension is not **corrected within
two minutes**, fetal bradycardia, acidosis and depression will follow (Hughes,
1992; Downing & Ramasubramanian, 1993). Clinically it may be difficult to
attribute fetal heart rate abnormalities to the direct action of the local anaesthetics or to maternal hypotension caused by drugs, although fetal acidosis
during Caesarean section is a recognized complication of local anaesthetics
(Steer, 1995).

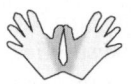 **Practice Points**

- If a fall in the blood pressure should occur, the woman should be turned on her left side, her legs elevated (Trendelenburg position) if possible and intravenous fluids administered. Medical advice must be sought immediately. If the blood pressure does not improve within two to three minutes, oxygen and ephedrine may be given (see below) (Davis, 1992).
- Following epidural anaesthesia, the functions of the sympathetic nervous system and blood pressure control may return **after** the return of sensation. It is therefore important that blood pressure monitoring is continued during this period.

Bupivacaine has more myocardial depressant action than lignocaine/lidocaine. This is important with both spinal and epidural administration. It is most severe if the parturient is acidotic or hypoxic. The cardiotoxicity threshold is lower in pregnancy. Cardiac arrests and maternal deaths have been reported. Therefore the use of the 0.75 per cent solution is absolutely contra-indicated in obstetrics (BNF, 2000). Bupivacaine is never used for intravenous anaesthesia since bupivacaine-induced cardiotoxicity is difficult to treat (Catterall & Mackie, 1996). Accidental intravenous administration of bupivacaine during epidural anaesthesia in labour has produced cardiovascular collapse (Kuhnert, 1993).

Box 4.1   Ephedrine

To correct hypotension, 3–6 mg ephedrine may be administered by a slow intravenous injection, repeated every three to four minutes if necessary, up to 30 mg (BNF, 2000).

Ephedrine has the potential to constrict uterine vessels (it is an alpha agonist [glossary]), but this is minimized if the drug is given slowly or as an infusion. Although this is considered safe for a full-term healthy fetus, a high risk fetus may not be able to tolerate this vasoconstriction (Hollmen, 1993) and therefore a lower dose (2.5 mg) is preferable (Hughes, 1992).

Several side effects associated with ephedrine, such as tachycardia and cardiac dysrhythmia, require monitoring. These are similar to the side effects of ritodrine (see Chapter 7, tocolytics). Like epinephrine (adrenaline), ephedrine may interact with oxytocin to cause severe hypertension.

Depression of smooth muscle

Uterine, gut and bladder contractions are depressed by local anaesthetics. Inhibition of the bladder usually produces retention of urine, but conversely urinary and faecal incontinence are possible (Karch, 1992). Epidural analgesia is associated with an increased risk of post-partum urinary retention (Olofsson et al, 1997). It is important not to underestimate the potential problems, short and long term, arising from repeated urinary catheterization (Mander, 1994).

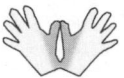 **Practice Point**

Since bladder sensation may be absent or diminished, the woman should be encouraged to micturate every two to three hours.

Studies (Howell & Chalmers, 1992; Thorp et al, 1993; Howell, 1995a; Steer, 1995; Halpern et al, 1998; McRae-Bergeron et al, 1998; Szal et al, 1999; Okojie & Cook, 1999; Walker & O'Brien, 1999) have indicated that when local anaesthetics are administered epidurally:

- the first and second stages of labour are more likely to be prolonged (the mean differences between epidural anaesthesia and parenteral opioids were 42 and 14 minutes (Halpern et al, 1998));
- cervical dilatation is slower;
- oxytocin is twice as likely to be used;
- fetal malposition is more common;
- Caesarean section for dystocia [glossary] is more likely;
- instrumental deliveries are two to four times more common.

Local anaesthetics prolong labour by:

- relaxing the pelvic floor muscles;
- diminishing the 'bearing down' reflexes;
- decreasing expulsive efforts;
- direct action on the uterine muscle reducing the muscle tone;
- diminishing the pulsatile release of oxytocin from the posterior pituitary gland.

Although studies offer no consensus (Dewan & Cohen, 1994; Fung, 2000), in a large study (n = 1250) the combined use of oxytocin, induction and epidural analgesia appeared to be additive in bringing about a higher rate of instrumental and operative deliveries (Carli et al, 1993). In a cohort study involving 1561 nulliparous parturients, Traynor et al (2000) found that the risk of Caesarean section increased threefold with the use of combined spinal epidural analgesia and 4.7 fold with the use of continuous infusion epidurals. The risk of Caesarean section is increased if two or more bolus doses of bupivacaine are administered (Hess et al, 2000) or if epidural analgesia is administered prior to either cervical dilatation >5 cm (Thorp et al, 1993) or engagement of the fetal head (Traynor et al, 2000).

Case Report

A woman had received an ineffective epidural in a previous pregnancy. She underwent a trial of labour with a breech presentation with effective epidural analgesia. However, when there was failure to progress in the second stage, it was decided to deliver the baby by Caesarean section. An additional 30 mls of 0.5 per cent bupivacaine was administered over 30 minutes, but this did not provide adequate anaesthesia for Caesarean section. During the induction of general anaesthesia, a hypoxic episode occurred, which led to death two days later (DOH, 1991:75)

Continuation of epidural analgesia into the second stage probably contributed to this woman's failure to progress.

Some authors recommend that epidural analgesia is not continued into the second stage of labour, due to increased incidence of malrotation of the presenting part, necessitating assisted vaginal delivery (Howell & Chalmers, 1992; Howell, 1995a). This discontinuation of epidural analgesia increases pain, which may have adverse psychological and physiological consequences, including hyperventilation and alkalosis (see p. 64).

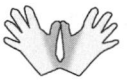 **Practice Point**

Women should be advised that although epidural analgesia is more likely to be effective than other methods of analgesia, its effects on the physiology of labour reduce the chances of a 'normal' vaginal delivery (Howell, 1995a).

Reduction in the muscle tone of the uterus may impair the contraction of the uterus after delivery and increase the risk of haemorrhage (Campbell & Lees, 2000).

Neuromuscular blockade

Loss of sensation and motor control

When administered by the intravenous, epidural or spinal routes, local anaesthetics affect the motor neurones as well as the sensory neurones. The recipient may feel weak and numb. Blockade of motor neurones of the lower spinal segments by epidural anaesthesia inhibits movement during labour. Paraesthesia or paralysis of the legs may occur, so that the woman is unable to stand or walk. This is less evident with bupivacaine or ropivacaine than lignocaine (Catterall & Mackie, 1996), and with 0.0625 per cent or 0.125 per cent rather than 0.25 per cent bupivacaine (Harms et al, 1999). Laxity of the pelvic floor muscles, due to the action of local anaesthetics, is the mechanism behind malrotation, malposition and shoulder dystocia [glossary] (Thorp et al, 1993; Howell, 1995a).

Some studies have linked bupivacaine with reduced neonatal muscle tone, suckling and reflex responses. Also, loss of sensation prevents the woman from feeling aware of uterine contractions and the birth process which may lead to dissatisfaction later (Brownridge, 1991).

An intraspinal nerve block in childbirth is intended to anaesthetize the spinal nerves below the 12th thoracic segment (innervation of the uterus). If the local anaesthetic rises above the tenth thoracic segment, too many nerves controlling the intercostal muscles will be inhibited, causing breathing difficulties. At the fourth thoracic segment, sympathetic nerves supplying the heart muscle will be depressed.

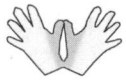   **Practice Point**

The level of skin sensation should be monitored regularly, and medical advice sought if necessary. Sensation at the level of the nipple represents the fourth thoracic segment and at the umbilicus the tenth thoracic segment, although some overlap exists (Tortora & Grabowski, 2000).

Respiratory failure

The intercostal muscles may be impaired by high spinal anaesthesia, causing over-reliance on the diaphragm. However, at term the diaphragm is 'splinted' by the uterus, and is less able to increase its movement to compensate for any inadequacies of the intercostal muscles. When these problems are compounded by the risk of medullary paralysis and the respiratory depression associated with spinal anaesthesia there is a possibility of inadequate ventilation and even arrest.

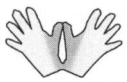 **Practice Points**

- It is important to monitor the rate and depth of respirations and check oxygenation by pulse oximetry if necessary.
- Pulse oximetry may not detect mild or moderate ventilatory depression (Herman et al, 1999).

Hypersensitivity reactions

Rare individuals are hypersensitive to local anaesthetics or their preservatives and some cross sensitivities occur. The clinical manifestations of hypersensitivity include:

- dermatitis;
- asthma;
- anaphylaxis;
- methaemoglobinaemia.*

Note: Both prilocaine, contained in EMLA® cream, and lignocaine/lidocaine may induce methaemoglobinaemia in rare, genetically susceptible individuals. Methaemoglobin is an oxidized form of haemoglobin which is unable to transport oxygen and is normally converted back to haemoglobin by various enzymes. Genetic deficiencies of these enzymes can be magnified by certain drugs, with disastrous consequences. Methaemoglobinaemia presents as cyanosis, accompanied by headache, weakness and breathlessness. Severe methaemoglobinaemia is incompatible with life (Bunn, 1991). Management of methaemoglobinaemia involves an intravenous injection of methylthioninium chloride (methylene blue) 1 per cent 1 mg/kg (BNF, 2000).

Effects on the neonate

Older studies have linked epidural anaesthesia with neonatal depression and neurobehavioural abnormalities at 24 hours post-partum (Catterall & Mackie, 1996). Epidural local anaesthetics may have subtle neurobehavioural effects on the neonate which are undetectable at 18 months (Kuhnert, 1993; Howell & Chalmers, 1992). The auditory system of the neonate may be transiently impaired (Reynolds et al, 1996). Halpern, et al (1999) suggest that any neu-robehavioural side effects are no impediment to breastfeeding, providng effec-tive support is offered.

The use of epidural analgesia increases the risk of neonatal hypoglycaemia, tachypnoea and a disturbance of lipid metabolism (Howell & Chalmers, 1992). Fetal acidaemia, without obvious clinical sequelae, was more likely when regional, particularly spinal, rather than general anaesthesia was used for Caesarean section (Roberts et al, 1995). Nevertheless, neonates generally fare better with epidural analgesia than with either general anaesthesia or systemic opioids (Reynolds et al, 1996). Neonates are less likely to have low APGAR scores at five minutes or to require naloxone after epidural analgesia than after intramuscular opioids (Halpern et al, 1998).

Box 4.2   Ropivacaine

This local anaesthetic has been developed to provide long lasting local anaesthesia without the cardiotoxicity of bupivacaine to which it is chemically related. While some authors consider these two agents to be equally effective (Muir et al, 1997; Irestedt et al, 1998), others have found that ropivacaine is less potent (Capogna et al, 1999; Fischer et al, 2000). Therefore ropivacaine may provide a less intense motor blockade than bupivacaine that could reduce the rate of instrumental deliveries (Cederholm, 1997) and improve ambulation and micturition (Campbell et al, 2000). In one study (n = 60), ropivacaine was found to have fewer neurobehavioural effects on neonates (Stienstra et al, 1995; Writer et al, 1998). However onset of action and termination of motor blockade following delivery may be slower than with bupivacaine (McCrae et al, 1995).

Cautions and contra-indications (see Box 4.3)

- Local anaesthetics should not be used in individuals where a previous allergy has occurred to any chemically related anaesthetic or other con-stituent of the preparation.
- Hypovolaemia must be corrected before intraspinal administration (BNF, 2000).
- Administration of local anaesthetics is not advised if the woman has had a recent haemorrhage as the cardiovascular responses to blood loss will be compromised (Beischer et al, 1997).
- Local anaesthetics should be applied cautiously, if at all, to inflamed areas.

Box 4.3   Cautions and contra-indications for local anaesthetics

Local anaesthetics are used cautiously in:
heart block or impaired cardiac conduction;
hypovolaemia and other forms of shock;
maternal bradycardia;
porphyria;
epilepsy;
respiratory impairment;
liver or kidney disease;
hyperthyroidism;
family history of malignant hyperthermia;
myasthenia gravis;
lactation.

Epidural anaesthesia is avoided in:
placenta praevia;
abruptio placenta;
haemorrhage or anticipated haemorrhage;
bacteraemia;
coagulation disorders, including:

> use of aspirin or heparin (see epidural haematoma below and Chapter 8);
> pre-eclampsia with bleeding abnormalities.

Spinal (intrathecal) anaesthesia is avoided in:
inflammatory conditions of the spine;
meningitis;
lumbar TB;
spinal metastases;
septicaemia.

Drug interactions

The unwanted effects of local anaesthetics may be enhanced by H_2 antagonists (cimetidine), anti-arrhythmics and other central nervous system depressants, including alcohol and prochlorperazine (Malseed et al, 1995).

● Regular use of alcohol increases the risk of therapeutic failure (Stockley, 1999).
● Beta blockers, cimetidine and possibly ranitidine, interfere with the hepatic clearance of bupivacaine. This increases the risk of toxicity (Kuhnert, 1993).

- Benzodiazepines may affect the clearance of local anaesthetics. Increased bupivacaine (but not lidcaine/lignocaine) concentrations have been reported in patients taking diazepam (Stockley, 1999).
- Tricyclic anti-depressants and phenothiazines (for example prochlorperazine) increase the risk of heart block, particularly if epinephrine/adrenaline is used.
- Calcium channel blockers (nifedipine, verapamil) enhance the cardiotoxicity of bupivacaine.

Implications for Practice: local anaesthetics

Problem	*Management*
Topical applications(EMLA)	
Contact dermatitis	Coolants available.
	Wear gloves.
Epidural or Spinal Anaesthesia	
Maternal	
Hypotension	Avoid supine position.
	Prehydration with intravenous fluids.
	Monitor BP, heart rate and rhythm and urine output.
	Assess skin and oxygen saturation with pulse oximeter.
	Ensure vasopressor agents available, for example ephedrine.
	Check histry and ECG for heart block.
	Check history for liver disease, malignant hyperthermia
	Ensure no signs of shock present.
	Use test dose.
Loss of uterine contractility	Monitor.
	Advise of possibility of prolonged second stage and increased incidence of instrumental deliveries.
Urine retention/incontinence	Monitor output and specific gravity.
	Catheterize if necessary.
Risk of fits	Diazepam available.
Loss of thermoregulation	Prevent shivering. Blankets should be available.
	Monitor maternal temperature and pre-empt non-infectious fever/pyrexia.
	Monitor infant for convulsions.
Hypersensitivity	Be aware of cross-sensitivity between local anaesthetics.
Methaemoglobinaemia	Recognize cyanosis. Have oxygen ready.
	Methylene blue antidote, if needed.

Implications for Practice: local anaesthetics (*continued*)

Problem	*Management*
Fetal/neonatal	
Depression of fetal heart rate	Monitor. Liaise with medical staff.
Depression of neonatal respiratory and suckling reflexes	Prepare to assist neonate to establish respirations.
	Give extra assistance to initiate breastfeeding.
Spinal anaesthesia	
Respiratory depression	Monitor rate and depth of respirations regularly.
	Ensure resuscitation equipment is available.

Routes of administration of local anaesthetics

Surface anaesthesia

EMLA (eutectic mixture of local anaesthetics) is a mixture of lignocaine/ lidocaine and prilocaine which may be applied to the skin surface to provide analgesia for venepuncture or cannulation. A thick layer under an occlusive dressing will provide analgesia if applied one to five hours before the procedure. Alternatively, amethocaine (tetracaine) gel may be similarly applied 30–45 minutes before venepuncture or cannulation. Application to mucous membranes, wounds or areas of atopic [glossary] dermatitis must be avoided (BNF, 2000).

Subcutaneous/intradermal injection

Local anaesthetics may be infiltrated directly into tissue, to varying depths, to anaesthetize relatively small areas. The addition of a vasoconstrictor (adrenaline/epinephrine) approximately doubles the duration of anaesthesia and reduces the peak concentration of local anaesthetic in plasma (Catterall & Mackie, 1996). However, vasoconstrictors carry an inherent danger of ischaemic necrosis. Due to potential cardiotoxicity, the total dose of adrenaline/epinephrine is limited to 500 micrograms (BNF, 2000).

When intradermal lignocaine/lidocaine is being administered to decrease the pain of perineal trauma or an episiotomy, accidental injection into the presenting part of the neonate may produce serious side effects: apnoea; loss of muscle tone; fixed dilated pupils.

Nerve block

A solution of local anaesthetic is injected into or around individual nerves or nerve plexuses. The onset of action is three minutes for lignocaine/lidocaine and 15 minutes for bupivacaine. The duration of actions are two to three hours and five to seven hours respectively, affecting motor as well as sensory modalities. A pudendal block may be performed prior to short procedures such as instrumental delivery, suturing or the manual removal of the placenta. This procedure may increase the administrator's risk from transmission of blood borne infections (Hughes, 1992).

Intraspinal analgesia

The term 'intraspinal' is used to refer to administration within the spinal column, that is to encompass epidural, spinal and combined spinal epidural administration (Wildsmith, 1996). The problems encountered with intraspinal analgesia are those attributed to the route of administration, plus the side effects of the drugs themselves. Comparisons of intraspinal analgesic regimens on the progress of labour, neonatal outcome and long term sequelae await the results of larger studies (*Drugs and Therapy Perspectives*, 1996).

Drugs administered intrathecally pass into the fetus to a limited extent; very low concentrations of opioids are found in the systemic circulation or cord blood following spinal opioid administration (Clyburn & Rosen, 1993). Drugs administered epidurally are administered in much larger doses and absorbed into the systemic circulation *via* the epidural veins, making side effects more likely.

Epidural anaesthesia

This entails injection into the fat in the narrow space between the dura and the bony canal. (see Fig. 4.3) The drug diffuses through the dura, where it acts on the nerve roots. There is also an effect at the intervertebral foramina. Sufficient local anaesthetic is injected to be absorbed into the circulation, *via* the epidural veins, in proportion to the total dose used. The local anaesthetic then passes into the fetus. Absorption is increased at delivery when the mother is spontaneously pushing and 'top up' injections are usually avoided at this time.

Following a test dose and initial administration, ongoing epidural analgesia may be by:

* bolus injection on request;
* patient controlled infusion;
* a constant infusion device;
* scheduled bolus injections (*Drugs and Therapy Perspectives*, 1996).

In most maternity units the anaesthetist will administer the initial bolus injection, with subsequent bolus doses given by midwives. Although scheduled bolus injections provide more effective analgesia, they call for more careful monitoring of the level of sensory blockade, and risk the administra-

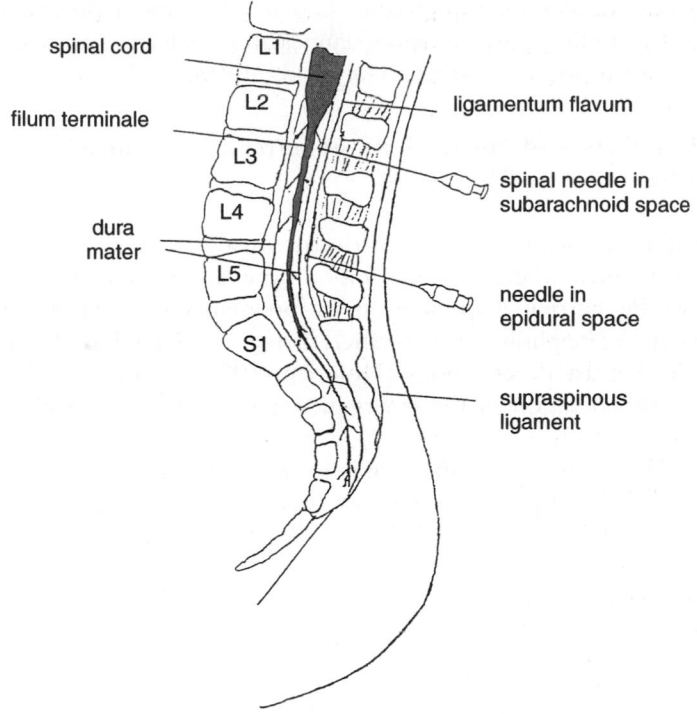

spinal cord

filum terminale

dura
mater

L1
L2
L3
L4
L5
S1

ligamentum flavum

spinal needle in
subarachnoid space

needle in
epidural space

supraspinous
ligament

Figure 4.3   Diagram of the lumbosacral spine to show needle placement for
subarachnoid and lumbar epidural analgesia
Source: Adapted from Hughes, 1992.

tion of higher doses (Howell, 1995b). Unfortunately, pre-set infusion devices
fail to take account of individual difference either in analgesic requirements
(Brownridge, 1991), or the need for increasing concentrations as labour
advances (Capogna et al, 1998). In one small study (n = 55), patient controlled administration of epidural analgesia resulted in less hypotension, possibly because the drugs were delivered more slowly (Al-Mufti et al, 1997).

Addition of adrenaline (epinephrine)   Adrenaline (epinephrine) may be
added to epidural analgesia to increase the duration and intensity of analgesia, for example with continuous epidural infusions (Clyburn & Rosen, 1993;
Norris et al, 1994). It may act directly on the pain pathways to enhance
analgesia. Bupivacaine is usually administered without adrenaline/epinephrine
(plain), but adrenaline/epinephrine is added to lignocaine/lidocaine if perineal analgesia is required quickly (Brownridge, 1991).

Adrenaline/epinephrine vasoconstricts the epidural venous plexus, thereby
reducing the systemic absorption of local anaesthetic (Catterall & Mackie,
1996). The addition of adrenaline/epinephrine to bupivacaine may increase

the placental transfer of bupivacaine, due to changes in protein binding. Therefore the addition of adrenaline/epinephrine reduces maternal, but not fetal, exposure to local anaesthetic (Reynolds, 1993b).

The side effects and interactions of adrenaline/epinephrine mitigate against its use:

● Adrenaline/epinephrine is a vasoconstrictor and reduces placental blood flow. In women where placental blood flow is already compromised, for example by chronic hypertension or pregnancy-induced hypertension, adrenaline/epinephrine may further jeopardize fetal blood supply and cause fetal heart decelerations (Hollmen, 1993). However this is a secondary consideration in the emergency management of anaphylaxis (see Chapter 1, p. 30).
● Adrenaline/epinephrine can precipitate cardiac dysrhythmias or alterations in maternal blood pressure which can decrease placental perfusion.
● Adrenaline/epinephrine may prolong the first stage of labour (Dounas et al, 1996).
● Adrenaline/epinephrine interacts dangerously with:

volatile general anaesthetic gases, causing dysrhythmias;
oxytocin, causing hypertension;
beta blockers, causing hypertension (BNF, 2000).

Case Report

A young primipara in normal labour received epidural analgesia containing adrenaline/epinephrine. When labour failed to progress, an oxytocin infusion was commenced. Over the next two hours, the woman became hypertensive, drowsy and comatose, and developed a hemiparesis. Following an emergency Caesarean section, the woman made a full but gradual recovery in intensive care. This involved transfer to a tertiary centre for several weeks.

If administering bupivacaine with adrenaline, professionals need to consider the intereactions of both components.

Spinal/intrathecal anaesthesia

This entails injection into the subarachnoid space, affecting the lower part of the spinal cord and the nerve roots which affords rapid pain relief (see Fig. 4.3) (Sheenan et al, 1995). Hypotension and headache occur more commonly with spinal than epidural analgesia (Reynolds et al, 1996). Low spinal anaesthesia, combined with epidural anaesthesia, is currently preferred to general anaesthesia for most Caesarean sections (Marx & Rabin, 1993; DoH, 1996).

Combined spinal-epidural (CSE) analgesia

Opioids and local anaesthetics may be administered epidurally or intrathecally, often in combination. The combined spinal-epidural technique allows lower doses of both drugs to be administered. When an opioid, usually fentanyl, is added to bupivacaine or ropivacaine, the dose of local anaesthetic is much less than with epidural administration. Some (not all) authors suggest that this may reduce the unpleasant motor blockade, paresis or paralysis of the lower body caused by the higher doses of local anaesthetics needed for epidurals, and permits ambulation during labour. Careful monitoring is required to avoid hypotensive episodes, which are potentially damaging to the fetus (Steer, 1995; Shennan et al, 1995).

Intrathecal opioids afford more rapid analgesia than epidural anaesthetics; for example fentanyl is effective within five minutes, compared to 30 minutes for bupivacaine. The addition of local anaesthetics overcomes the short duration of action of intrathecal opioids. In a large study (n = 1000), the use of 0.125 per cent bupivacaine with sufentanil was associated with reduced administration of oxytocin and fewer Caesarean sections when compared to 0.25 per cent bupivacaine with adrenaline/epinephrine (Olofsson et al, 1998).

However CSE analgesia has some disadvantages when compared to traditional epidural analgesia: the incidence of hypotension and headaches is not improved by the addition of opioids (Norris et al, 1994); the rates for Caesarean section are not improved (Traynor et al, 2000); the common side effects of opioids, such as nausea, vomiting and itching, may still be troublesome; the potential for local problems, such as meningism, is increased. Also, the onset of analgesia is only shortened by two minutes when opioids are added to both epidural and intrathecal analgesia (Nickells et al, 2000).

Opioids Administered by intraspinal injection   Advantages of intraspinal opioids over local anaesthetics include:

- no blockade of the sympathetic nervous system but hypotension remains a problem.
- no motor blockade, therefore movement and ambulation are unaffected.
- minimal effect on other sensory systems.
- reversal of shivering induced by local anaesthetics (Reynolds et al, 1996).

Some of the problems associated with intramuscular opioids such as constipation are diminished. However many of the opioid side effects remain (Kan and Hughes, 1995):

- pruritus/itching, which is more troublesome at higher doses (Lyons et al, 1997);
- nausea and vomiting;
- respiratory depression or even arrest;

- hypotension;
- fetal heart rate changes;
- sedation, slurred speech;
- retention of urine;
  (Arkoosh, 1991; Armand et al, 1993; Norris et al, 1994)

When opioids are administered epidurally or intrathecally, hypotension is likely to occur within 30 minutes of administration, particularly with meperidine (pethidine). This may be accompanied by severe fetal bradycardia (Richardson, 2000). Following the administration of normal doses, maternal respiratory depression, apnoea and sedation may occur 30 minutes later or be delayed up to 16 hours, presumably due to the gradual spread of the drugs (Clyburn & Rosen, 1993; Catterall & Mackie, 1996; Hall, 1996; Arkoosh, 1991).

Case Reports

Epidural or intrathecal opioids may cause sudden, profound maternal respiratory depression.

Case 1. 1 mg of morphine was administered intrathecally during labour. Apnoea occurred seven hours later, after delivery. It was merely fortuitous that apnoea did not occur during labour.

Case 2. 100 micrograms of fentanyl were administered extradurally for Caesarean section. Profound respiratory depression occurred one hundred minutes later.

These cases, cited by Clyburn and Rosen (1993) show the effects of delayed respiratory depression on the mother.

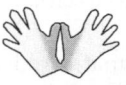 **Practice Points**

- It is important that vital signs continue to be monitored up to 16 hours after administration of intraspinal opioids (Hall, 1996).
- If the spinal (intrathecal) anaesthetic has 'worn off', administration of other opioids, for example meperidine (pethidine) intramuscularly, may intensify respiratory depression (Arkoosh, 1991).

Recurrence of *Herpes simplex* infections have been reported with spinal administration of opioids (Bowdle, 1998).

Morphine

Intraspinal morphine induces pruritus and emesis in the majority of women (Richardson, 2000).

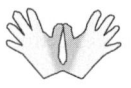 **Practice Point**

Anti-histamines do not always relieve this pruritus, but naloxone in low doses is often effective (Bowdle, 1998).

There are case reports of intrathecal morphine or diamorphine worsening pain, due to the unopposed action of a metabolite (morphine-3-glucuronide) in the CNS (Twycross, 1994). Nalbuphine may be more effective than naloxone at reversing the side effects of epidural morphine in post-Caesarean patients. Nausea and pruritus are less frequent with the more lipid-soluble opioids such as fentanyl, alfentanil and sufentanil which are superseding morphine in combined spinal epidurals (CSE) (Kan & Hughes, 1995; Bem et al, 1996). However these drugs have the potential to cause respiratory depression in mother and fetus in the absence of maternal sedation (Herman et al, 1999).

Fentanyl

This lipid-soluble opioid can be administered by several routes: transdermal, transmucosal, intrathecal. Since it is 80 times more potent than morphine, relatively small volumes are required. The rapid action of fentanyl (within five minutes) and longer duration of action (80–90 minutes) offer a considerable advantage over morphine (Kan & Hughes, 1995). The lipophilic [glossary] properties of fentanyl make it more likely to remain in the spinal cord and less likely to spread to the medulla and cause respiratory depression (Clyburn & Rosen, 1993). There is less reliance on the kidneys for elimination, making it more suitable in pre-eclampsia and for long term administration, but fentanyl may accumulate in the occasional patient (Bem et al, 1996). Fentanyl administered via the epidural route passes into the fetus, and has the potential to produce neonatal depression, which is not always detected by the APGAR score (Reynolds, 1993b). Passage of fentanyl into colostrum is very low (Dailland, 1993).

Fentanyl may reduce the heart rate of mother and fetus, and even cause asystole if the mother is intubated. Although reductions in blood pressure are usually minor, severe hypotension has been reported. Increases in heart rate and blood pressure occur in a minority of patients (Bowdle, 1998). Since fentanyl provokes less histamine release than morphine, this gives the following advantages:

- reduced incidence of pruritus (66% incidence);
- less hypotension;
- less risk of asthma attack.

Fentanyl requirements are increased in women regularly taking anti-convulsants.

The fentanyl analogues are relatively new drugs. Alfentanil and sufentanil are less likely to induce hypotension than fentanyl (Marshall & Longnecker, 1996), but late hypotension has been reported with sufentanil (Gautier et al, 1997). Their distinguishing features are outlined below.

Sufentanil

Sufentanil is more potent than fentanyl. Duration of action may vary from 30–300 minutes. Onset of analgesia is within five minutes of intrathecal administration (Kan & Hughes, 1995; Harsten et al, 1997). However the rapid passage into the brain may increase the risks of opioid myoclonus or muscular rigidity (Bowdle, 1998) or swallowing difficulties (Richardson, 2000). Itching was reported by 44 per cent of women receiving intrathecal sufentanil (Norris et al, 1994). Sufentanil gives a longer duration of both analgesia and pruritus than fentanyl (Gaiser et al, 1998). Placental transfer of sufentanil is lower than other opioids and neonates studied have not demonstrated any adverse effects following the epidural administration of 50 micrograms, although a dose of 80 micrograms has caused neonatal respiratory depression (Armand et al, 1993).

Alfentanil

Alfentanil has shorter onset and duration of action than sufentanil but is more likely to cause nausea (Scholz et al, 1996; Bowdle, 1998). Neonatal elimination of this drug is delayed (Clyburn & Rosen, 1993) with cases of neonatal hypotonia being reported (Armand et al, 1993).

The implications for practice associated with intraspinal opioids are considered in association with administration of CSE and intraspinal analgesia.

Administration of intraspinal analgesia

The technical complexities of administration and the need for specialist skills and support counterbalance the advantages of intraspinal analgesia (Reynolds, 1993a). The use of 'test doses' is mandatory. It is suggested that the administration of large bolus doses of local anaesthetics 'will sooner or later lead to a catastrophe' (Hughes, 1992: R21). Epidurals are more likely to fail if: the first dose fails; presentation is posterior; pain occurs during placement; the epidural is given for less than one hour or more than six hours (Le Coq et al, 1998).

Common technical problems associated with intraspinal analgesia include:

- Failure to flex the spine;
- Kinking of lines;
- Accidental removal of lines;
- Infection;
- Systemic absorption;
- Intravascular injection;
- Dural puncture.

Complications of intraspinal administration

Intravascular injection The prominent venous plexus in the epidural space makes **inadvertent intravascular injection** a potential hazard of epidural analgesia (Catterall and Mackie, 1996). An accident of this type may cause cardiac toxicity and profound hypotension.

Dural puncture Headache, sometimes with tinnitus and photophobia, is the most common complaint following intraspinal anaesthesia. It is attributed to the puncture of the dura by the spinal needle or accidentally by the epidural needle (Reynolds et al, 1996). This may cause a leak of CSF, reducing intracranial pressure; this may take a few weeks to resolve (McKenry & Salerno, 1995). Headache is more likely to follow spinal anaesthesia if large needles (greater than 25 gauge or without pencil point tips) are used or if the woman does not remain supine during the immediate post-partum period. In one series (n = 924), 2.7 per cent of parturients suffered unintended dural puncture. This was more likely when either the parturient was suffering severe labour pains, and therefore unable to maintain a constant position, or combined spinal-epidural analgesia was administered (Norris et al, 1994).

Severe post-dural puncture headache, which is hindering mobilization, may require an epidural **'blood patch'** (Tay et al, 1994; Wildsmith, 1996). This is the epidural injection of 15 20 ml of the patient's own blood. If a blood patch is performed to treat a headache, the epidural needle must be reintroduced; this prospect may deter some women from accepting the treatment. Prophylactic blood patch is the administration of 15 ml blood after delivery but before removal of the epidural needle. This has been shown to reduce, but not eliminate, the need for a second procedure (Howell, 1995c).

Both epidural and spinal anaesthesia are associated with headache and **backache**. Prolapsed intervertebral disc has been reported in association with epidural analgesia (Forster et al, 1996). The relationship between new long term backache and epidural analgesia during labour remains controversial.

Studies suggest that 18 per cent of women who receive epidural analgesia suffer long term neurological or orthopaedic problems, compared to 10 per cent of those receiving other forms of analgesia (Howell & Chalmers, 1992; Mander, 1994). Whereas retrospective studies have indicated that this association exists (MacArthur et al, 1990; Russell et al, 1993), a prospective randomized study of 599 women found no association between new onset, long term backache and either the use of epidural analgesia or the dose of bupivacaine administered. Previous backache was significantly associated with new onset, long term backache (Russell et al, 1993; Butler & Fuller, 1998). Attention to posture before, during and after labour may reduce long term backache (Reynolds, 1993a).

Epidural haematoma   An epidural haematoma may form if insertion of the intraspinal needle causes bleeding and bruising. This can compress vital structures, for example in the spinal cord.

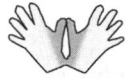 **Practice Point**

To reduce the risk of epidural haematoma, the woman should be examined for signs of bleeding (see Chapter 8) and coagulation and platelet count should be checked before the procedure if:

• HELLP syndrome is even a remote possibility (Yerby, 2000);
• anticoagulants have been administered;
• low molecular weight heparin has been administered within the last 24 hours;
• other haematological disorders are present.

Spinal analgesia is hazardous if the woman has disseminated intravascular coagulation (Richardson, 2000).

Neurological deficit   It is estimated that serious neurological complications arise in around one in 2530 women receiving epidural analgesia in childbirth (Holdcroft et al, 1995). Neurological deficit may arise from either accidental damage to nerve roots during injection or chronic inflammatory reactions to impurities injected. There have been rare cases of incomplete recovery from the blockade of sensory, motor and sympathetic neurones. Septic and aseptic meningitis and reversible bilateral hearing loss have been reported (Karch, 1992; McKenry & Salerno, 1998; Reynolds et al, 1996).

Case Report

This case illustrates the rare complication of septic meningitis.

A healthy 22 year-old primigravida received epidural analgesia with fentanyl. Following uncomplicated delivery, she was discharged 24 hours post-partum with a healthy infant. She returned 48 hours later, vomiting and febrile but alert and complaining of headache. She rapidly deteriorated and developed neck rigidity. Despite treatment, she died four weeks later.

The skin is not sterilized prior to intraspinal analgesia. Puncture of the skin and dura may allow entry of micro-organisms into the cerebro-spinal fluid that in very rare cases can bring about infection (Choy, 2000).

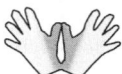 **Practice Points**

- Vomiting, headache and fever alert practitioners to possible serious complications.
- New long term headache requires urgent attention (Reynolds, 1993a).
- To minimize the potential for error, all intraspinal drugs must be:
  - double-checked;
  - freshly prepared;
  - administered slowly;
  - sterile.
- Some intraspinal drug regimens are complex, and involve more detailed calculations than are normally performed in hospital practice. The possibility of error should be reduced if all intraspinal infusions are:
  - prepared in the pharmacy under sterile conditions;
  - standardized;
  - prescribed on charts reserved for spinal infusions;
  - accompanied by charts detailing the clinical monitoring required (Cousins, 1996).
- *Monitoring must include:*
  - maintaining maternal non-supine position;
  - BP, HR every five minutes for first 30 minutes, every 15 minutes until at least two hours post-partum and hourly for 16 hours if opioids are administered;
  - maternal respirations;
  - the height of sensory block;
  - the height of motor block until complete recovery;
  - continuous fetal heart monitoring;
  - pulse oximetry if needed

(Norris et al, 1994; Brownridge, 1991; Stienstra et al, 1995; *Drugs and Therapy Perspectives*, 1996; DoH, 1996; Hall, 1996; Arkoosh, 1991).

Use of intravenous fluids

During intraspinal analgesia, fluids are infused to maintain maternal blood pressure and to prevent a fall in placental blood flow, with subsequent fetal distress (Hofmeyr, 1995). The administration of intraspinal analgesia requires skilled and experienced personnel. When life threatening incidents have occurred, they have usually been associated with lapses in standards of administration and management (Brownridge, 1991; DoH, 1996, 1998). Maternal death has also occurred from circulatory overload during induced labour (DoH, 1996:26), indicating the importance of careful monitoring.

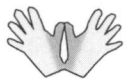 **Practice Points**

- To ensure safety, protocols for management of complications (however rare) must be in place, and experienced personnel must be available. The necessary equipment, including facilities for resuscitation and 'rescue drugs' such as ephedrine, must be in place and checked daily (Brownridge, 1991; *Drugs and Therapy Perspectives*, 1996).
- In view of the risk of complications, all women receiving intraspinal analgesia must have intravenous access established.

Conclusion: intraspinal analgesia

Although epidurals have been associated with a failure rate of 8–20 per cent (Howell & Chalmers, 1992; Mander, 1994; Le Coq et al, 1998), intraspinal analgesia offers more effective and satisfactory pain relief than other methods of obstetric analgesia, particularly intramuscular opioids (Philipsen & Jensen, 1990; Reynolds, 1993a; Thorp et al, 1993; Steer, 1995; Halpern et al, 1998); these benefits persist 24 hours after delivery (Sheiner et al, 2000). Epidural and combined spinal epidural anaesthesia for Caesarean section carry a lower mortality rate than general anaesthesia (Reynolds, 1993a; Dewan & Cohen, 1994; DoH, 1998).

Although epidural anaesthesia with local anaesthetics is the most effective available method for relieving the pain of labour (Armand et al, 1993), the benefits of epidural anaesthesia are tempered not only by side effects but also by increases in: the duration of labour; the need for oxytocin augmentation; the incidence of malrotation; the incidence of instrumental deliveries and Caesarean sections. The problems associated with instrumental deliveries, such as vaginal lacerations, should be considered when evaluating epidural analgesia (Okojie & Cook, 1999). Carli et al (1993) and Thorp et al (1993) suggest that epidural anaesthesia may be responsible for the current 'epidemic' of instrumental deliveries and Caesarean sections in primagravidae. The rising rates of Caesarean section may be attributed to many factors, including fear of the complications of instrumental delivery (Drife, 1996).

Interpretation of the studies in this area can be confusing because: variables such as posture and fluid management are not always mentioned; individual differences exist between patients; some studies do not compare equivalent groups of parturients; dystocia may cause painful and protracted labour, and may therefore be the cause, not the effect, of epidural administration (Hess et al, 2000). Possibly the women with the highest risks of prolonged labour and complications will require the most invasive analgesic regimens which complicates any assessment of the risks of side effects (Traynor et al, 2000). Considering the widespread use of intraspinal analgesia during labour, and the potential for adverse reactions, the absence of large randomized controlled trials is surprising and should be rectified.

Conclusion

All pharmacological methods of pain relief have side effects which may adversely affect the mother, the fetus, the neonate or the progress of labour. The midwife should discuss with the woman all the options available, while taking into account her medical and obstetric history (Findley and Chamberlain, 1999). The information given should include the relevant side effects. Non-disclosure of serious risks is not acceptable to women (Pattee et al, 1997).

There may be advantages in selecting analgesia which permits ambulation and mobility during labour, as this, by itself, may shorten labour and reduce the need for analgesia (de Jong et al, 1997; Al-Mufti et al, 1997; Larimore & Cline, 2000). Mobility is obviously hindered by sedation or motor block-ade of the legs. Psychologists suggest that perception of 'loss of control' in labour may be linked to poor adjustment post-partum (Czarnocka & Slade, 2000).

Dissatisfaction with childbirth may be linked to the experience of pain (Waldenstrom, 1999). However it is not always necessary to achieve complete analgesia during normal childbirth. Many women will be satisfied if the pain is made 'tolerable'. While this reduces the amount of drug administered, the greater risk of analgesic failure requires closer supervision and more frequent dosage adjustments.

The current regional variations in pharmacotherapy indicate the need for practice guidelines (Williams et al, 1998). In the majority of cases, the midwife will be administering these drugs on her own responsibility, either as initial or subsequent doses. It is essential that the midwife makes a careful assess-ment of the woman, the condition of the fetus and the parameters of the labour to ascertain whether it is clinically appropriate to administer any drug before doing so. Knowledge of the potential side effects of the drug administered will empower the midwife to monitor for adverse reactions and to take timely remedial action.

Further Reading

Jordan, S. (1992) Drugs for Severe Pain. *Nursing Times*:88:2: 24–6.

Reynolds, F. (ed.) (1993) *Effects on the Baby of Maternal Analgesia and Anaesthesia*. London, Saunders.

Yerby, M. & Page, L. (eds) (2000) *Pain in Childbearing*, Edinburgh, Bailliere Tindall.

CHAPTER 5

Anti-Emetics

SUE JORDAN

This chapter discusses metoclopramide, phenothiazines (prochlorperazine) and anti-histamines. Brief mention is made of other anti-emetics, ondansetron, pyridoxine and cannabinoids.

Chapter Contents

▦ The physiology of nausea and vomiting

▦ Emesis in early pregnancy

▦ The pharmacological management of emesis

▦ Dopamine antagonists (metoclopramide and prochlorperazine)

▦ Drug Interactions

▦ Anti-histamines (cyclizine, promethazine)

▦ Other anti-emetics (anti-muscarinics, serotonin antagonists, pyridoxine, cannabinoids)

▦ Conclusion

In midwifery, emesis is encountered in early pregnancy, labour and the post-operative period. It is not only distressing, but may lead to serious physiological consequences. The term '*hyperemesis gravidarum*' is applied when vomiting results in fluid, electrolyte or nutritional deficiencies (Friedman & Isselbacher, 1991).

The physiology of nausea and vomiting

Vomiting is usually, but not always, associated with nausea. Nausea is the conscious recognition of subconscious excitation of the vomiting centre or an area close to it in the medulla (Guyton, 1996). Vomiting is a complex series of movements which rids the gut of its contents when any part of it is irritated or distended. The sensory and motor components of the vomiting reflex

121

are governed by the autonomic nervous system. This brings about the emotion of 'feeling sick'.

Causes of vomiting

Many stimuli act directly on the vomiting centre (VC) or the chemoreceptor trigger zone (CTZ). The chemoreceptor trigger zone lies outside the blood/brain barrier in the medulla, close to but distinct from the vomiting centre. The vomiting centre receives inputs from: the higher centres of the brain, the chemoreceptor trigger zone, the vestibular apparatus of the inner ear and the whole body via the autonomic nervous system.

Nausea and vomiting depend on the interaction of many factors including drugs administered, emotional state, pain, tissue damage, motion or changes in homeostasis. To prevent vomiting, the midwife must keep in mind all the factors affecting the vomiting centre (see Box 5.1). In labour, gastric stasis, pain and pressure on the stomach combine to cause emesis.

Description of vomiting

Vomiting is usually accompanied by secretion of saliva, sweating, pallor, drop in blood pressure, tachycardia and irregular respirations, as well as subjective feelings. Gastric stasis usually precedes vomiting. To remove the gut contents, the lower oesophagus and upper stomach relax while the duodenum and lower stomach contract. The stomach is squeezed between the diaphragm and the abdominal wall. A deep breath is taken, and the glottis and the back of the nostrils are closed. However, there may be no time for deep inspiration if the urge to vomit is overwhelming.

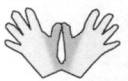 **Practice Points**

- If reflexes are dulled by sedation, there is a risk of aspiration of vomit. In recent maternal deaths (DoH, 1994), Adult Respiratory Distress Syndrome has been subsequent to aspiration of vomit. Therefore, labouring women who receive opioids should not eat.
- Fainting may occur if BP drops; therefore, a woman likely to vomit should not be left unattended, for example after administration of opioids (Torrance & Jordan, 1996).

Box 5.1   Causes of vomiting (with some examples)

The VOMITING CENTRE is affected by:

- The CTZ (chemoreceptor trigger zone) which detects:

    CIRCULATING CHEMICALS such as oestrogens, alcohol, nicotine, opioids, iron, anaesthetics, thyroid hormones,

    ELECTROLYTE IMBALANCE (low sodium, including Addison's diease)

    WITHDRAWAL FROM REGULAR USE OF ALCOHOL;

    PRODUCTS of TISSUE DAMAGE released into the circulation on injury.
- The VESTIBULAR NUCLEUS* which detects:

    motion, including ambulation and sudden movements, for example after labour or an operation.
- HIGHER CENTRES which detect:

    tastes, smells, sights, emotion, pain, fear, anxiety, anticipation, individual factors.
- The AUTONOMIC NERVOUS SYSTEM which detects:

    IRRITATION TO GUT, THROAT or PERITONEUM such as gastric stasis or distension (for example migraine, pain, labour), liver disease, some foods, alcohol, NSAIDs, obstruction of gastrointestinal tract, constipation;

    PHYSIOLOGICAL DISTURBANCES such as changes in BP, pH, blood gases, blood glucose, pain, shock, ketoacidosis, uraemia, organ damage, infections, UTI, intercurrent illness (for example, asthma, gall stones);
- RAISED INTRACRANIAL PRESSURE (for example, pre-eclampsia/eclampsia).

* This input may be direct to vomiting centre (Mitchelson, 1992a; Friedman Isselbacher, 1991).

Consequences of vomiting

It is important that emesis is managed effectively because of the potentially serious consequences:

- dehydration and, consequently, increased risk of thromboses;
- electrolyte imbalance (sodium and potassium loss) and, consequently, weakness;
- pH imbalance;
- ketone formation;

- loss of oral medication;
- risk of aspiration of vomit and Adult Respiratory Distress Syndrome;
- risk of hypotension, reduced placental blood flow, syncope, shock, circulatory collapse;
- psychological distress;
- hyperemesis gravidarum may result in vitamin deficiency or, rarely, liver failure;
- risk of trauma to gastrointestinal tract (Mallory-Weiss tears);
- long term: malnutrition, dental caries.

There is a danger that the symptoms of acute illness may be dangerously masked by the use of anti-emetics, impeding the diagnosis of serious pathology, such as rising intracranial pressure in severe pre-eclampsia (Brunton, 1996).

Emesis in early pregnancy

In early pregnancy, nausea and vomiting are very common, and may even have a physiological role in encouraging the woman to eat more (Huxley, 2000). In pregnancies where there is no nausea, the risk of spontaneous abortion or premature labour is higher (Beischer et al, 1997). Non-pharmacological approaches to the problem are usually preferable to the use of drugs. Women often benefit from the assurance that the problem rarely persists beyond 12–14 weeks of pregnancy. It may be helpful to consider the following:

- Specific causes of nausea should be considered, such as iron tablets, UTI, anxiety (see Box 5.1), multiple or molar pregnancy.
- Rest and intake of bland carbohydrate, such as a biscuit or cereal, may be effective.
- Small, frequent, bland meals are advised (Chamberlain, 1975). Hypoglycaemia may aggravate emesis, and it is inadvisable to miss meals.

Table 5.1 Summary of actions of commonly used anti-emetics: side effects expected with commonly administered anti-emetics

DRUG	dopamine antagonism (causes movement disorders)	histamine antagonism (causes sedation)	anti-muscarinic [glossary] properties (for example, drying of secretions; see Table 5.3)
promethazine	+	+	+
prochlorperazine	++	+	+
chlorpromazine	++	++	++
metoclopramide	++	–	–
haloperidol	+++	little	very little
cyclizine	–	+	+

symbols: – no appreciable action, + action important, ++ action prominent; +++ action very prominent

- Distension of the stomach will be reduced if fruit and liquids are taken separately from meals.
- Women are advised to avoid: sudden movements; eating late at night; eating spicy, fatty, greasy or acidic food; swallowing food without chewing thoroughly (Rogers, 1995).
- Peppermint after a meal relaxes the lower oesophagus and reduces gastric distension which may relieve nausea after meals. However peppermint may worsen constipation or induce 'heartburn', particularly if used before lying down.
- Intake of herbal teas must be limited since their affects on pregnancy are uncertain: for example, fennel is contra-indicated in pregnancy (see Rogers, 1995). A ginger biscuit may be helpful.
- Self-administered acupressure has been shown to reduce nausea but not vomiting when compared to placebo (Howden, 1995).

Pharmacological management of emesis

A wide variety of drugs are used as anti-emetics, both in labour and in hyper-emesis gravidarum. The pattern of use varies between centres. The diversity of drugs used for emesis may be explained by the complexity of the neural pathways affecting the vomiting centre. If vomiting is severe, single agents are not always completely effective. The neurotransmitters involved in vomiting that can be modified by the actions of drugs include: dopamine, acetylcholine, histamine, serotonin, benzodiazepines and cannabinoids.

The anti-emetics commonly used in childbirth fall into two main groups:

- the dopamine (D_2) antagonists/blockers, such as metoclopramide and prochlorperazine;
- the histamine (H_1) antagonists, such as cyclizine, promethazine.

For each drug, side effects depend on the neurotransmitters affected. For example, all histamine (H_1) antagonists can cause sedation, and all dopamine (D_2) antagonists can cause movement disorders. Some drugs such as promethazine (Avomine®, Phenergan®) and prochlorperazine (Stemetil®) are both histamine and dopamine antagonists; while they have the anti-emetic actions of both drug groups, they also have the side effects of both groups. Table 5.1 aims to clarify this complicated situation.

Dopamine (D_2) antagonists (mainly metoclopramide and prochlorperazine)

D_2 antagonists include metoclopramide (Maxalon®), haloperidol, domperidone and the phenothiazines such as chlorpromazine and prochlorperazine (Stemetil®) (see Implications for Practice). In actions, side effects, cautions and contra-indications, prochlorperazine is very similar to chlorpromazine (BNF, 2000). Promethazine is a phenothiazine, but its predominant actions are those of anti-histamines; it is therefore considered below under the anti-histamines. Metoclopramide is a substituted benzamide, not a phenothiazine. It is therefore free of anti-muscarinic side effects such as constipation. Its anti-emetic properties are due to actions on both dopamine and serotonin receptors (Mitchelson, 1992a).

Uses of D₂ antagonists

These drugs are prescribed to counter emesis in a variety of situations:

- to counteract the emetogenic effects of opioids and ergotamine;
- to counteract the emesis of labour itself (although this is rarely necessary);
- prior to anaesthesia;
- post-operative emesis;
- Meniere's disease, radiation sickness, cytotoxic therapy;
- any situation with gastric stasis, for example labour, migraine, pain, gastric paresis due to diabetes.
- Metoclopramide has been used in hyperemesis gravidarum; however the manufacturer advises 'use only when compelling reasons' (BNF, 2000).

D_2 antagonists are ineffective in motion sickness. Therefore they offer little protection to the mobilizing woman who has used opioids. Phenothiazines are important in the management of psychotic illness, usually in higher doses than for emesis (see Chapter 16).

How the body handles phenothiazines, for example prochlorperazine

Prochlorperazine acts within 10–20 minutes of intramuscular injection, and anti-emetic actions last for 12 hours (Joshua & King, 1997). Phenothiazines cross the placenta, and may lead to movement disorders in the neonate. They are eliminated by metabolism in the liver and excretion by the kidneys. Phenothiazines pass into breast milk in small amounts, and drowsiness of infants has been reported. Animal studies indicate that prolonged use of phenothiazines, in early pregnancy or when breastfeeding, may affect the infant's nervous system.

These drugs are eliminated in a complex way, with considerable individual variation: for example the half-life of chlorpromazine varies from 2–30 hours. This means that, with repeated doses, the drugs will build up in some people, but not in others. There is also a diurnal variation in plasma concentration (Mitchelson, 1992a).

How the body handles metoclopramide

The onset of action of metoclopramide is within minutes of injection, and within one hour of oral ingestion. This drug is eliminated rather quickly from the body (half-life 4–8 hours) which necessitates frequent dosing. Therefore metoclopramide is most effective if given by continuous intravenous infusion (Michelson, 1992a).

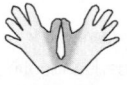 **Practice Point**

The rapid elimination after a single dose is useful if the mother wishes to breastfeed. The concentration of metoclopramide is higher in breast milk than in plasma (Brunton, 1996). Although the amount of drug in breast milk is likely to be small, authorities advise against breastfeeding with regular use.

Actions of D_2 antagonists

Drugs which block the action of dopamine (D_2 antagonists) relieve vomiting by their actions in the gut wall, vomiting centre and chemoreceptor trigger zone. By inhibiting the actions of dopamine, drugs in this group have the potential to:

- reduce emesis and increase appetite;
- alter gastrointestinal motility;
- depress the central nervous system;
- disturb posture and movement;
- disturb the cardiovasular system;
- trigger syndrome inappropriate ADH (SIADH) and water retention. (Chapter 6);
- increase prolactin production (Chapter 16);
- suppress the symptoms of schizophrenia and schizo-affective disorders (Chapter 16).

Side effects of D_2 antagonists (mainly metoclopramide and prochlorperazine)

Gastrointestinal tract

In addition to central anti-emetic actions, these drugs increase gastric emptying, This prokinetic action on the stomach and intestine counteracts the gastric stasis induced by pain, labour, migraine or opioids. Diarrhoea is a recognized side effect of metoclopramide. If stimulation of gastrointestinal motility would be dangerous, for example if the gastro-intestinal tract is obstructed or traumatized, metoclopramide is contra-indicated (Spencer, 1993a). Intestinal hurry interferes with absorption from the gut, not only of food, but also of other drugs (see below).

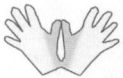 **Practice Point**

Alteration in food absorption may interfere with control of diabetes. If metoclopramide or a phenothiazine are used, diabetics must have glucose levels closely monitored because insulin requirements will be altered (Malseed et al, 1995; Brunton, 1996).

In contrast, phenothiazines such as prochlorperazine cause constipation due to their anti-muscarinic properties. They do not interfere with absorption of food but increase insulin resistance in the long term. They may be a better choice for short term use in diabetic women.

Central nervous system depression

Dopamine antagonists, particularly phenothiazines (prochlorperazine), usually cause sedation, depressed mood or blunting of emotions. There is an increased risk of seizures in women with epilepsy. They also depress the functions of the brain stem such as thermoregulation, thirst, respiration and the cough reflex.

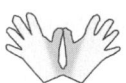 **Practice Points**

- The mother may feel cold until the drug has been eliminated. Extra care should be taken to protect the neonate from hypothermia.
- Depression of the **respiratory centres** impedes the establishment of normal respirations in the neonate and increases the chances of a post-operative chest infection in the mother, particularly if she is dehydrated.
- If mother and infant are sedated, they are less able to initiate effective **breastfeeding**. For women receiving prochlorperazine, this problem is likely to persist for up to 24 hours. Drowsiness and difficulties in feeding are likely to persist for longer in neonates. The midwife should offer explanations and encouragement during this time.
- These effects on the central nervous system are compounded by co-administration of opioids.
- D_2 antagonists increase the likelihood of fits. They are used with caution in people with epilepsy (Karch, 1992; Malseed et al, 1995).

Posture and movement disorders

These serious side effects are rare at normal doses but are more likely with higher doses and in young people. Posture and movement disorders (including extra-pyramidal side effects) are associated with all the D_2 antagonists due to their actions on the basal ganglia:

- acute dystonia (abnormal muscle tone and spasms);
- pseudo-parkinsonism;
- akathisia (restlessness and involuntary movements);
- tardive dyskinesia (involuntary movements of the face or limbs – this can occur with prolonged administration (BNF, 2000);
- the neuroleptic malignant syndrome (see Chapter 16).

Acute dystonic reactions

Oculogyric crises (spasms of the muscles controlling the eyeballs), torticollis (spasm and twisting of the neck muscles), severe swelling of the tongue or facial grimacing usually occur within the first 48 hours of use. These very dramatic and distressing side effects are rare but occur more commonly in women under 20 when higher doses are used (particularly metoclopramide in doses over 0.5 mg per kg) (McLaughlin & Thompson, 1995), or if viral infection is present. Acute dystonic reactions may be mistaken for hysteria; however, unlike hysteria, they involve the tongue (Rascol et al, 1995).

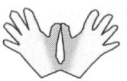 **Practice Points**

- During an acute dystonic reaction, it is important that the patient is not left alone, not only because these reactions are terrifying to experience but also because the airway may be jeopardized (Baldessarini, 1996).
- An antidote is administered as quickly as possible; this is usually procyclidine 5 mg im, repeated if necessary 20 minutes later. Relief may not be obtained for up to 30 minutes (BNF, 2000).
- If dopamine antagonists are likely to be administered, the midwife should seek a specific history of adverse reactions to these drugs.
- Because of the risks of acute dystonia, the BNF (2000) imposes severe restrictions on the use of metoclopramide in those under 20 years of age. Advice should be sought before administering metoclopramide to women younger than 20. Prochlorperazine is not restricted in this way.

Prochlorperazine given intramuscularly is associated with a high incidence of dystonic reactions, and is therefore used with caution in childbirth in the US (Brunton, 1996).

Parkinsonian side effects

Masklike facies, bradykinesia (paucity of movement), tremor and rigidity may develop gradually over the first few days or weeks of administration. This reaction may be mistaken for signs of depression in a woman suffering from hyperemesis.

Akathisia

This presents as restlessness, inability to keep still, anxiety, insomnia or confusion. Drowsiness or restlessness occurs in 20 per cent of recipients of D_2 antagonists (Mitchelson, 1992a). If these drugs are administered rapidly iv, feelings of anxiety and agitation are particularly likely (Spencer, 1993).

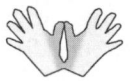 **Practice Point**

It is important that these side effects are recognized and explained to women, rather than attributed to psychological factors.

With continuous use in the last three months of pregnancy, D_2 antagonists can cause prolonged movement disorders in neonates (Cox & Nicholls, 1996). This may occur in women with mental health problems or in women suffering from hyperemesis.

The neuroleptic malignant syndrome

This is usually associated with anti-psychotic medication and has been reported with metoclopramide and prochlorperazine (Blair & Dauner, 1992). This rare but serious side effect is described in Chapter 16.

Cardiovascular side effects

D_2 antagonists are associated with cardiac dysrhythmias, particularly when given rapidly by the intravenous route (Spencer, 1993a). Cardiac dysrhythmias are particularly likely in women who are potassium depleted, for example due to prolonged vomiting, co-administration of corticosteroids, ritodrine or diuretics. Cardiac dysrhythmias may also occur as a result of drug interactions (see p. 134).

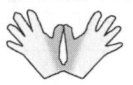 **Practice Points**

- An intravenous injection of metoclopramide should be given over one to two minutes (BNF, 2000).
- With prolonged administration of anti-emetics, signs of dysrhythmia may be detected by monitoring the pulse and ECG.

Metoclopramide may cause tachycardia and elevation of blood pressure, which should be monitored. It has the potential to mimic the action of aldosterone, causing loss of potassium and retention of sodium and water. It is therefore not a good choice of drug for women with fluid retention or potassium depletion (Govoni & Hayes 1990; Spencer, 1993a).

Phenothiazines (for example prochlorperazine) inhibit the vasoconstrictor actions of noradrenaline (norepinephrine) on the peripheral blood vessels. The resultant vasodilation reduces BP, makes the patient feel the cold and may cause **orthostatic hypotension**. In young women, this inability to adjust the peripheral blood vessels causes dizziness on sudden standing. More importantly, hypotension may decrease placental blood flow. Therefore if phenothiazines are prescribed during pregnancy, close fetal monitoring is required. In labour, blood pressure must be closely observed, particulalry if intraspinal analagesia or opioids are co-administered.

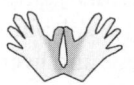 **Practice Point**

To prevent falls, advice on standing slowly should be given and orthostatic hypotension should be assessed (Karch, 1992).

Syndrome inappropriate ADH (SIADH)

SIADH [glossary] is a rare side effect of several drugs (including phenothaizines, opioids and anaesthetics). The clinical picture is of water intoxication (Chapter 6).

Anti-muscarinic side effects

Both the phenothiazines (including prochlorperazine) and anti-histamines may cause anti-muscarinic (anti-cholinergic) side effects. These result in dry

Table 5.2   Anti-muscarinic side effects (prochlorperazine, promethazine)

Potential Problem	Patient care
Short term (for example in labour)	
dry mouth	dental hygiene, mouth care
glaucoma	avoid these drugs if acute angle glaucoma present; cautious use with relevant family history, or other types of glaucoma (Malseed et al, 1995)
retention of urine, dysuria	assess output
blurred vision	short term use – advise
Longer term (for example post-operation)	
drying of bronchial secretions	breathing exercises
chest infection	advise cessation of smoking
raised heart rate	monitor, be alert for signs of myocardial ischaemia
Longer term (for example emesis in pregnancy)	
dry eyes	artificial tears if needed, protect eyes from wind
constipation, ileus	long term use: monitor output and bowel sounds
confusion	avoid driving, operating machinery
dry skin	skin care using emollients if needed
reduced ability to sweat	avoid raised temperatures, for example fever, high environmental temperatures
reduced libido	

mouth, retention of urine, constipation. These problems are described with the anti-histamines (see Table 5.2).

Hypersensitivity responses

Rash, bronchospasm, periorbital oedema and methaemoglobinaemia [glossary] have been reported with metoclopramide (Spencer, 1993a). All phenothiazines have been implicated in cases of hepatitis, agranulocytosis and liver dysfunction.

Cautions

- Due to the dangers of acute dystonic reactions, administration of metoclopramide to people under 20 is restricted to premedication, intubation and intractable vomiting associated with cancer therapies. The daily dose should not exceed 500 micrograms per kg body weight per day, or 5 mg three times per day in those under 20 and weighing under 60 kg (pre-pregnancy body weight is normally taken) (BNF, 2000).
- D_2 antagonists are potentially toxic to the fetus. Use in pregnancy is controversial, particularly in the first trimester, and particularly metoclopramide and domperidone: metoclopramide has been linked with neural tube defects in experimental animals (McLaughlin & Thompson, 1995; Pfaffenrath & Rehm, 1998; Pangle, 2000). However metoclopramide,

given intramuscularly, is the most effective drug for women hospitalized with hyperemesis gravidarum (*Drugs and Therapy Perspectives*, 1993a).

- D_2 antagonists enter breast milk and are not usually advised during lactation (Malseed et al, 1995; Pangle, 2000).
- D_2 antagonists complicate the management of some common diseases such as diabetes and epilepsy.
- Metoclopramide should be avoided if ileus or gastro-intestinal obstruction is suspected.
- All these drugs require healthy liver and kidneys for elimination. Therefore problems are likely if these organs are impaired, for example in pre-eclampsia. Renal elimination is reduced in dehydration which intensifies the drugs' side effects.
- Masking of emesis is dangerous when raised intracranial pressure is suspected, for example severe pre-eclampsia.
- Cross allergy with procainamide (Spencer, 1993a).
- Phenothiazines should not be administered to women with hypertension.

Other cautions are listed in Appendix 1.

Drug interactions

A wide variety of drugs interact. Some drug combinations will require modification of dosage.

- *Movement disorders*
  When two or more D_2 antagonists are co-administered, the risk of movement disorders increases. Therefore women taking anti-psychotic medication, lithium, methyldopa or some non-sedating anti-histamines (astemizole, terfenadine) may experience serious CNS side effects if metoclopramide or prochlorperazine are also administered. A young woman experienced an acute dystonic reaction and respiratory obstruction when metoclopramide was administered after prochlorperazine (Stockley, 1999).

- *Increased sedation*
  When two or more sedatives are co-administered, their effects are magnified. D_2 antagonists increase the CNS depression of all sedatives including alcohol, opioids, barbiturates, anti-histamines, benzodiazepines and anaesthetics. The combination of meperidine (pethidine) and phenothiazines (including prochlorperazine) increases the risk of respiratory depression, sedation, CNS toxicity and hypotension (Stockley, 1999).

- *Loss of effect*
  The relief of gastric stasis by D_2 antagonists is counteracted by opioids.

- *Lowering seizure threshold*
  The protective effects of anti-convulsants may be reduced.

METOCLOPRAMIDE only
- *Altered absorption from gut*
  Metoclopramide increases the absorption of several drugs: aspirin, para-cetamol, alcohol, cyclosporin, tetracyclines, and decreases the absorption of others: digoxin, atovaquone, fosfomycin, cimetidine. Changes in the absorption of food may affect the response to insulin. Dosages will be modified by the prescriber.

PHENOTHIAZINES only
- *Risk of hypotension*
  Hypotension is more likely with anti-hypertensives, diuretics, opioids, anaesthetics, tricyclic anti-depressants. Co-administration of epinephrine (adrenaline) may induce hypotension and tachycardia (Karch, 1992).
- *Potentiation of muscle relaxants*
  This may result in prolonged apnoea. Therefore, this drug combination is usually avoided.
- *Risks of cardiac dysrhythmias*
  Drugs used in mental illness, drugs used for cardiac dysrhythmias, some non-sedating anti-histamines (astemizole, terfenadine), some anti-malarials (halofantrine) and potassium depletion increase the likelihood of cardiac dysrhythmias.
- *Accumulation*
  Cimetidine (but not ranitidine) reduces the hepatic elimination of phenothiazines and intensifies side effects. Phenytoin may accumulate and cause sedation if prochlorperazine is administered (Stockley, 1999).

Anti-histamines

This term is used to refer to H_1 receptor antagonists. These are divided into:

- Sedating anti-histamines (for example brompheniramine, cinnarizine, meclozine, trimeprazine, cyclizine, promethazine, chlorpheniramine). Promethazine hydrochloride is available as Phenergan ®. Promethazine theoclate is marketed in 25 mg tablets as Avomine ®. These drugs are sometimes used to relieve the symptoms of emesis in early pregnancy, during labour or post-anaesthesia.
- Non-sedating antihistamines (for example cetirizine, terfenadine, acrivastine and loratadine). Sedation is less pronounced but still important with the 'non-sedating' antihistamines (BNF, 2000). They are used to relieve the symptoms of allergic disorders, such as hayfever and urticaria. These are not included in this book, since manufactuers advise to avoid use in pregnancy and lactation.

Anti-histamines are available in a variety of over-the-counter products; accidental overdose by infants is not uncommon.

The anti-emetic effects of these drugs are due to their actions on histaminic and muscarinic receptors in the vomiting centres.

Uses of anti-histamines

- Anti-emetics, in association with opioids, anaesthesia or motion sickness.
- Relief of pruritus or urticaria caused by opioids, for example following intraspinal analgesia.
- Emergency management of anaphylaxis and angioedema after epinephrine (adrenaline) administration (BNF, 2000).
- Hypersensitivity responses, including drug allergies, pruritus, urticaria, insect stings, hayfever. Administration before release of histamine is important, for example at the start of the hayfever season.
- Premedication and sedation, for example promethazine, trimeprazine.
- Insomnia from over-the-counter preparations, for example promethazine.
- Relief of coughs and colds from over-the-counter preparations, for example tripolidine, diphenhydramine (Benylin ®).

How the body handles anti-histamines

These drugs work within 15–60 minutes of oral administration, are maximally absorbed within one to two hours and last three to six hours. They cross the blood/brain barrier and the placenta and pass into breast milk. They are cleared by the liver and the kidneys.

Role of histamine

Histamine is found in most tissues, especially lungs, skin, brain and gut. Histamine is involved in CNS function, gastric acid secretion and smooth muscle contraction. It is also an important chemical mediator in anaphylaxis, allergy and inflammation. Several histamine receptor types have been extensively studied. Drugs acting on H_1 and H_2 receptors are widely used. The H_2 receptor antagonists (such as ranitidine and cimetidine) are discussed in Chapter 12, gastric acidity.

Actions of histamine via H_1 receptors

- smooth muscle contraction, in lungs, gut and uterus;
- vasodilation;
- inflammation. Intra-dermal histamine causes reddening, weals and flare due to vasodilation of the microvasculature and increased permeability of venules;

- itch;
- central nervous system regulation; histamine-containing neurones are found in all parts of the central nervous system, including the cerebral cortex and the spinal cord.

Side effects of anti-histamines

The sedating anti-histamines cause side effects related to inhibition of both histamine and acetylcholine. These side effects are shared with the phenothiazine anti-emetics such as prochlorperazine.

Central nervous system

Both stimulation and depression of the CNS are possible side effects of H_1 antagonists. The usual effects are sedation, somnolence, diminished alertness, delayed reaction times, confusion, fatigue, depression, weakness or heaviness of the hands and impaired co-ordination, including diplopia. All these make driving hazardous.

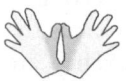 **Practice Points**

- Administration of an anti-emetic, such as promethazine or prochlorperazine in labour, may make the neonate too drowsy to initiate breast feeding efficiently.
- Drowsiness is compounded by co-administration of other sedatives, including alcohol and opioids. Cyclizine is less sedating than other drugs in this class (McLaughlin & Thompson, 1995).
- If a nursing mother takes anti-histamines, the breastfed infant may become sedated, fail to feed and fail to gain weight adequately. Sedation may also impair fluid and nutrient intake in adults.

Although sedation is the usual response, the occasional patient will become restless, nervous and insomniac on the conventional dose (Babe & Serafin, 1996). Convulsions are possible, especially in neonates and children, and caution is advised in epilepsy (BNF, 2000; Malseed et al, 1995). Other manifestations of CNS excitation include: dizziness, headache, tinnitus, euphoria, tremor, irritability. Some anti-histamines (for example promethazine) are structurally related to the phenothiazines and can cause posture and movement disorders.

Cardiovascular system

Histamine is a potent vasodilator. This effect is reversed by anti-histamines. This action is life-saving in anaphylaxis and angioedema. However, anti-histamines can act on the H_1 receptors to cause vasodilation, leading to hypotension, orthostatic hypotension, sweating and headache (Malseed et al, 1995).

Gut and liver disturbance

Some people experience loss of appetite, abdominal pain, constipation, diarrhoea, nausea or vomiting when taking anti-histamines. Soreness of mouth and tongue are occasional problems. Taking the drugs with milk or food can be an effective strategy (Lucas, 1992). Occasionally, appetite increase and weight gain may occur (Babe & Seraffin, 1996).

Anti-muscarinic side effects

All the drugs which antagonize histamine have anti-muscarinic (anti-cholinergic) properties. While these enhance the anti-emetic actions, they add further side effects, which are summarized in Table 5.2. This group of side effects is common to all anti-emetics with the exception of metoclopramide. They are caused by the drugs blocking the actions of the parasympathetic nervous system throughout the body.

All anti-muscarinic medications inhibit the mucus-secreting glands, which moisten all the epithelial linings of the body such as the linings of the digestive, respiratory and genitourinary tracts, and the conjunctiva. This dries the tissues, causing discomfort and thirst. Drying of the respiratory tract may facilitate the formation of mucus 'plugs', which may impede airflow and allow the development of infection or worsen asthma.

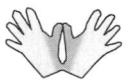 **Practice Points**

- The midwife must monitor carefully any asthmatic women receiving anti-histamines long term.
- If the patient is dehydrated, the drying and discomfort of the mucous membranes will be intensified.

Hypersensitivity responses (rare) include rash, urine discolouration, photosensitivity, bronchospasm and, rarely, anaphylaxis. Bone marrow depression is very rare. Overdose may present as fits, involuntary movements, ataxia, excite-

ment, hallucinations and coma, with fixed dilated pupils. Unintentional overdose by toddlers can be life-threatening. Other, rarer side effects are listed in
Appendix 1.

Cautions

- As with all drugs, previous hypersensitivity contra-indicates use.
- Anti-histamines are potentially hazardous to the breastfed infant (Lucas,
  1992). A single dose administered to the mother may sedate the breastfed
  infant. Repeated doses may cause lethargy, failure to feed and weight gain.
- Abrupt discontinuation of anti-histamines after regular use can cause withdrawal symptoms, such as nervousness, ataxia, muscle spasms and excitability, particularly in the neonate exposed to these drugs *in utero* (McKenry
  & Salerno, 1995).
- Use in pregnancy should be on specialist advice, when the potential benefits have been weighed against the known but small risks.

Effects of anti-emetics on the fetus

Since midwives are often asked for advice on emesis in early pregnancy, the
available evidence has been summarized.

- Anti-histamines are considered the safest anti-emetics in early pregnancy
  (Mazzotta & Magee, 2000), but they are often ineffective. Since the
  studies are conflicting, and the drugs have been widely used in the past, it
  is likely that the risk to the fetus is low when treatment is limited to one
  or two doses. Also, stress itself is linked to fetal malformations (Hansen
  et al, 2000).
- Promethazine theoclate (Avomine®) is usually the first choice anti-emetic,
  given at bedtime (Po & Po, 1992). However it has been associated with
  congenital hip dysplasia.
- Cyclizine (Valoid®) has been associated with some congenital abnormalities, but this has not been substantiated in prospective controlled studies.
- Meclozine (Sea-legs®) may carry an increased risk of cleft palate or congenital eye defects (Howden, 1995).
- Dimenhydrinate (Dramamine®) has been associated with spontaneous
  abortions (Rayburn & Conover, 1993).
- The sedative anti-histamine brompheniramine (Dimotane®) ingested
  during the first trimester has been associated with birth defects (Pangle,
  2000).
- Some over-the-counter anti-emetics and analgesics contain appreciable
  amounts of caffeine, which, in daily doses over 600 mg, has been associated with low birth weight (McKenry & Salerno, 1998).

- Used in the last trimester, paticularly the last two weeks, anti-histamines have been linked with increased incidence of retrolental fibroplasia in premature babies (Rayburn & Conover 1993; Pangle, 2000).

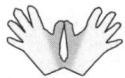 **Practice Point**

If any anti-emetic is used in pregnancy, it is important that a specialist is consulted if symptoms do not settle within 24–48 hours (BNF, 2000).

Drug interactions

The side effects of anti-histamines are compounded by drugs with similar actions.

- Administration of other sedatives, such as alcohol or opioids, will greatly enhance sedation.
- Concurrent use of another drug with anti-muscarinic actions, such as phenothiazines or tricyclic anti-depressants, will produce significant drying of the mouth, tachycardia and other side effects.
- If anti-histamines are combined with drugs which damage the vestibulo-cochlear (auditory) nerve, such as furosemide (frusemide), gentamicin or salicylates, any damage to this nerve will be masked and therefore remain undetected, increasing the risk of irreversible damage.

Other anti-emetics

Anti-muscuarinics, serotonin antagonists, pyridoxine (vitamin B_6), cannabinoids, benzodiazepines and corticosteroids (particularly dexamethasone) are also useful anti-emetics in some circumstances. Oral methylprednisolone has been used to good effect in hyperemesis gravidarum (Safari et al, 1998), but adrenocorticotropic hormone is ineffective (Jewell & Young, 2000). Corticosteroids are considered in Chapters 7 and 15 and benzodiazepines in Chapters 16 and 19.

Anti-muscarinic drugs

Anti-muscarinics, such as atropine and hyoscine (scopolamine), are generally second choice anti-emetics after anti-histamines. Hyoscine hydrobromide (Kwells®) is an important over-the-counter drug for motion sickness, but it is very sedating. The side effect profile for these drugs is as described for anti-histamines.

Serotonin antagonists

Serotonin (5-hydroxytryptamine, 5HT) is a neurotransmitter found through-out the brain which has many different receptors and actions. The receptors involved in vomiting are mainly the $5HT_3$ receptors, but other classes ($5HT_4$) are involved. These are found in the vomiting centre, the chemoreceptor trigger zone and the gut wall; when stimulatated, they cause emesis.

Antagonists of serotonin ($5HT_3$), such as ondansetron (Zofran®) and granisetron (Kytril®), are effective anti-emetics. The half-life of ondanse-tron is between 3–5.5 hours. In midwifery, ondansetron is most likely to be used post-operatively, particularly when other, cheaper, drugs have failed, or if the woman has a history of emesis or migraine. Granisetron was found to be more effective than metoclopramide or droperidol in reducing nausea and vomiting following spinal anaesthesia for Caesarean section (Fujii et al, 1998).

Although ondansetron is generally well tolerated (Mitchelson, 1992a), there are occasional side effects: headache, flushing, sedation, dry mouth, shiv-ering, hypotension, retention of urine, hypersensitivity reactions, visual dis-turbances, raised liver enzymes, gastro-intestinal disturbances and, rarely, cardiac dysrhythmias or fits. In women of reproductive age, the side effects are usually confined to a mild headache, drowsiness and dryness of mouth. No information is available in the BNF (2000) on the use of these drugs in pregnancy and breastfeeding, but the manufacturers advise against use.

Pyridoxine

Pyridoxine has been used as an anti-emetic for 40 years and may be a safe and effective agent in early pregnancy (Mitchelson, 1992b; *Drugs and Therapy Perspectives*, 1993a; Vutyavanich et al, 1995; Mazzotta & Magee, 2000). In a small, double blind, placebo controlled trial of 342 women attending ante-natal clinic, pyridoxine 30–200 mg per day reduced nausea over five days; no adverse effects were reported (Vutyavanich et al, 1995). The dose used was 15–100 mg twice daily which is well above the daily vitamin requirement (2 mg/day), but lower than the 2 g/day (2000 mg/day) known to produce neurological symptoms (Mitchelson, 1992a).

At 2 g/day pyridoxine causes peripheral neuropathy (numbness, paraesthae-sia, unsteady gait). This indicates that the recommended dose should not be exceeded. Sale of products administering a daily dose of more than 10 mg of pyridoxine is restricted. The BNF 2000 includes the pre-menstrual syndrome, but not pregnancy sickness, under the indications for pyridoxine. Pyridoxine (vitamin B_6) was one ingredient of Debendox® (dicyclomine, doxylamine and pyridoxine) which was prescribed for emesis in early pregnancy until it was suddenly withdrawn by the manufacturers in 1983 on suspicion of causing congenital abnormalities (Howden, 1995).

Cannabinoids

Cannabis is used by disseminated sclerosis sufferers to reduce pain and emesis. Nabilone was developed to incorporate the anti-emetic effects of cannabis, without the euphoriant actions. All cannabinoids may cause sedation, dry mouth, loss of appetite, sleep disturbance, hallucinations, psychosis, dizziness and loss of orientation. Nabilone is likely to be superseded by dronabinol, which has a lower incidence of these side effects. However, all cannabinoids (prescribed or otherwise) are contra-indicated in pregnancy and lactation (BNF, 2000).

Implications for Practice: anti-emetics

- Vomiting is potentially dangerous to mother and fetus. No one should be left alone while vomiting.
- Ideally, no anti-emetics should be administered to pregnant or lactating women. Non-pharmacological measures should be employed to minimize emesis. if these fail, specialist advice should be sought.
- If anti-emetics are administered, the midwife must undertake to monitor the client, according to the drug prescribed.

Monitoring for all D_2 antagonists (metochlopramide and prochlorperazine)

Potential problem	Management
Acute dystonic reaction	Procyclidine should be available

Movement disorders
    Signs of restlessness
	Monitor, be prepared to withhold further
	    doses

CNS depression, sedation	Monitor all intake, respirations, sedation in
	    mother and neonate
	Protect neonate from hypothermia
	Provide extra help with breastfeeding
	Avoid other sedatives, for example alcohol,
	    opioids

Hypo or hypertension	Monitor BP, stand gradually
Interference with blood glucose	Monitor blood glucose in diabetics
Cardiac dysrhythmias	Monitor for palpitations
Drug accumulation	Monitor for dehydration, check urine output
Breast tenderness	advise client

Withdrawal reaction	Following prolonged administration:
	    taper dose over several weeks; observe
	    neonate for signs of restlessness

Risk of seizures	Avoid dopamine antagonists in epileptics

If a phenothiazine is administered, the monitoring described under anti-histamines and anti-muscarinics should be added (see Table 5.2).

Conclusion

The consensus on the management of emesis in early pregnancy is described above, although further large scale trials are needed to establish the true efficacy and incidence of adverse effects on mother and foetus (Mazzotta & Magee, 2000; Jewell & Young, 2000). Unfortunately, no such consensus exists on the management of emesis in labour. The widespread, prophylactic use of sedating drugs such as prochlorperazine, often in combination with opioids, impedes the mother's participation in labour. The prolonged action of prochlorperazine means that both mother and infant are sedated at a time when breastfeeding should be initiated, reducing the chances of success. Some US authors advise against the intramuscular administration of prochlorperazine, due to the high incidence of side effects (Brunton, 1996). The shorter half-life of metoclopramide makes this drug a more acceptable alternative, but it is not recommended for women under 20 years of age, due to its potentially serious side effects (BNF, 2000). Many of the side effects of anti-emetics are subtle, and easily overlooked or attributed to co-administered analgesics. Not all women will experience emesis following opioid administration; the 'normal' vomiting of labour is usually transient, and less distressing than the side effects of anti-emetics. Therefore, the authors see little place for the prophylactic use of anti-emetics in 'normal' labour.

Further Reading

Mazzotta, P. & Magee, L. (2000) A risk-benefit assessment of pharmacological and non-pharmacological treatments for nausea and vomiting of pregnancy. *Drugs*:59:781–800.

Pangle, B. (2000) Drugs in Pregnancy and Lactation. In: Herfindal, E. & Gourley, D. (eds) *Textbook of Therapeutics: Drug and Disease Management*, 7th edition. Philadelphia, Lippincott Williams & Wilkins.

CHAPTER 6

Drugs Increasing Uterine Contractility/Oxytocics

SUE JORDAN

This chapter considers the drugs commonly used for induction of labour and in the active management of the third stage of labour.

Chapter Contents

- Uterine contractility
- Oxytocics
- Prostaglandins
- Oxytocin
- Conclusions: the induction/augmentation of labour
- Ergometrine
- Conclusions: the third stage of labour and post-partum haemorrhage

---

The contractility of the uterus is influenced by a number of physiological and pharmacological factors. While many drugs affect the smooth muscle of the uterus, certain oxytocic agents are used in the medical management of labour specifically to increase uterine contractility.

Uterine contractility

The smooth muscle of the uterus has considerable spontaneous activity which can be modified by the administration of drugs. Smooth muscle contractions are triggered by waves of electrical excitation that rapidly spread from cell to cell Electrical activity is initiated by 'spike' potentials arising spontaneously in pacemaker areas throughout the myometrium. The force of uterine contraction depends on the number of gap junctions and the frequency and duration of the electrical activity in 'pacemaker' areas of the uterus. The responsiveness of the uterus varies with the period of gestation, the degree of uterine stretch and the region of the myometrium. Electrical activity, and therefore contractility, is influenced by:

- **Oxytocin:** Fetal and maternal oxytocin play an important facilitatory role in childbirth; secretion of both increases during labour. The number of oxytocin receptors in the uterus increases over a hundred times during pregnancy.
- **Sympathetic nervous system:** Stimulation of alpha$_1$ receptors excites the uterus while stimulation of beta$_2$ receptors inhibits contractions. If a woman experiences fear or anxiety, endogenous epinephrine (adrenaline) may reduce uterine contractions, and postpone or prolong labour (Hoffman & Lefkowitz, 1996). This is more likely if women are exposed to unfamiliar staff, surroundings and technologies (Niven, 1992).
- **Steroid hormones:** Progesterone plays a role in maintaining the pregnancy by reducing uterine contractility. The falling concentration of progesterone, coupled with the rising concentration of oestrogen towards term, is generally considered to be responsible for the corresponding increase in oxytocin sensitivity.
- **Relaxin** inhibits uterine activity throughout pregnancy.
- **Prostaglandins** and related substances, such as platelet activating factor, are important regulators of childbirth. Production of prostaglandins by fetal membranes increases in the last month of pregnancy. The release of prostaglandins is stimulated by vaginal examination and membrane rupture (Kelsey & Prevost, 1994).
- **Serotonin** is an important neurotransmitter in all smooth muscle. It increases uterine contractility. Its action is mimicked by the ergot alkaloids, for example ergometrine.
- **Uterine stretch** increases the number of oxytocin receptors and contractility.
- **Mechanical stimulation** of fetal membranes or the cervix can induce labour.
        (Guyton, 1996; Ganong, 1999; Rang et al, 1999; Graves, 1996).

Oxytocics

Oxytocics are widely used for induction and augmentation of labour, prevention and treatment of post-partum haemorrhage, control of bleeding due to incomplete abortion, active management of the third stage of labour. The oxytocics used in the UK are prostaglandins E and F, oxytocin, ergometrine. Syntometrine® is a combination of oxytocin and ergometrine. Ergometrine acts on the inner region of the myometrium, whereas oxytocin and prostaglandins act on the outer myometrium (de Groot et al, 1998).

Prostaglandins

The prostaglandins are a group of chemically related compounds made *in vivo* from the phospholipids of cell membranes in a variety of tissues. They are important as 'local hormones'.

Endogenous prostaglandins in childbirth

The process of parturition has two essential components:

- cervical ripening (prostaglandins)
- uterine contractions (oxytocin + prostaglandins).

The formation of prostaglandins by the amnion increases towards the end of pregnancy, raising the concentration of prostaglandins in amniotic fluid, umbilical cord blood and maternal blood. These prostaglandins may be important in the normal initiation of labour (Graves, 1996). Uterine sensitivity to prostaglandins increases progressively throughout pregnancy. During the last month of pregnancy, the cervix normally 'ripens' under the influence of PGE_2 (prostaglandin E_2) which increases the production of enzymes that break down and loosen cervical collagen.

Four types of endogenous prostaglandins play a role in parturition. The letters assigned to them denote the chemical structure of the ring part of the molecule.

- PGE_1 ripens the cervix
- PGE_2 causes uterine contractions from late second trimester onwards and ripens the cervix
- PGI_2 ensures blood flow from mother to fetus and maintains a patent ductus arteriosus
- $PGF_{2\alpha}$ causes uterine contractions at all times (unlike oxytocin). It is also important in menstruation, when it causes vasoconstriction and uterine contraction

Synthetic prostaglandins prescribed in childbirth

In the UK, the prostaglandins commonly used in midwifery are:

- Dinoprostone (PGE_2), for cervical priming and induction of labour, is usually administered vaginally. An overview of studies suggests that the time between induction and delivery is shortened by the use of prostaglandins (Dawood, 1995). It may be administered intravenously in cases of missed abortion or hydatidiform mole (Reynolds et al, 1996).

- Carboprost (15 methyl $PGF_{2\alpha}$, a synthetic derivative) for post-partum haemorrhage is given by deep im injection. This is usually given after other agents have failed to stop a haemorrhage, but may be the drug of choice if the woman is hypertensive (Gulmezoglu, 2000).
- Gemeprost (an analogue of PGE_1), to assist with uterine evacuation, is administered vaginally.
- Misoprostol (an analogue of PGE_1), has been used for induction and augmentation, and for management of the third stage of labour (Adair et al, 1998; Hofmeyr et al, 1998; Amant, 1999; Lumbiganon et al, 1999; Ngai et al, 2000). It is also used for the termination of pregnancy (Orioli & Castilla, 2000). However, neither oral nor intravaginal misoprostol is currently licensed for use in obstetrics and uncertainty persists regarding optimum dose, route of administration and safety (Hofmeyr et al, 2000; Hofmeyr & Gulmezoglu, 2000).

Prostaglandins, like oxytocin, increase uterine contractions. They also facilitate oxytocin in the induction of labour, thereby reducing the amount of oxytocin required (Darroca et al, 1996). There would seem to be no advantage gained by using repeated applications of prostagandins for induction of labour (Nuutila & Kajanoja, 1996; Rix et al, 1996). A large randomized study (n = 5041) by Hannah et al (1996) found that the use of vaginal prostaglandin E2 gel was not associated with an increased rate of Caesarean section. Overall, the literature offers no consensus on the influence of prostaglandins on the rates of: failed induction; Caesarean section; instrumental deliveries (Dawood, 1995).

How the body handles prostaglandins

Vaginal or cervical administration of prostaglandin pessaries or gels reduces but does not abolish systemic absorption and side effects.

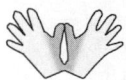 **Practice Points**

- These routes of administration permit ambulation during labour, which encourages efficient uterine activity (Mahmood et al, 1995).
- Upjohn (1995) suggests that following vaginal administration the woman should remain lying down for 30 minutes to improve absorption.
- Prostaglandin pessaries, unlike tablets, can be removed if problems occur.

Dinoprostone acts within about ten minutes of vaginal insertion. The rate of absorption through the walls of the vagina differs between tablets and gels, with gels being absorbed more rapidly than tablets. In one small study, fewer insertions of prostaglandins were needed for gels than pessaries (Dharmasena et al, 1995).

Intracervical administration is more likely to be effective than intravaginal administration if the cervix is unfavourable, with a Bishop score of less than three (Dawood, 1995; Darroca et al, 1996). Intracervical dinoprostone gel must be inserted carefully, because insertion into the extra-amniotic space may cause uterine hyperstimulation (Upjohn, 1990b).

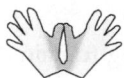 **Practice Points**

- The doses of the various dinoprostone preparations are related to the site of administration. For example, if vaginal gel is given by the intracervical route this could result in dangerous overdose (Reynolds et al, 1996).
- Different formulations also have different storage requirements and different bioavailabilities [glossary]. Tablets and gels are not bioequivalent.

Normally, prostaglandins are inactivated at their site of action (Graves, 1996). If they enter the circulation, which usually only occurs with synthetic prostaglandins, they are cleared by the lungs, liver and kidneys.

Misoprostol may be administered orally. Peak plasma concentration is seen within an hour, but onset of peak uterine activity occurs five to seven hours later (Ngai et al, 2000). When administered as prophylaxis in the third stage, some authors consider this too slow to prevent early blood loss (Amant et al, 1999), but others disagree (El-Refaey et al, 2000).

Actions and side effects of prostaglandins

Prostaglandins act on a number of distinct prostaglandin receptors. They affect many systems and cause a variety of side effects:

- smooth muscle contraction – gut, uterus, blood vessels, bronchioles;
- vasodilation and hypotension;
- pyrexia;
- inflammation;
- sensitization to pain;
- diuresis + loss of electrolytes;
- central nervous system effects (tremor is a rare side effect);

- release of pituitary hormones, renin and adrenal steroids;
- inhibition of autonomic nervous system responses;
- increase in intraocular pressure.

Problems are most likely to occur when high doses are used, as in the control of post-partum haemorrhage or evacuation of the uterus, rather than in induction of labour. See 'Implications for Practice'.

Smooth muscle contraction

Intensified uterine contractions

Uterine contractions may become abnormal and too intense, leading to pain, fetal compromise or rupture of the uterus or cervix, with or without previous Caesarean section; these problems are intensified if misoprostol is substituted for dinoprostone (Hofmeyr et al, 2000). In one study (n = 118) the incidence of Apgar score <9 at one minute, but not at five minutes, was increased by the use of intracervical prostaglandins (Darroca et al, 1996). The fetal problems are similar to those produced by oxytocin: heart beat coupling; hypertonus and tetany. Uterine hyperstimulation occurred in 3 per cent of women following insertion of vaginal prostaglandins (Blair et al, 1998) and in 8 to 10 per cent of women following intracervical prostaglandins. Uterine rupture, typically through the lower posterior wall, may occur at any stage of gestation. To prevent this, salbutamol may be administered should uterine hyperstimulation occur (Dawood, 1995). Particular care is required if oxytocin and prostaglandins are administered sequentially.

Case Reports

The Report on Confidential Enquiries into Maternal Deaths in the UK (DoH, 1996) cites cases where substandard care led to fatalities. These cases illustrate the danger of uterine rupture following the administration of prostaglandins:

1. Labour was induced by prostaglandins at 42 weeks in a woman aged over 35, who had had four previous deliveries. After delivery, the woman died of post-partum haemorrhage, due to rupture of the uterus. (p. 41)

2. A grand multiparous woman was booked into a GP maternity unit. Post-term, labour was induced with prostaglandin pessaries. Following vaginal delivery, the woman became unable to breathe and collapsed. A rupture of the lower uterine segment was found at autopsy. (p. 84)

Use of prostaglandins in grand multiparous women is hazardous because the uterus is already weakened by previous deliveries, and more likely to rupture. In addition the administration of prostaglandins is unduly hazardous if there are no facilities on site to manage emergencies such as rupture of the uterus.

Misoprostol, administered vaginally, has been associated with uterine ruptue in women with no previous Caesarean sections (Hofmeyr & Gulmezoglu, 2000).

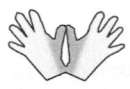 **Practice Points**

- Uterine contractility and fetal heart rate should be monitored continuously initially then regularly. Women should be informed that this will be necessary.
- The woman should not be left alone for at least 20–30 minutes after vaginal administration (Chamberlain & Zander, 1999).

Increased contractility of the gastro-intestinal tract

This causes diarrhoea, vomiting, bile reflux, abdominal cramps, hiccups, or a choking sensation. These problems are less likely with vaginal administration than with other routes (Mahmood et al, 1995). The incidence of vomiting following insertion of intracervical prostaglandins was reported as up to 5 per cent in large trials (Dawood, 1995) compared to 0.2 per cent with intravaginal dinoprostone (Reynolds et al, 1996). When prostaglandins are used as abortifacents, the incidence of emesis (60 per cent) and diarrhoea (20 per cent) is very high, and anti-emetic and anti-diarrhoeal agents are often needed and may be prescribed prophylactically (Olsen & D'Oria, 1992; Malseed et al, 1995). Such problems currently preclude the use of prostaglandins for the routine prophylactic management of the third stage of labour (Gulmezoglu, 2000).

Constriction of the bronchioles

This may induce wheezing, cough and asthma; women with asthma are particularly sensitive to $PGF_{2\alpha}$ (similar to carboprost (Hemabate®)) (Campbell & Halushka, 1996).

Vasoconstriction

Vasoconstriction caused by $PGF_{2\alpha}$ and 15 methyl $PGF_{2\alpha}$ (carboprost) may result in hypertension up to two hours after injection. Hypertension is more likely in pre-eclamptic/eclamptic patients. Occasionally, $PGF_{2\alpha}$, may cause an increase in pulmonary artery pressure, which alters the perfusion of the lungs, resulting in pulmonary oedema, dyspnoea, reduced partial pressure of oxygen and increased partial pressure of carbon dioxide [glossary] (Hayashi, 1990). Coronary artery spasm, associated with myocardial infarction (Gulmezoglu, 2000) and a fatal myocardial infarction in a high risk woman have been reported (Reynolds et al, 1996).

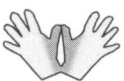 **Practice Point**

Women receiving carboprost should be monitored for hypoxia, using a pulse oximeter, and administered oxygen if necessary. Problems are more likely if there is pre-existing heart or lung disease (Upjohn, 1990a).

Vasodilation

In contrast, PGE_2 (dinoprostone) causes vasodilation, which usually occurs within 30 minutes of administration (Dawood, 1995). The consequences of vasodilation are:

- sweating, flushing and dizziness;
- cranial vasodilation causing headache;
- a reduction in blood pressure, resulting in increased heart rate and contractility which may induce cardiac dysrhythmias (Reynolds et al, 1996);
- cases of cardiovascular collapse are on record (Upjohn, 1990a).

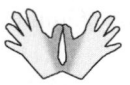 **Practice Point**

Women receiving prostaglandins should have regular blood pressure monitoring.

Pyrexia

Prostaglandins normally act on the hypothalamus to induce fever during infection. Pyrexia appears within minutes or hours after prostaglandin administration and may be accompanied by shivering, chills and leucocytosis [glossary]. Distressing shivering in 42 per cent of women (n = 200) detracts from the use of oral misoprostol for prophylaxis (Amant et al, 1999). A pyrexia of more than 1°C occurred in over 12 per cent of patients receiving intramuscular carboprost (Malseed et al, 1995) and in 34 per cent of women receiving oral misoprostol for prevention of postpartum haemorrhage (Amant et al, 1999). These effects are usually transient, and disappear within several hours of the last administration (Upjohn, 1990a).

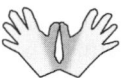 **Practice Points**

- Following administration of oral misoprostol for prophylactic management of the third stage, some women shiver for 20–30 minutes, during which time they are unable to hold or feed their babies (El-Refaey et al, 2000).
- This pyrexia should not be mistaken for a sign of infection. However, it is important not to overlook the possibility of infection.

The inflammatory response and pain

Prostaglandins are part of the normal response to tissue damage, producing pain and inflammation and therefore may cause pain and redness at the injection or administration site. Vaginal administration is associated with localized pain and irritation. Local infection may follow intra or extra-amniotic administration (Reynolds et al, 1996), and vaginal application may introduce ascending infection if membranes are ruptured (Tan & Hannah, 2000). Backache is reported as a side effect of prostaglandins. This increase in pain from uterine contractions would appear to be related to the dose of dinoprostone (Tan & Tay, 1999).

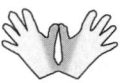 **Practice Point**

Pelvic inflammatory disease, particularly endometriosis, may be worsened by prostaglandin administration.

Central nervous system

Tremor or seizures may be due to pyrexia or direct stimulant effects of prostaglandins on the central nervous system.

Loss of fluids and electrolytes

This occurs due to impairment of renal tubular reabsorption. It may cause cramps and contribute to hypotension.

Raised intraocular pressure

Prostaglandins may cause eye pain or even precipitate acute glaucoma.

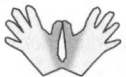 **Practice Point**

Prostaglandins should be used cautiously, if at all, in women with a history (or strong family history) of glaucoma (BNF, 2000).

Contra-indications and cautions

Prostaglandin induction is contra-indicated in the presence of ruptured membranes (Alberta Medical Association, 1993; BNF, 2000). Prostaglandins are used cautiously, if at all, in any of the following conditions likely to impede vaginal delivery or predispose to uterine rupture:

- previous uterine scar – a vertical scar is a contra-indication;
- major cephalo-pelvic disproportion;
- placenta praevia;
- malpresentation – particularly transverse lie;
- grand multiparity (4+);
- multiple pregnancy;
- history of difficult or traumatic delivery or hypertonic uterine contractions;
- polyhydramnios or oligohydramnios.

If the fetus is already compromised, prostaglandin administration is likely to worsen this. Many existing maternal diseases will be acutely exacerbated by the administration of prostaglandins. These include cardiac disease, pulmonary disorders, asthma, hypo- or hypertension, epilepsy, glaucoma or raised intraocular pressure, acute pelvic inflammatory disease, active genital herpes. In addition, women with liver or kidney insufficiency will be unable to eliminate prostaglandins as rapidly as normal.

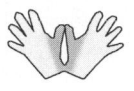 **Practice Point**

Health care professionals should avoid skin contact or inhalation of prostaglandins to avoid possible hypersensitivity responses (Reynolds et al, 1996).

The administration of prostaglandins is covered by some restrictions: for example the manufacturers advise the administration of only two doses (2 × 3 mg) of dinoprostone as Prostin E2 ® vaginal tablets (Upjohn, 1995).

Storage

Parenteral prostaglandin preparations should always be kept in a refrigerator. Many of these products have a short shelf life. The exact requirements differ for the various preparations and midwives should consult the manufacturer's data sheet for each preparation. Misoprostol tablets can be stored without a refrigerator, and have a long shelf life.

Interactions

Oxytocin: if two uterine stimulants are administered concurrently, hyper-stimulation may occur. Therefore, oxytocin is usually not given until 6–12 hours after the last dose of prostaglandin (Kelsey & Prevost, 1994).

Case Report

A woman had labour induced with prostaglandins because of post-maturity. This was later augmented with oxytocin. Fetal distress developed, and delivery was by forceps. The patient collapsed quickly due to haemorrhage from a tear in the lower uterine segment (DoH, 1966: 63).

The combination of prostaglandins plus oxytocin may over-stimulate the uterus which may lead to rupture. Therefore this drug combination requires careful surveillance.

Aspirin and other non-steroidal anti-inflammatory drugs antagonize the production of prostaglandins, thus dealying or prolonging labour. Paracetamol does not interact. **Alcohol** antagonizes the action of dinoprostone.

Implications for Practice: prostaglandins

In the event of emergencies, appropriate 'rescue therapies' and staff must be available.

Potential Problem	Management
Dysfunctional uterine contractility	Before administration, check for disproportion and fetal distress.
	Avoid prostaglandin induction if the uterus is likely to rupture when tone is increased or if the fetus is already stressed.
	Monitor uterine contractions and fetal heart, particularly for the first hour after insertion. Do not leave unattended.
	Limit administration, *both dose and duration*, as advised by manufacturers for different preparations.
	Ensure tocolytic therapy is available (Chapter 7).
	Ensure facilities are available for prompt delivery, in the event of uterine hypertonus.
	Allow six hours between dinoprostone insertion and planned induction.
Respiratory distress, asthma	Monitor breathing patterns, shortness of breath or chest tightness. Avoid in women with asthma, if possible.
Fever	Monitor temperature, assess whether infection present. Sponge to prevent hyperthermia, if necessary.
Shivering	Offer blankets. Be prepared to assist mother to hold and feed baby for up to 30 minutes, particularly after misoprostol administration.
Cardiovascular collapse	Monitor BP and HR. Hypotension is a danger with dinoprostone.
Worsening of pelvic inflammatory disease	Before administration, check for history of pelvic inflammatory disease.
Parenteral preparations are chemically unstable, and may become inactivated over time.	Check storage instructions, shelf life and temperature of the refrigerator used for storage on a regular basis.

Conclusion

When compared to oxytocin for induction of labour, dinoprostone intravaginal gel is equally effective and less likely to cause post-partum haemorrhage and neonatal jaundice. It is also less invasive, and therefore more popular with mothers (Reynolds et al, 1996). While prostaglandins administered topically are generally safe, it is important to remember that they are not without side effects and inherent dangers. Women should be informed of these. Prostaglandins speed up the induction of labour, and reduce the need for oxytocin administration. Their ability to influence the outcomes of labour remains a subject for further large scale investigation. Their role in managment of post-partum haemorrhage is likely to become increasingly important.

Oxytocin

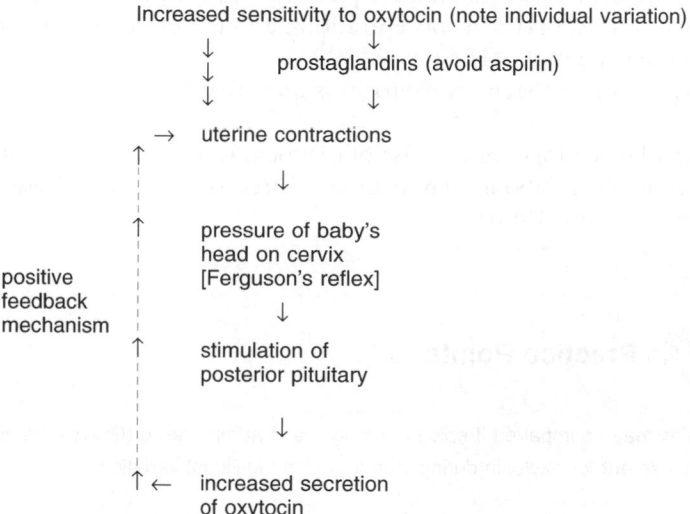

The onset of normal labour depends on a positive feedback mechanism, whereby an initial change is intensified until completion of the process. To summarize, the pressure of the baby's head on the cervix causes the release of oxytocin, which stimulates uterine contractions and further increases the pressure on the cervix, intensifying the release of oxytocin. This feedback loop repeats until the baby is delivered.

Figure 6.1   Diagram to indicate the role of oxytocin in normal labour
Source: adapted from Ganong, 1999.

Actions of oxytocin (see Figure 6.1)

Oxytocin, in association with other factors, plays a pivotal role in labour and milk ejection. Oxytocin acts on oxytocic receptors to cause:

- uterine contraction at term both by direct action on smooth muscle and by increased prostaglandin production;
- constriction of umbilical blood vessels;
- contraction of myoepithelial cells (milk ejection reflex).

Oxytocin acts on antidiuretic hormone (ADH) receptors* to cause:

- a sudden increase or decrease in blood pressure (particularly diastolic) due to vasodilation;
- water retention.

Note: Oxytocin and antidiuretic hormone have very similar structures which explains the overlap in functions.

Other actions of oxytocin include: uterine (Fallopian) tube contraction to assist sperm transport; luteolysis (involution of the corpus luteum); other neurotransmitter roles in the central nervous system. Oxytocin is synthesized in the hypothalamus, the gonads, the placenta and the uterus. From 32 weeks' gestation onwards, oxytocin concentrations, and therefore uterine activity, are higher during the night (Hirst et al, 1993).

The release of endogenous oxytocin is increased by:

- labour. (The endogenous release of oxytocin is pulsatile. The positive feedback controls of labour culminate in a surge of oxytocin release (see Fig. 6.1 and Guyton, 1996));

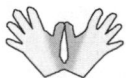 **Practice Points**

- This reflex may be impaired if epidural analgesia is administered (Graves, 1996).
- The requirement for oxytocin during labour shows individual variation.

- cervical, vaginal or breast stimulation;
- circulating oestrogens;
- increased plasma osmolality/concentration [glossary];
- low circulating fluid volume;
- Stress. Stress in labour can initiate precipitate labour, known as the 'fetal ejection reflex'. Stress caused by a baby crying will stimulate milk production.

The release of oxytocin is suppressed by:

- alcohol (This may impair the establishment of breastfeeding.);
- relaxin;

- decreased plasma osmolality (concentration);
- high circulating fluid volume (Graves, 1996).

Synthetic oxytocin

Oxytocin (Syntocinon®) is manufactured to reproduce the structure and actions of the natural hormone. The secretion of endogenous oxytocin is *not* suppressed by a negative feedback mechanism. This means that artificial syntocinon will not suppress the release of endogenous oxytocin.

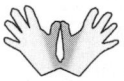 **Practice Point**

It follows that there is a danger that the combined actions of natural oxytocin and artificially administered oxytocin can easily lead to overstimulation of the uterus. In view of this, the midwife must be alert for the onset of active labour during oxytocin infusion, as the combined effects of two sources of oxytocin may lead to uterine hyperstimulation and a potentially dangerous situation (Shyken & Petrie, 1995) (see below: uterine rupture).

How the body handles synthetic oxytocin

Oxytocin may be administered intramuscularly, intravenously, sublingually or intranasally. Infusion pumps are recommended for intravenous infusions (Xenakis & Piper, 1997). Oxytocin acts within one minute of intravenous administration; increased uterine contractions begin almost immediately, stabilize within 15–60 minutes of commencing intravenous infusion and last for 20 minutes after discontinuation. Estimates of half-life range from 1–20 minutes, although more recent pharmacological data indicate a value of 15 minutes (Gonser, 1995). Oxytocin is eliminated 30–40 minutes after administration (Clayworth, 2000).

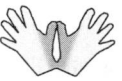 **Practice Points**

- Uterine action should be constantly monitored for at least the first hour of the intravenous infusion and following dosage adjustment. It is recommended that this is every 15 minutes during infusion and for 20 minutes after discontinuation.
- If dosages are adjusted too frequently, within less than 40–60 minutes, it will not be possible to assess the effect of the infusion, as fewer than three to five half-lives will have elapsed (Gonser, 1995; Shyken & Petrie, 1995; Clayworth, 2000) (see Chapter 1).

Pulsatile administration has been investigated, but the technology is not readily available (Shyken & Petrie, 1995). Although the extent to which oxytocin crosses the placenta is uncertain (Graves, 1996), oxytocin is rapidly eliminated by the liver, kidneys and placental enzymes. Sublingual oxytocin may help to establish and augment breastfeeding, but further studies are needed to clarify its clinical role (Renfrew et al, 2001). Absorption via the intranasal route may be erratic, and therefore these preparations are considered ineffective (Renfrew et al, 2000).

Side effects of oxytocin

When synthetic oxytocin is administered, its physiological actions may be intensified, leading to potentially dangerous side effects. (See Implications for Practice.) The side effects can be grouped:

- overstimulation of the uterus;
- contraction of umbilical blood vessels;
- anti-diuretic actions;
- actions on blood vessels (constriction and dilation);
- nausea;
- hypersensitivity responses.

Overstimulation of the uterus

During the last nine weeks of pregnancy, the responsivity of uterine muscle to oxytocin increases by a factor of eight (Graves, 1996). When oxytocin is administered, both the frequency and force of smooth muscle contractions are increased, intensifying the pain of labour (Olah & Gee, 1996). Women report that contractions induced by oxytocin are more painful than those of spontaneous labour (Bramadat, 1994; Fraser et al, 1998). Augmentation of labour with oxytocin carries an inherent risk of uterine hyperstimulation: since some individuals are hypersensitive to oxytocin, infusion always entails some danger of a tetanic or spasmodic uterine contraction, however low the dose (BNF, 2000).

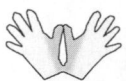 **Practice Points**

- Following induction or augmentation both uterine action and the fetal heart rate must be continuously monitored (Reynolds et al, 1996), with a midwife in constant attendance (Chamberlain & Zander, 1999). (See Gibb & Arulkumaran, 1997.)
- If signs of fetal distress or uterine hyperstimulation appear, the oxytocin infusion should be discontinued immediately (BNF, 2000) and oxygen and a tocolytic administered (Stock, 1992; Graves, 1996).
- In the US, magnesium sulphate is kept available during oxytocin administration to produce myometrial relaxation if needed (Stock, 1992).

Oxytocin administration impairs the application of the fetal head to the cervix (Allman et al, 1996). If the cervix has neither softened nor dilated, labour cannot progress and in these circumstances violent, prolonged and forceful uterine contractions may have serious consequences:

- **Trauma to neonate and mother** If the baby is forced through an incompletely dilated cervix, maternal soft tissues may be extensively lacerated.
- **Uterine rupture** Uterine rupture is less likely in nulliparous women, but has occurred (DoH, 1996). Oxytocin is contra-indicated in women with a high risk of uterine rupture, for example grand multiparae, multiple pregnancies, polyhydramnios or those with uterine scars (BNF, 2000).

Case Report

A grand multipara was managed by artificial rupture of membranes combined with low dose oxytocin at 37 weeks' gestation, resulting in a spontaneous vaginal delivery. Laparotomy was undertaken to ascertain the cause of persistent post-partum haemorrhage and longitudinal lateral rupture of the uterus was revealed. Despite resuscitative measures, the patient died (DoH, 1994).

This woman was clearly a 'high risk', due to her age and parity. Grand multiparity is listed as a contra-indication to oxytocin use (BNF, 2000).

- **Post-partum haemorrhage** This has occurred, but may have been attributable to obstetric complications or uterine rupture rather than uterine hyperstimulation (Reynolds et al, 1996).
- **Pelvic haematoma** This may arise from violent contractions. If this is extensive, clotting factors will be depleted, leading to **disseminated intravascular coagulopathy (DIC)**, coagulation failure and bleeding.
- **Placental abruption** Placental abruption has been attributed to violent uterine contractions and implicated in maternal death (DoH, 1991).

Case Report

This case illustrates the need to be alert to the possibility of placental abruption when oxytocin is administered.

In this case Syntocinon was infused for 21.5 hours before delivery. Towards the end of labour, clotting studies became abnormal. A blood loss of 300 ml was recorded at delivery. Twenty minutes after delivery, the patient collapsed with an unrecordable blood pressure. Death followed the next day, despite intensive treatment (DoH, 1991:37).

Clotting factors were consumed in the placental bed, leaving the woman unable to coagulate and vulnerable to bleeding. Prolonged infusion requies very careful monitoring due to the risks involved.

- **Amniotic fluid embolism** This may be precipitated by tumultuous labour, particularly if the amniotic fluid is stained with meconium or death *in utero* has occurred. In the *Report on Confidential Enquiries* (DOH, 1991) six out of nine deaths from amniotic fluid embolism were associated with either prostaglandin or oxytocin administration.
- **Fetal hypoxia** During uterine contraction, blood vessels are compressed, impairing the delivery of oxygen to the uterus, placenta and fetus. Normally, oxygenation is restored during relaxation, preventing the accumulation of lactic acid. However if the uterus is over-stimulated and relaxation too brief, fetal hypoxia and acidosis will follow (Kulb, 1990). Uterine tetany or spasm may reduce uterine blood flow to a point where the fetus is asphyxiated, with the possibility of intracranial haemorrhage or death. It is therefore important to continuously monitor the fetal heart rate to detect early signs of fetal distress. Higher doses of oxytocin have been associated with increased rates of assisted deliveries for fetal bradycardia and more neonates with APGAR scores below 7 (Shyken & Petrie, 1995). Studies in the developing world have highlighted the increased risk of fetal intracranial heamorrhage associated with oxytocin infusion where facilities for fetal and uterine monitoring are suboptimal (Ellis et al, 2000).

Constriction of umbilical blood vessels

If this physiologically protective mechanism is activated prematurely, the fetus will become starved of oxygen. Fetal hypoxia may lead to bradycardia, cardiac dysrhythmia and even death (Reynolds et al, 1996). Any pre-existing fetal distress is likely to be worsened by oxytocin infusion.

Anti-diuretic hormone actions and SIADH (syndrome inappropriate ADH)

The main action of anti-diuretic hormones is to conserve water by acting (mainly) on the collecting ducts of the renal tubules (via the V_2 receptors). Due to structural similarities, oxytocin also causes water retention, resulting in:

- reduced urine output;
- increased osmolality (and specific gravity) of urine;
- plasma dilution;
- hyponatraemia [glossary].

When synthetic oxytocin is administered, particularly in high doses, the actions of anti-diuretic hormone are mimicked. In the absence of careful monitoring, this may produce dangerous fluid retention (Reynolds et al, 1996). Any water retained passes, by osmosis, from plasma into tissue fluids, and thence into the cells of the body which swell. Water retention may increase the volume of tissue fluid. This in turn causes dependent oedema, raised jugular venous pressure and even pulmonary oedema which impairs breathing and oxygenation.

It is possible that water retention will lead to **water intoxication** (cells swelling); however, *not all cases of water intoxication are preceded by signs of fluid retention* (Reynolds et al, 1996). Water intoxication is more likely if hypotonic infusions, such as glucose (dextrose), are administered.

If water intoxication occurs, the cells of the cardiac conduction system may be disturbed, giving dangerous cardiac dysrhythmias, particularly premature beats, which the woman may experience as 'palpitations'. Cardiac dysrhythmias reduce cardiac output, thus jeopardising the blood supply to the placenta. Water intoxication also affects the cells of the brain. Initially, the woman becomes confused, drowsy, disorientated, uncoordinated and 'loses touch with reality'. Headache and vomiting may be the presenting features (Stock, 1992), but these problems may be attributed to other drugs administered or mistaken for pre-eclampsia.

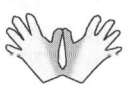 **Practice Point**

It is important that the midwife recognizes the early signs of water intoxication because cerebral dysfunction may progress to twitches, fits, and eventually brain damage and death (Fraser & Arieff, 1990).

Neonatal convulsions following maternal water retention have been reported (Kulb, 1990).

The danger is greatest with administration of prolonged high doses of oxytocin, accompanied by infusions of large volumes of electrolyte-free or hypotonic fluids such as 5 per cent glucose (BNF, 2000). In all the reported cases of water intoxication, more than 3.5 litres of fluid had been infused (Reynolds et al, 1996).

Case Report

Despite deteriorating pre-eclampsia, a planned emergency Caesarean section was cancelled because the fetus died in utero. Induction of labour lasted 26 hours and circulatory overload and death from adult respiratory distress syndrome followed (DoH, 1996).

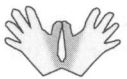 **Practice Points**

- Prolonged infusions should contain electrolytes (Kulb, 1990; Reynolds et al, 1996, BNF, 2000).
- Early recognition of water intoxication is important because no specific antidote exists.
- During oxytocin infusions it is important that:
  - accurate fluid balance records are kept;
  - urine output is monitored and specific gravity checked;
  - intake by mouth is restricted and monitored;
  - no more than three litres of fluid are administered (Reynolds et al, 1996);
  - lung bases are checked for pulmonary oedema (Stock, 1992);
  - furosemide (frusemide) should be available, as this may be required to induce a diuresis in an emergency (Stock, 1992).

Neonatal jaundice

Oxytocin crosses the placenta and has an anti-diuretic action in the fetus, leading to a dose dependent increase in red cell fragility, haemolysis and hyper-bilirubinaemia (n = 12 461; n = 90) (Friedman et al, 1978; Buchan, 1979). It is thought that glucose injection used to mix oxytocin may have aggravated this problem in the past (Reynolds et al, 1996).

Actions on blood vessels

Oxytocin may either raise or lower blood pressure, depending on the circumstances of infusion and individual responsiveness.

Vasoconstriction

Oxytocin acts on the antidiuretic hormone (V_{1A}) receptors in the blood vessels to produce vasoconstriction. This may lead to a sudden, severe rise in blood pressure, to above 200/120 mm Hg which could produce either a hypertensive crisis or a subarachnoid haemorrhage and maternal deaths have occurred (Reynolds et al, 1996).

Case Report

A multigravida was admitted with a blood pressure of 185/105 mm Hg, oedema, 3+ proteinuria, headache, epigastric tenderness, hyper-reflexia and vomiting. Over the telephone, the consultant advised induction. Within 2.5 hours, an eclamptic fit had occurred. Following an emergency Caesarean section, a second fit occurred and DIC developed. The patient remained in the labour ward, where she was over-transfused, and eventually died of ARDS (DoH, 1996:28).

The effects of oxytocin on fluid balance may be fatal, particularly if pre-eclampsia/eclampsia is present.

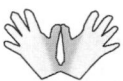 **Practice Points**

- The hazards of oxytocin administration are increased when a degree of vasoconstriction is already present, as in pre-eclampsia, renal impairment and heart failure.
- Close monitoring of blood pressure is essential. The midwife should be alert to such warning signs as severe headache, visual disturbances and epistaxis (Stock, 1992).
- If vasopressors (such as epinephrine/ adrenaline or ephedrine) have been administered with local or regional anaesthesia, the likelihood of a hypertensive crisis is increased (BNF, 2000).

Transient vasodilation

Oxytocin may lower, rather than raise blood pressure, with the potential for equally catastrophic results, including cardiac arrest (Shyken & Petrie, 1995). The administration of large amounts of oxytocin may produce a sudden but marked vasodilation, with a consequent fall in blood pressure, particularly the diastolic. Cardiac output may be reduced, provoking a reflex tachycardia.

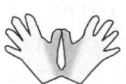 **Practice Points**

- The increased blood flow to the limbs may cause sweating, headache, dizziness or tinnitus. These effects are more pronounced if the woman is anaesthetized or hypovolaemic (Kulb, 1990; Graves, 1996). For these reasons the BNF (2000) advises against rapid intravenous injection.
- Particular care is needed if ten units of oxytocin are infused for the management of postpartum haemorrhage.

Nausea and vomiting

This may be due to either contraction of the smooth muscle of the gut or direct action on the chemoreceptor trigger zone and vomiting centre in the medulla.

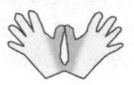 **Practice Point**

It is important not to dismiss the nausea caused by hypertension, water intoxication or other causes of raised intracranial pressure as a side effect of oxytocin.

Anaphylactoid reactions

Hypersensitivity responses, including anaphylaxis have been reported.

Cautions and contra-indications

- Oxytocin is contra-indicated if the uterus is already contracting vigorously, or if there is a mechanical obstruction to delivery such as placenta praevia or cephalopelvic disproportion. If the cervix is unfavourable, cervical ripening should be performed prior to the administration of oxytocin (Shyken & Petrie, 1995).
- Despite its commonplace use in a large number of obstetric centres, the potential disruption to fluid balance and blood pressure makes oxytocin unsuitable for women with pre-eclampsia, cardiovascular disease or those aged over 35 years.
- Oxytocin infusions are contra-indicated in women who are at risk from vaginal delivery, for example those with malpresentation or placental abruption or at high risk of uterine rupture. Persistence with oxytocin infusion in the face of uterine resistance and inertia is contra-indicated (BNF, 2000).
- Starved uterus. Muscle contraction requires both glucose and oxygen. If either of these are not supplied to the contacting muscle, due to starvation or inadequate blood supply, the response to oxytocin will be inadequate, and dose increments will be ineffective. This situation is most likely to arise in prolonged labour (Clayworth, 2000).

Storage should be away from light, between 4–22°C, for example, in a refrigerator (Sandoz, 1995).

Drug interactions – oxytocin

Vasopressors (sympathomimetics)

If oxytocin is administered with another vasoconstricting agent, there is a danger of a catastrophic rise in BP, leading to a cerebro-vascular accident. This may occur if **adrenaline** (epinephrine) is added to a local anaesthetic, for example with a caudal block, or if **ephedrine** is administered to correct hypotension induced by epidural anaesthesia. **Ergometrine** and oxytocin act synergistically and are often co-prescribed in the management of the third stage of labour. **Inhalational anaesthetics** may further lower blood pressure or induce cardiac dysrhythmias. **Prostaglandins, oestrogens:** if more than one agent promoting uterine contractility is administered, uterine overstimulation is more likely to occur.

Case Report

Labour was induced at 42 weeks with prostaglandin pessaries followed by an oxytocin infusion. The oxytocin constricted the umbilical arteries, causing fetal distress in the second stage, necessitating forceps delivery, and augmented uterine contractions to such an extent that the uterus ruptured, resulting in an amniotic fluid embolism. The woman collapsed after delivery and died 24 hours later (DoH, 1996).

In this case, the combination of oxytocin with prostaglandins induced vigorous contractions, leading to a uterine tear. The BNF (2000) cautions against the use of this drug combination.

Opioids and phenothiazines: water retention and hyponatraemia are potential problems with oxytocin, opioids and phenothiazines (for example prochlorperazine), increasing the hazards of co-administration (Reynolds et al, 1996). **Blood, plasma or metabisulphite** will inactivate oxytocin if infused in the same intravenous giving set (Sandoz, 1995).

Implications for Practice: oxytocin

- It is essential to gain informed consent from the woman and document the reasons for induction or augmentation of labour. Fetal maturity and presentation must be documented to avoid iatrogenic prematurity and malpresentations (Kulb, 1990).
- Because of the inherent dangers and the intensive monitoring required, it is important that anyone receiving an infusion of oxytocin is never left alone (Graves, 1996).
- Protocols should be in place to terminate the infusion if uterine hyperstimulation, precipitous labour, abnormal vaginal bleeding, water intoxication, alterations in BP or fetal asphyxia occur (Kulb, 1990).
- It is prudent to use Y-tubing for infusions, since the port not in use will afford intravenous access should any emergency arise.

Implications for Practice (*continued*)

Potential Problem	Management
BP ↑ or ↓	Monitor every 15 minutes. Administer slowly.
HR ↑	Monitor every 15 minutes.
Overstimulation of uterus	Monitor contractions every 15 minutes.
	Discontinue oxytocin if frequency > every two minutes and duration > one minute or >50 mm Hg.
	Uterine resting tone should be below 20 mm Hg.
	Oxygen and a tocolytic should be available.
	Avoid if there is a risk of uterine rupture.
	Avoid concurrent use of prostaglandins.
	Be prepared to decrease or discontinue oxytocin infusion when the active phase of labour begins.
Fetal asphyxia	Monitor fetal heart rate.
	Avoid maternal supine position.
Water retention	Fluid balance, restrict fluid intake (maximum three litres in 24 hours).
	Check lung bases, respiration rate and oedema of dependent parts.
	Check jugular venous pressure and distension.
	Avoid in women with pre-eclampsia.
	Administer in electrolytes, such as 0.9% sodium chloride (Reynolds et al, 1996).
Water intoxication	Check level of consciousness and/or confusion.
	Monitor for cardiac dysrhythmia, ECG if necessary.
Unresponsive uterus	Avoid prolonged labour with inadequate oxygenation and energy supply.

Conclusions: the induction/augmentation of labour

Although prolonged labour is commonly assumed to be deleterious (Nkata, 1996), the outcome may not be improved by the use of oxytocics. In many nulliparous women, the reasons underlying delay in progress in labour are unclear, and may be due to causes other than failure of the myometrium to contract (Olah & Gee, 1996). The available randomized clinical trials show that oxytocin augmentation does not improve Caesarean section rates, operative vaginal delivery rates or neonatal outcomes: rather, it increases pain, hyperstimulation and fetal heart rate declerations with all the attendant dangers (Bramadat, 1994; Spencer, 1995; Olah & Gee, 1996; Fraser et al, 1998).

In a randomized trial (n = 405), high dose oxytocin reduced duration of labour by an average of 1.7 hours (Rogers et al, 1997), and oxytocin can shorten prolonged labours (Blanch et al, 1998; Sadler et al, 2000). However early use of oxytocin and 'active management' of labour in nulliparae were found to confer no advantage in larger randomized controlled trials (n = 2000, n = 306) (Frigoletto et al, 1995; Cammu & Eeckhout, 1996). The non-selective use of amniotomy and oxytocin have been shown to offer no benefits over conservative regimens (Thornton, 1996). In a prospective randomized trial (n = 196), the durations of the first and second stages of labour were similar when amniotomy alone was performed compared with amniotomy plus oxytocin infusion (Moldin & Sundell, 1996).

To many women and health care professionals induction and augmentation of labour epitomize the use of technology in childbirth. Their use is associated with reduced satisfaction with childbirth when compared to sponateous delivery (Bramadat 1994). In the UK, the use of oxytocin for low risk primiparous women is around 38 per cent and shows wide variation between centres (Willaims et al, 1998). Concerns over the use and management of induction of labour were a prominent feature of the first *Confidential Enquiry into Stillbirths and Deaths in Infancy* (Neale, 1996) which are echoed in subsequent editions (for example MCHRC, 1997). Further research is needed to clarify the optimum strategy for induction of labour and indications for the use of oxytocin infusions (Busowski & Parsons, 1995; O'Connor 1995), as well as protocols for administration and monitoring.

Ergometrine

Ergot is a fungus which grows on rye, wheat and other grasses. Since mediaeval times, ergot poisoning, from eating infected rye bread, has been associated with abortion, mental disturbances and gangrene. Several pharmacologically active substances are derived from ergot; these are known as the ergot alkaloids and include ergometrine (ergonovine in the USA), ergotamine, lysergic acid, methylsergide and bromocriptine (Rang et al, 1999). Historically, ergometrine has played an important role in reducing maternal mortality from post-partum haemorrhage. However the use of ergot alkaloids for induction and augmentation of labour was found to be extremely hazardous in the last century (van Dongen & de Groot, 1995). In view of this, use prior to delivery is now firmly contra-indicated (Kulb, 1990; BNF, 2000).

Ergometrine, used alone, is important in the management of acute post-partum or post-abortion haemorrhage. As one of the constituents of Syntometrine®, it is widely used prophylactically for the active management of the third stage of labour. Ergometrine may be administered intravenously, intramuscularly or orally (BNF, 2000). Oral preparations are unreliable due to difficulties with storage and bioavailability [glossary] (de Groot et al, 1998). Onset of action is within one minute of intravenous administration, three to seven minutes with intramuscular administration and up to ten minutes if given orally. If intramuscular injections are placed in the subcutaneous fat, they will not be absorbed adequately. Half-life is three hours and duration of action is three to eight hours (Malseed et al, 1995). Excretion is via the kidneys.

Actions and side effects of ergometrine

Like other ergot alkaloids, ergometrine interacts with serotoninergic, noradrenergic (alpha$_1$) and dopaminergic receptors in a complex manner. Actions on alpha$_1$ and serotonin receptors are thought to underlie the uterine and gut contractility brought about by ergometrine.

Contraction of the uterus

Ergometrine has a rapid stimulant effect on the uterus, particularly at term. The resultant contractions are unco-ordinated and in rapid succession (de Groot et al, 1998).

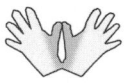 **Practice Point**

There is a danger that the uterus will fail to relax between contractions (Malseed et al, 1995). Therefore ergometrine is **never** administered before the delivery of **all** fetuses (Kulb, 1990; Soriano et al, 1996).

The contractions may be so painful or cramping that women will require analgesia post-partum, and so powerful that the risk of retained placenta is increased. This may be caused by excessive contraction of the lower segment of the uterus hindering placental separation (Yuen et al, 1995).

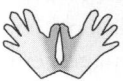 **Practice Point**

Administration prior to delivery of the placenta may result in entrapment, unless the placenta is removed by controlled cord traction as soon as it is perceived to have separated from the uterine wall (Steer & Flint, 1999a).

Retention of placental fragments may account for the reported association with increased problems with bleeding in the first six weeks post-partum (Begley, 1990a).

Diarrhoea and vomiting

Ergometrine mimics the actions of dopamine, frequently causing nausea and vomiting in 20–32 per cent of parturients, depending on dose administered (Begley, 1990a). Mild or moderate diarrhoea may result from increased contractility of the GI tract.

Vasoconstriction

Ergometrine acts on alpha$_1$ (noradrenergic) receptors in arterioles and veins to bring about vasoconstriction and venoconstriction. This raises total peripheral resistance, causing hypertension (daistolic >95 mmHg) in 5 per cent of parturients with intravenous administration (Begley, 1990a). This may lead to:

- reflex bradycardia and reduced cardiac output;
- a hypertensive crisis and cerebral haemorrhage;
- post-partum eclamptic fits;
- raised central venous pressure;
- coronary artery spasm.

Cerebral vasoconstriction may cause sudden severe headache, tinnitus, dizziness, sweating, confusion, retinal detachment, cerebrovascular acident or seizures.

Case Report

Two women given 500 micrograms ergometrine iv for active management of the third stage of labour suffered eclamptic seizures within four hours of delivery, despite no previous history or record of high blood pressure in pregnancy or labour.

This was attributed to ergometrine (Begley, 1990a).

Vasoconstriction may also affect the peripheral circulation, making the hands and feet cold; occasionally the woman may experience numbness, paraesthe sae, pain, weakness or even gangrene.

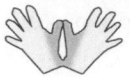 **Practice Points**

- To minimize the risks, the midwife should:
  - check the temperature and circulation of hands and feet;
  - monitor blood pressure during and after the third stage of labour;
  - be alert for symptoms of chest pain or palpitations.

Vasospasm of coronary arteries may cause chest pain, cardiac dysrhythmias and even cardiac arrest.

A thorough assessment of cardiovascular risks is essential before administration of ergometrine for prophylactic management of the third stage of labour.

Case Reports

A 27-year-old woman was known to have familial hypercholesterolaemia. She smoked 20 cigarettes per day. After an uncomplicated pregnancy, at 41 weeks she had an unplanned vaginal delivery at home. After delivery, the midwife administered an intramuscular injection of oxytocin (5 units) and ergometrine (500 micrograms). Five minutes later, the woman complained of acute chest pain. She was then rushed into hospital, where an acute myocardial infarction was diagnosed and treated (Mousa et al, 2000).

A 20-year-old woman sustained a permanent hemiparesis following a heart attack related to post-partum administration of 200 micrograms of ergometrine, intramuscularly. The only risk factor was a history of migraine. This catastrophic outcome was related to the failure of staff to recognize and treat the signs and symptoms of coronary artery spasm (Taylor & Cohen, 1985).

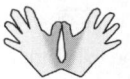 **Practice Points**

- Because of the dangers of cerebrovascular or cardiovascalar accidents and cardiac dysrhythmias ergometrine is:
  - only given intravenously in emergencies (Malseed et al, 1995);
  - not used if the woman has pulmonary, hypertensive or cardiovascular disorders (including pre-eclampsia and anaemia);
  - only administered in emergencies to women with a sensitivity to coronary artery spasm such as migraine and Raynaud's phenomenon.

Inhibition of prolactin production

Ergot alkaloids act on dopamine receptors to suppress prolactin production and lactation. One drug in this group, bromocriptine, is prescribed to manage galactorrhoea and, occasionally, to suppress lactation post-partum. Intramuscular methylergonovine, 200 micrograms after delivery of the placenta, inhibits the normal post-partum rise in serum prolactin (Weiss et al, 1975). Oral ergometrine, 600 micrograms daily for seven days, reduces serum prolactin and progressively inhibits lactation with some individual variation (Canales et al, 1976). Intravenous ergotamine, 500 micrograms,* was associated with a statistically non-significant reduction in serum prolactin concentration 48–72 hours post partum, after suckling (n = 132) (Begley, 1990b). In this study, use of intravenous ergometrine for active management of the third stage of labour gave a statistically significant increase in the number of women supplementing and ceasing breastfeeding by one and four weeks post-partum, mainly because lactation was inadequate for the infants' needs (Begley, 1990b; 1990c). Midwives need to consider that ergometrine, particularly repeated doses, may adversely impact on breastfeeding.

* *Note: This dose is twice that recommended for intravenous administration. Current recommendation is 500 micrograms with 5 units of oxytocin (Syntometrine®) to be given intramuscularly with or after the delivery of the shoulders (BNF, 2000:363).*

Effects on the neonate

Ergometrine is linked to hyperthermia, increased muscle tension, respiratory problems and convulsions in neonates (de Groot et al, 1998). Cases (n = 7) are reported where ergometrine or syntometrine have been mistaken for intramuscular injections of vitamin K and accidentally administered to neonates. All infants convulsed, and most required cardiorespiratory support in special care units. Feeding was initially problematic. However most infants recovered within four days and no long term sequelae were reported (Dargaville & Campbell, 1998).

Hypersensitivity

A range of hypersensitivity responses have been reported, including anaphylactic shock, weak and rapid pulse, pulmonary oedema and dyspnoea (McKenry & Salerno, 1998). Ergometrine can induce bronchospasm in asthmatic women and should be avoided outside emergency situations (Campbell & Lees, 2000). Puerperal psychosis may be linked to ergometrine administration (de Groot et al, 1998).

Cautions and contra-indications

The vasoconstrictor properties of ergometrine make it unsuitable for women with pre-existing pulmonary, cardiac or vascular disorders including pre-eclampsia, eclampsia, migraine, Raynaud's phenomenon. If sepsis, renal or hepatic failure are present, sensitivity to ergometrine is increased (McKenry & Salerno, 1995). Repeated use of ergometrine is rarely justified due to the increased risk of side effects.

Case Report

Use of ergometrine is extremely hazardous in pre-eclampsia or eclampsia.

Administration of syntometrine following delivery precipitated eclampsia in one woman, who eventually died (DoH, 1996:29).

Ergometrine raises BP and contracts circulating volume, exacerbating the effects of pre-eclampsia. Ergometrine must be avoided in *all* cases of pre-eclampsia unless there is severe haemorrhage (DoH, 1996).

Storage: ergometrine must be stored in a cool, dark place, prefereably in a refrigerator, and expiry dates checked regularly. Loss of potency after one year of storage may be 90 per cent (El-Refaey et al, 2000). The tablets are unstable in all conditions, particularly high humidity, and therefore not recommended (de Groot et al, 1998),

Interactions with Ergometrine

The effectiveness of ergotmetrine may be compromised if the woman is hypocalcaemic; this can be rectified by the intravenous administration of calcium salts (McKenry & Salerno, 1998). Nicotine, other oxytocics, general anaesthetics, beta blockers, summatriptan and erythromycin intensify the actions of ergometrine. Women should be advised to refrain from using tobacco for three hours following administration.

Implications for Practice: ergometrine

Problem	Management
Abdominal cramps	Assess, discontinue if excessive.
Vomiting and diarrhoea	Warn, prior to administration.

Implications for Practice (*continued*)

Problem	Management
Hypertension	Monitor BP and HR, take a careful history to exclude cardiovascular disease and pre-eclampsia. Be alert for warning signs, such as headache or emesis.
Lack of effect	Ensure bladder is empty. Monitor vaginal blood loss, uterine tone. Blood test for calcium levels.
Chest pain	Take a careful history to exclude pre-existing cardiovascular risk factors. Recognize association with myocardial infarction. Arrange ECG. Withhold further doses.
Signs of peripheral vasoconstriction	Monitor temperature of hands and feet regularly. Withhold further doses.
Hypersensitivity	Monitor breathing patterns, BP. Ensure protocol for anaphylaxis is in place.
Difficulties with breastfeeding	Support and reassurance that this will be easier when the effects of ergometrine have worn off.

Conclusions: the third stage of labour and post-partum haemorrhage

The risk of post-partum haemorrhage, including severe events, is reduced (by about 40 per cent or a relative risk of 2.42) by active management of the third stage of labour, including the administration of oxytocics. The incidence of anaemia (Hb < 10 g/dL) post-partum is also reduced (Nordstrom et al, 1997; Rogers et al, 1998). In low risk women, blood loss associated with 'physiological management' of the third stage may depend on the technique employed by the midwife (Begley, 1990a). Although active management shortens the third stage of labour, it is associated with an increase in vomiting and hypertension (Prendiville et al, 2000).

Randomized controlled trials (n = 3497, 2189) of oxytocin alone (intramuscular or intravenous) *versus* oxytocin plus ergometrine indicate that oxytocin (5 or 10 units) used alone causes significantly less nausea, vomiting, headache, sweating, shortness of breath, chest pain, blood pressure elevation and bradycardia, and is equally effective in preventing blood loss greater than one litre (McDonald et al, 1993; Khan et al, 1995; Soriano et al, 1996; McDonald et al, 2000). However, the optimum dose of oxytocin requires further study (de Groot et al, 1998).

Due to the differences in the side effect profiles of the drugs, several authors (Kelsey & Prevost, 1994; Rogers et al, 1998; de Groot et al, 1998; Steer &

Flint, 1999a) assert that oxytocin is the prophylactic drug of choice for the prevention of post-partum haemorrhage, and ergometrine should be used only if this is found to be ineffective, or in high risk cases. However, oxytocin is not currently licensed for intramuscular administration (BNF, 2000), and many women do not have intravenous access established. Therefore, the BNF (2000) recommends ergometrine 500 micrograms plus 5 units oxytocin by intramuscular injection for the routine management of the third stage. Use of this regimen necessitates the careful exclusion of women who should not receive ergometrine, for example those with pre-eclampsia. In contrast, 5 units of oxytocin can be administered following most normal labours (Nordstrom et al, 1997).

If refrigeration is not readily available, misoprostol tablets may be an acceptable and effective alternative to traditional oxytocics for the management of the third stage of labour (El-Refaey et al, 2000; Walley et al, 2000). However using a lower dose of misoprostol than other investigators (400, rather than 600 or 500 micrograms), Cook et al (1999) found that misoprostol was less effective than the traditional oxytocic agents in reducing blood loss after delivery.

The author suggests that the management of the third stage of labour is discussed with clients as part of the birth plan. The pharmacological options and the associated side effect profiles should be discussed with all women so that informed choices can be made. Women receiving ergometrine may require extra help, understanding and support to establish and continue breastfeeding, particularly if sedating analgeics and anti-emetics have been co-administered.

Severe postpartum haemorrhage is a life-threatening emergency for which all units have established protocols. In the event of post-partum haemorrhage, the BNF (2000:365) recommends oxytocin (5 units) by slow intravenous injection, followed, if necessary, by intravenous infusion of 5–20 units in 500 ml of 5 per cent glucose solution. Ergometrine, either alone or combined with oxytocin, is an alternative, providing pre-eclampsia/hypertension can be excluded. Carboprost is generally reserved for severe haemorrhage.

Further Reading

Begley, C. (1990a) A comparison of 'active' and 'physiolgocial' management of the third stage of labour. *Midwifery*:6:3–17.

Begley, C. (1990b) The effect of Ergometrine on breast feeding. *Midwifery*:6:60–72.

Gibb, D. & Arulkumaran, S. (1997) *Foetal Monitoring in Practice*, 2nd edition. Oxford, Butterworth-Heinemann.

Graves, C. (1996) Agents that cause contraction or relaxation of the uterus. In: Hardman, J., Limbard, L., Molinoff, P., Ruddon, R. & Goodman Gilman, A. (eds) *Goodman & Gilman's: The Pharmacological Basis of Therapeutics*, 9th edition. New York, McGraw-Hill.

CHAPTER 7

Drugs Decreasing Uterine Contractility/Tocolytics

SUE JORDAN

This chapter considers the tocolytic agents most widely used. The newest agent, atosiban, is mentioned briefly. Nifedipine is included in this chapter, as it is now more widely used as a tocolytic than as an anti-hypertensive.

Chapter Contents

- Beta$_2$ adrenoreceptor agonists (ritodrine)
- Calcium channel blockers (mainly nifedipine)
- Atosiban
- Conclusions: tocolytics
- Corticosteroids and tocolysis

Several classes of drugs have tocolytic properties, including, beta$_2$ adrenoreceptor agonists (such as ritodrine), magnesium sulphate, calcium channel blockers (such as nifedipine), prostaglandin synthetase inhibitors (such as indomethicin, sulindac), oxytocin antagonists (for example atosiban), alcohol; glycerol trinitrate (Graves, 1996). Some of these are under investigation for use in premature/preterm labour. Current UK practice favours the beta$_2$ adrenoreceptor agonists (BNF, 2000; Steer & Flint, 1999) or calcium antagonists (for example nifedipine), with indomethicin reserved as second line treatment due to fetal toxicity (Reynolds et al, 1996). Larger studies are needed to address the issues of fetal outcomes (Steer, 1999) (see Chapter 9 for magnesium).

Bed rest and hydration are traditionally the first line of management for premature labour, but tocolytics have a limited role in prevention of premature labour in women of 24–33 weeks' gestation (BNF, 2000). Earlier premature labour is likely to be due to fetal malformation and therefore medical intervention is considered inappropriate (Graves, 1996). Administration of tocolytics is seen as useful in postponing labour long enough to allow:

- transfer to specialist centres for operative delivery if emergencies arise such as cord prolapse, breech presentation or partial premature detachment of the placenta (Graves, 1996);
- time (at least 48 hours) for the administration of corticosteroids to hasten fetal lung maturation (BNF, 2000; Reynolds et al, 1996).

Beta$_2$ adrenoreceptor agonists

This group of sympathomimetics includes ritodrine, terbutaline, salbutamol and adrenaline.

How the body handles beta$_2$ adrenoreceptor agonists

These drugs may be administered by the intravenous, intramuscular, subcutaneous or oral routes. Intravenous administration of ritodrine is effective within five minutes, with peak concentration and side effects occurring after 50 minutes (Olsen & D'Oria, 1992). Because of the danger of pulmonary oedema, intravenous administration in minimum volumes of 5 per cent w/v dextrose is recommended (BNF, 2000; DoH, 1996), and saline is avoided (Lamont, 2000). It is important that these guidelines are observed because dextrose (unlike saline) is distributed into all the body's fluid compartments rather than being confined to the extracellular compartments where a build-up may cause oedema (Chapter 2). Intravenous ritodrine should be administered via a controlled infusion device, preferably a syringe pump (DoH, 1996).

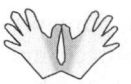 **Practice Point**

A large vein should be used for cannulation to reduce the risk of drug extravasation. Should this emergency arise, 10–15 ml of normal saline containing phentolamine may be administered (Olsen & D'Oria, 1992).

The conventional dosage regimen involves incremental dose adjustments, according to uterine activity and side effects; however a loading dose was associated with fewer adverse effects in one study (n = 203) (Holleboom et al, 1996). Maintenance therapy is no longer recommended (Sanchez-Ramos et al, 1999; BNF, 2000). The short acting beta$_2$ agonists, for example ritodrine, salbutamol or terbutaline, are effective for about four hours. Therefore the drug must be administered every four hours, or even more frequently (two to three-hourly) during periods of uterine activity (McKenry & Salerno, 1998).

Beta$_2$ adrenoreceptor agonists cross the placenta and enter breast milk, thus neonates may experience side effects. Beta$_2$ adrenoreceptor agonists are eliminated by liver and kidneys, but due to the complexities of the triphasic half-lives of these drugs, elimination may be delayed and cardiovascular symptoms may recur up to 12 hours after terbutaline discontinuation (Olsen & D'Oria, 1992).

Actions of beta$_2$ adrenoreceptor agonists

These drugs act, like adrenaline, by stimulating the beta$_2$ receptors which are present in the liver and the smooth muscle and glands of many organs, including the uterus, lungs and gut. There is also pronounced action on the beta$_1$ receptors, which stimulate the heart, in a manner similar to adrenaline/epinephrine and noradrenaline (norepinephrine). Due to individual differences, doses are adjusted according to response and side effect monitoring (see Implications for Practice).

Side effects of beta$_2$ adrenoreceptor agonists

Serious and even fatal side effects have occurred with these agents. Perry et al (1995) found that 0.54 per cent of women receiving continuous intravenous terbutaline infusion experienced serious cardiopulmonary problems (n = 8709). It is acknowledged that these are related to the total dose, but dose changes (Holleboom et al, 1996) and individual susceptibility (MacKay & Evans, 1995) are also contributory factors. Neonatal cardiovascular and metabolic problems have been reported (Hill, 1995).

The side effects of tocolytics/uterine relaxants follow from the stimulation of the beta$_2$ adrenoreceptors affecting the:

- cardiovascular system;
- renin-angiotensin system;
- central nervous system;
- smooth muscle of many organs;
- mucus-secreting glands;
- metabolic processes.

Cardiovascular stimulation

Beta$_2$ adrenoreceptor tocolytics are related to the hormones used to drive the cardiovascular system in 'fright, flight or fight' situations. This involves increasing the heart rate, pulse pressure and cardiac contractility via $beta_1$ receptors. On administration of tocolytics, maternal heart rate normally rises by 20–40 beats per minute and neonatal tachycardia also occurs. Tachycardia may be more common with ritodrine than other drugs of this group (McKenry & Salerno, 1998).

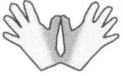 **Practice Points**

- Careful monitoring is required because an excessive rise in heart rate is associated with myocardial ischaemia, cardiac dysrhythmia, reduced cardiac output and pulmonary oedema (Reynolds et al, 1996; Vesalainen et al, 1999).
- Patients should be asked to report any palpitations, chest pains or shortness of breath.

In addition to a rise in heart rate, the work of the heart is further increased by the rise in pulse pressure, normally:

- systolic BP rises about 10 mmHg;
- diastolic BP falls about 10–15 mmHg (MacKay & Evans, 1995).

Any sudden rise in blood pressure has the potential to trigger a cerebro-vasacular accident. The putative link between maternal blood pressure fluctuations and periventricular-intraventricular haemorrhage in preterm infants requires further investigation (Holleboom et al, 1996).

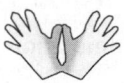 **Practice Point**

The effect of maternal blood pressure changes on uterine blood flow is reduced by placing the woman on her left side (McKenry & Salerno, 1998).

Vasodilation

Beta$_2$ adrenoreceptor agonists relax the vascular smooth muscle and dilate the blood vessels. This reduces the diastolic blood pressure in mother and fetus which is most marked if the woman is hypovolaemic (Olsen & D'Oria, 1992). Dilation of the blood vessels increases the blood flow to peripheral tissues, including the uterus. The drug is therefore not advised for use where antepartum haemorrhage has occurred.

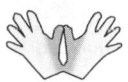 **Practice Points**

- Increased uterine blood flow increases the tendency to (uterine) bleeding. This is problematic if Caesarean section is performed (BNF, 2000).
- Dilation of the peripheral blood vessels increases the blood flow to the skin, causing redness, sweating or a rash. The colour of the skin should be noted before and during therapy.
- Dilation of the pulmonary vessels affects the ventilation/perfusion imbalance. The increased flow of blood to the lungs may result in a transient fall in pO_2 (Hoffman & Lefkowitz, 1996).
- The woman should be advised to get up slowly due to the fall in diastolic blood pressure and the consequent risk of postural hypotension (Malseed et al, 1995).
- Increased cerebral blood flow gives rise to a headache, which is a common side effect of these drugs.

Activation of the renin-angiotensin system

Beta$_2$ adrenoreceptor agonists stimulate the renin–angiotensin–aldosterone axis. This normally maintains blood pressure, both by regulating fluid balance and by constricting arterioles. Combined with the expanded cardiovascular volume of pregnancy, stimulation of the renin-angiotensin system may lead to **pulmonary oedema** (Lamont, 2000).

Overstimulation of the renin-angiotensin-aldosterone axis may be life-threatening due to:

- pulmonary oedema, secondary to acute fluid retention, which may or may not be accompanied by bloating;
- fluid retention, bloating and congestive cardiac failure (Reynolds et al, 1996);
- hypertension;
- hypokalaemia.

The precipitous decline in potassium levels is caused by uptake of potassium ions into skeletal muscle due to the stimulation of beta$_2$ adrenoreceptors (Ganong, 1999). This results in weakness, cramps, bradycardia and cardiac dysrhythmias. Over several hours, potassium is lost from the body by the actions of aldosterone on the renal tubules.

Case Report

This case illustrates the need for careful monitoring and rigorous protocols as outlined in Implications for Practice.

A young woman in premature labour at 33 weeks' gestation was given intravenous rito- drine for three days, before being converted to oral ritodrine. At this point, she developed a persistent tachycardia and fetal distress. Following Caesarean section, pulmonary oedema developed. This led to lung damage, fibrosis and acute respiratory distress syn- drome which proved fatal.

Ritodrine was the probable cause of pulmonary oedema in this case. The long half-life of ritodrine caused accumulation. When the drug was discontinued, it could not be quickly eliminated. Therefore, vigilance should have been maintained despite drug discontinuation (DOH, 1996).

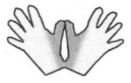 **Practice Points**

To **prevent pulmonary oedema**, it is essential that:
- Accurate fluid balance is maintained; fluid input is restricted to 2.5 L/24 hrs (MacKay & Evans, 1995);
- The lung bases are regularly auscultated;
- Warning signs such as shortness of breath (inability to finish a sentence), dry cough, chest pain and tachycardia are heeded;
- Sodium chloride infusions are avoided, as they remain within the extracellular compartments;
- The maximum infusion rate of the drug is **never** exceeded – 350 micrograms/minute (DoH, 1996);
- Adminsitration is avoided if maternal infection is present (Reynolds et al, 1996);
- The supine position is avoided (Lamont, 2000).

Due to the potentially serious sequelae, such as adult respiratory distress syn- drome (ARDS), if pulmonary oedema occurs, the tocolytic infusion should be discontinued immediately and diuretics administered (Reynolds et al, 1996). Pulmonary oedema may occur subsequently in the woman or fetus (Olsen & O'Dria, 1992).

Case Report

A young woman in premature labour at 33 weeks' gestation was given intravenous rito- drine in normal saline. Tachycardia and patient anxiety prompted dose reduction after 36 hours. On transfer to the ante-natal ward the woman became short of breath. This was treated as bronchospasm and worsened. The woman was transferred to ICU. A Caesarean section was performed for fetal distress. The woman developed acute respiratory distress syndrome and died of a myocardial infarction.

The use of normal saline contributed to this death. The **absence** of fluid balance charts and a written protocol for administration of ritodrine indicated to the assessors that care was suboptimal (DoH, 1996).

Central nervous system

The effects of beta$_2$ adrenoreceptor agonists on the CNS are well known: tremor, tension, headache (10–15 per cent with iv use), anxiety, nervousness, insomnia, irritability, emotional lability, dizziness, hallucinations and even paranoia. In addition, retinopathy has been observed in premature babies following use of ritodrine or salbutamol (Reynolds et al, 1996).

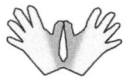 **Practice Point**

Orientation should be checked before and during therapy.

Smooth muscle inhibition

Inhibition of the smooth muscle of the GI tract/gut may cause gastric stasis, leading to loss of appetite, nausea and vomiting. With intravenous use 10–15 per cent of patients will experience nausea. Gastric reflux may cause heartburn. After two to three days of use, the patient may experience constipation and paralytic ileus may occur in the fetus (Olsen and D'Oria, 1992). Inhibition of the smooth muscle of the genito-urinary system reduces uterine activity but also depresses bladder and ureteric contractility, possibly causing retention of urine and dysuria.

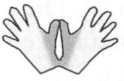 **Practice Point**

An accurate record of fluid output will highlight any problems.

Drying of mucus secretions

Beta$_2$ adrenoreceptor agonists inhibit mucus secretion which may cause:

- dry mouth, which requires frequent water rinses;
- drying of lung secretions, which may lead to chest infections. The risk can be minimized if dehydration is avoided and deep breathing exercises are followed.

Metabolic side effects

The administration of beta$_2$ adrenoreceptor agonists produces hyperglycaemia. If the woman is diabetic, there is an appreciable risk of keto-acidosis and subsequent fetal loss. Hyperglycaemia, and other side effects, are more common with terbutaline (McKenry & Salerno, 1998). Hyperglycaemia may stimulate over-production of fetal insulin, resulting in neonatal hypoglycaemia. Hypocalcaemia in the neonate has been reported (Olsen & D'Oria, 1992).

Hypersensitvity responses include:

- bronchospasm;
- rash in 3–4 per cent of recipients;
- depletion of white cells after several weeks' administration;
- liver enzyme elevations/abnormalities (De Arcos et al, 1996);
- anaphylaxis.

Cautions and contra-indications

Safety in pregnancy has not been established and neonatal side effects have been reported; in view of this, use in the first and second trimesters is contra-indicated (BNF, 2000). Beta$_2$ adrenoreceptor agonists are considered particularly dangerous for women with cardiac disorders (either congenital or acquired), hyperthyroidism or hypertension, including pulmonary hypertension (Lamont, 2000). In addition, pre-existing diabetes, hypokalaemia or acute angle glaucoma may be dangerously worsened. The use of tocolytic therapy is precluded if the fetus is jeopardized, for example by cord compression. Although severe pre-eclampsia precludes tocolytic therapy, mild pre-eclampsia is considered a relative contra-indication (BNF, 2000). Other tocolytic agents, such as nifedipine, may be acceptable if beta$_2$ adrenoreceptor agonists are contra-indicated (van Dijk et al, 1995) (see above).

Storage must be in a cool dry place and away from light (Solvay Health Care, 1995). The infusion pump must be kept away from moisture, even if administration is within the home (McKenry & Salerno, 1998). Discoloured, cloudy or precipitated solution should be discarded (Malseed et al, 1995).

Interactions

- Hypokalaemia may be intensified by drugs and conditions which danger-ously increase the loss of potassium such as steroids, theophylline, diuret-ics, digoxin or hypoxia. If pulmonary oedema should arise, it should be treated with diuretics (BNF, 2000). In this situation, hypokalaemia (involv-ing cardiac dysrhythmias) is a real danger which must be closely monitored.
- The risks of cardiac dysrhythmia, fluid overload and pulmonary oedema may be compounded by co-administration of corticosteroids (Vesalainen et al, 1999).
- The risks of cardiac dysrhythmias are increased by addition of other sympathomimetic drugs [glossary], such as: over-the-counter cold cures, amphetamines, cocaine, anti-depressant medication, drugs prescribed for asthma such as salbutamol or terbutaline.

Implications for Practice: beta$_2$ adrenoreceptor agonists

Potential Problem	Management
Myocardial infarction, tachyarrhythmia, chest pain or heart failure	Monitor maternal pulse/HR at least every 15 minutes. ECG if suspicions arise. Be aware that problems may arise despite a normal ECG. Do not increase the infusion rate if HR > 135/140.
	Monitor pulse before each dose and withhold doses if HR > 110 or 120. Monitor fetal heart rate; this should remain <170–180 bpm.
Maternal hypertension, leading to cerebro-vascular accident	Monitor BP every 15 minutes.
Maternal hypotension, impairing uterine perfusion	Left lateral position during infusion.
Hyperglycaemia, leading to neonatal hypoglycaemia or (rarely) maternal or neonatal ketoacidosis	Four-hourly blood glucose measurements such as BM stix.
Pulmonary oedema, leading to hypoxia and ARDS	Strict fluid balance records. Limit intake to 2.5 litres/24 hours. Observation for shortness of breath, inability to finish sentences. Listening to lung bases with a high quality stethoscope.
	Body weight before and during therapy. Diuretics and potassium monitoring available.

Implications for Practice: beta₂ adrenoreceptor agonists (*continued*)

Potential Problem	Management
Hypokalaemia, leading to cardiac dysrhythmia, or arrest, and muscle weakness, impairing respiration	Venous blood sample for urea and electrolytes at least every 24 hours. ECG at least every 24 hours.
GI tract stasis	Assess bowel movements. Be prepared for client to feel nauseous and vomit. Maintain adequate fluid intake.
Premature labour, despite tocolytic therapy	Monitor uterus. Facilities for premature delivery should be in place.
Increased uterine bleeding, should Caesarean section be needed	Beta blockers should be available to counter this emergency.

Calcium channel blockers (mainly nifedipine)

The actions, side effects and interactions of nifedipine are described here, although they are equally relevant to the management of hypertension. While emergency administration of nifedipine is usually for tocolysis, prolonged administration is more likely to be associated with hypertension in the UK.

Calcium channel blockers (calcium antagonists) are prescribed for tocolysis and hypertension (see Figure 7.1). Nifedipine is as effective as beta₂ agonists (for example ritodrine) in inhibiting premature uterine contractions (Graves, 1996). Since it may have fewer maternal side effects (Lockwood, 1997), longer postponement of delivery and a lower incidence of neonatal morbidity (Papatsonis et al, 2000), nifedipine is now the first line agent in some units. Nifedipine is more suitable than ritodrine for women with diabetes (van Dijk et al, 1995). Long term effects on the infant are unknown, but the manufacturers offer no reassurance (Sibai, 1996; Bayer, 1995).

For the control of hypertension in pregnancy, nifedipine (in a modified release preparation) is usually reserved for those who do not respond to, or cannot tolerate, methyldopa (Nelson-Piercy, 1996). Nevertheless, nifedipine is becoming increasingly popular for management of hypertension antenatally (see Chapter 9). However, nifedipine is not currently licensed for this (BNF, 2000). Due to the variety of preparations on the market, each with its own bioavailability [glossary], in long term therapy it is important that the same brand of nifedipine is prescribed each time (BNF, 2000).

How the body handles nifedipine

Unlike other tocolytics, nifedipine is administered orally (Smith et al, 2000). Nifedipine acts within 30–60 minutes when taken orally as tablets or capsules.

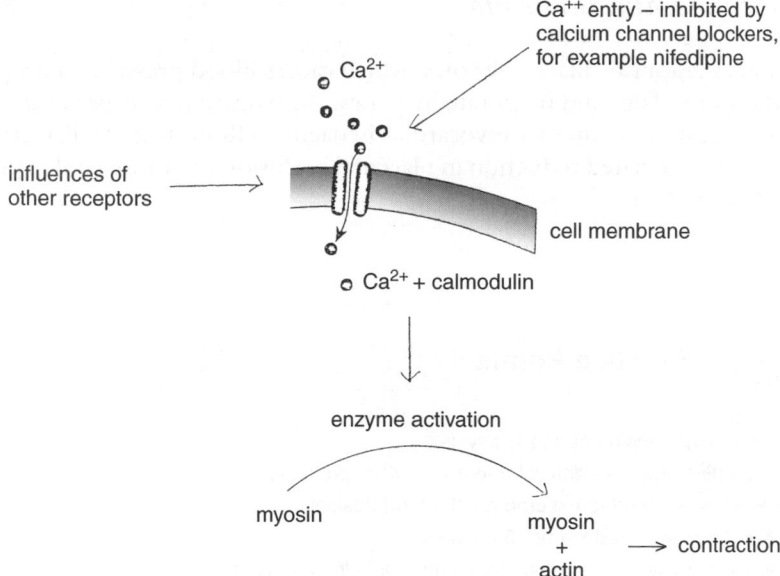

Figure 7.1 Diagram to illustrate the actions of calcium channel blockers on smooth muscle cells

Food increases absorption of nifedipine from tablets but decreases absorption from capsules (Reynolds et al, 1996). The short half-life (1.2–3.8 hours) of standard preparations may allow potentially dangerous oscillations of BP when nifedipine is prescribed regularly; therefore, sustained release preparations are in common use (Oates, 1996). Nifedipine is extensively metabolized by the liver, therefore lower doses are prescribed for those with liver disease (for example alcoholism, HELLP syndrome). Some authorities consider sublingual capsules to be unsafe as they can cause severe hypotension, leading to maternal cardiovascular events and fetal death (Grossman et al, 1996).

Actions and side effects of nifedipine

Calcium channel blockers inhibit the passage of calcium ions into smooth and cardiac muscle cells, reducing their contractility (see Fig. 7.1). The smooth muscle cells of the walls of the arterioles depend on the entry of calcium ions for their contractility. It is this contractility which maintains blood pressure. Nifedipine also depresses the action of the heart but less than other currently available drugs in this class (Robertson & Robertson, 1996).

The myometrium, like other smooth muscle, depends on calcium ion influx for its contractility. Nifedipine reduces uterine contractility, inhibiting labour and increasing the rate of Caesarean section which is a problem if it is used as an anti-hypertensive (Reynolds et al, 1996).

Hypotension and ischaemia

Calcium antagonists dilate arterioles, which causes blood pressure to drop. As blood pressure falls, and heart rate increases, the woman may experience chest pain or palpitations due to myocardial ischaemia (Robertson & Robertson, 1996). The associated reduction in placental perfusion can cause fetal hypoxia, acidosis and death.

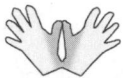 **Practice Points**

To minimize hypotension during tocolysis:
- Intravenous fluids are administered as a 500 ml preload;
- The woman is asked to assume a left lateral position;
- BP & HR are recorded every 15 minutes;
- Evidence of symptomatic (dizziness, lightheadedness) hypotension is sought regularly;
- Infusions are adjusted according to signs and symptoms;
- Strict fluid balance is maintained.

Symptomatic hypotension may necessitate the use of an alternative tocolytic.

Pulmonary oedema

This may be caused by dilution of the plasma due to vasodilation, combined with the infusion of intravenous fluids and loss of protein in the urine (in pre-eclampsia). Pulse oximetry and urine monitoring are indicated during tocolysis (Hill, 1995).

Vasodilation

Whether prescribed for hypertension or tocolysis, **nifedipine lowers BP** by relaxing arteriolar smooth muscle, bringing about general vasodilation. This may predispose the woman to peri-operative or post-partum blood loss (Davis et al, 1997). Vasodilation causes flushing, dizziness, oedema, headache, tinnitus and nausea, causing about 10 per cent of women to discontinue long term medication. Localized oedema may lead to blurred vision or nasal congestion (stuffiness). Gravitational oedema may develop 10–14 days after starting nifedipine, and must be distinguished from signs of pre-eclampsia.

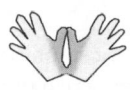 **Practice Points**

- For ambulatory clients, postural hypotension is a significant problem which must be assessed.
- These problems are lessened by the use of sustained release preparations (Oates, 1996).

Gastro-intestinal problems

Nifedipine relaxes the smooth muscle of the gut, causing nausea, constipation and gastro-oesophageal reflux with heart burn. With long term use, gingival hyperplasia may occur. This can be avoided with scrupulous attention to dental hygiene.

CNS side effects

A variety of CNS side effects are reported with nifedipine including depression, somnolence, lethargy, weakness, insomnia and agitation (Karch, 1992).

Hypersensitivity responses

Hypersensitivity responses have occasionally occurred, including rashes, telangiectasia and maternal hepatotoxicity. Liver function tests are probably indicated (Hill, 1995).

Effects on the fetus

Animal testing has raised concern over adverse effects in the fetus. Reduction in BP may be excessive, jeopardizing the blood flow to the placenta and the fetus; this may explain possible associations with IUGR and prematurity (Reynolds et al, 1996). However, comparisons with other tocolytic agents in human infants to date have not been unfavourable (Hill, 1995); US pregnancy category C (McKenry & Salerno, 1998).

Breastfeeding

Manufacturers advise that nifedipine should be avoided during breastfeeding (BNF, 2000).

Cautions and contra-indications

Abrupt withdrawal of calcium channel blockers may precipitate chest pain, palpitations or even a myocardial infarction; therefore the dosage is usually tailed off gradually (McKenry & Salerno, 1998). The contra-indications to tocolytic therapy are discussed above.

Storage should be in airtight containers and away from the light.

Interactions with nifedipine

Concurrent use of other antihypertensives, particularly magnesium salts and alpha receptor antagonists (for example labetolol), may provoke a profound hypotension (Oates, 1996). Alcohol also has hypotensive effects and is best avoided. Stockley (1999) suggests that there is a potential for profound hypotension to arise should bupivacaine be inadvertently administered into a vein (rather than the epidural space) of a patient receiving nifedipine.

Magnesium sulphate combined with nifedipine may induce a profound neuromuscular blockade (Hill, 1995; Magee et al, 1999) or cardiac depression and even arrest (Davis et al, 1997). Therefore many clinicians prefer to avoid nifedipine if there is any chance that the woman will develop eclamptic seizures.

Case Report

Where two drugs have the same action, they may dangerously potentiate each other.

A woman of 32 weeks' gestation received nifedipine for premature uterine contractions. However, 12 hours later, contractions returned and intravenous magnesium sulphate was administered for tocolysis. The woman developed jerky movements in the extremities (tetany), difficulty in swallowing, paradoxical respirations and muscle weakness so intense that she was unable to lift her head from the pillow. Magnesium was discontinued, and the woman recovered within the next 25 minutes (Stockley, 1999:412).

This case illustrates the hazards of drug interactions, particularly in units where certain agents are rarely needed.

Grapefruit juice, erythromycin, cimetidine, ranitidine, fluoxetine (Prozac®) and some antifungals inhibit the liver enzymes responsible for the elimination of nifedipine, prolonging its action and causing profound hypotension (Karch, 1992; Dresser et al, 2000). Anecdotal reports suggest that raw grapefruit can have a similar effect.

Atosiban

This oxytocin antagonist has recently been introduced in the UK. It is indicated for tocolysis, with the same restrictions as other agents: administration is restricted to 48 hours. Side effects include vomiting, hypertension, headache, hyperglycaemia, injection site reactions (BNF, 2000). However US authors report that atosiban is generally well tolerated (Valenzuela et al, 2000).

Conclusions: tocolytics

The use of pharmacological tocolytic agents has not yet been shown to improve perinatal outcome (BNF, 2000; Reynolds et al, 1996; Kinsler et al, 1996; Gyetvai et al, 1999; Katz & Farmer, 1999); therefore their administration cannot be considered as evidence based practice.

The most widely used tocolytic is ritodrine, but terbutaline and salbutamol have similar actions. These drugs may be administered intravenously in an acute situation to inhibit premature labour and then continued for 12–48 hours after cessation of uterine contractions (BNF, 2000). Following certain clinical incidents, the DOH (1996) recommends that the daily dose of ritodrine should not exceed 120 milligrams, and the maximum infusion concentration should not exceed 350 micrograms/minute. Alternative tocolytics, nifedipine and magnesium sulphate, also cause very similar cardiovascular problems (Vesalainen et al, 1999).

A patient receiving uterine relaxants must be closely monitored both for side effects and the failure of tocolysis. If premature labour continues, despite maximum tolerated doses, the drugs should be discontinued and preparations made for the care of a premature neonate (Solvay Healthcare, 1995).

Corticosteroids and tocolysis

Since 1994, corticosteroids have been increasingly employed in the management of preterm labour. For premature infants born within seven days of administration, corticosteroids reduce the incidence of neonatal respiratory distress syndrome, intraventricular haemorrhage and death (NIH Consensus, 1995; Crowley, 1999). Both dexamethasone and betamethasone are prescribed. Betamethasone is a more potent steroid and associated with more maternal side effects (Mulder et al, 1997) but may be safer for the infant (Klinger & Koren, 2000).

Fetal lung maturation

Infants born prior to 34 weeks' gestation have insufficient surfactant in their lungs to breathe effectively. Production of surfactant can be induced by maternal administration of corticosteroids. This reduces the incidence of respiratory distress syndrome in infants born at 29–34 weeks' gestation, and reduces its severity for those born at 24–28 weeks' gestation.

Administration of corticosteroids

Intramuscular injection may be associated with a lower rate of neonatal intraventricular haemorrhage and sepsis than oral administration (Egerman et al, 1998). Dexamethasone and betamethasone readily cross the placenta. The transfer to the fetus is rapid, and some benefit may be derived even if delivery occurs within 12 hours of administration (Wallace et al, 1997).

One commonly prescribed regimen is four doses of 6 mg dexamethasone by intramuscular injection every 12 hours which should be started 24 hours before delivery, if possible. This will remain effective for seven to ten days (Lougher, 1999; personal communication).

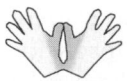 **Practice Points**

- Intramuscular injections of dexamethasone are inadvisable if the woman has purpura due to thrombocytopenia (low platelets), for example in association with pre-eclampsia or regular steroid therapy (Malseed et al, 1995).
- Care of the injection site is essential, since steroid injections are associated with swelling, tingling, numbness, pain and sterile abscess (McKenry & Salerno, 1998).
- Each injection site should be used once only and documented, as repeated injections may cause scarring, induration, necrosis and tissue atrophy.
- Dexamethasone should be administered deeply into the gluteal muscle. The deltoid muscle is too small for steroid injections (Fowler, 1998).
- With intravenous injection, women should be warned to expect a 'tingling' sensation in the perineal area.

Actions and side effects of corticosteroids

Dexamethasone and betamethasone act as endogenous corticosteroids. This accounts for both their actions and their side effects (see Chapter 15, Implications for Practice; Ganong, 1999).

Side effects can be summarized:
Side effects likely to arise immediately:

- Cardiovascular problems;
- metabolic disturbances – hyperglycaemia;
- central nervous system problems.

Side effects likely to arise in the longer term:

- anti-inflammatory actions – infection;
- metabolic disturbances;
- adrenal suppression.

The short term problems are considered here. The long term problems are considered in Chapter 15, asthma (see also Appendix 1). However the potential side effects of corticosteroids may be encountered in any situation where they are prescribed.

Cardiovascular side effects

All steroids increase sodium reabsorption in the kidneys in exchange for potassium or hydrogen ions. This promotes fluid retention, weight gain and hypertension. Cerebral oedema has been reported (BNF, 2000). An independent association between oral corticosteroids and pre-eclampsia was found in one study (n = 1502) but was not associated with adverse outcomes (Schatz et al, 1997). Hypertension was more common in women receiving a complete course of corticosteroids for fetal lung maturity than in controls (Wallace et al, 1997).

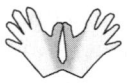 **Practice Point**

- Women prescribed corticosteroids for any acute condition (premature delivery, asthma) should be monitored for fluid retention, hypertension and potassium loss (see implications for practice of tocolytic therapy).

Corticosteroids increase the production of erythropoietin, causing polycythaemia, and increase the clotting tendency of the blood.

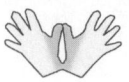 **Practice Point**

- If corticosteroids are administered, it is important to maintain vigilance for thrombosis and mobilize early.

Fetal heart rate variability is affected by corticosteroid administration (Mulder et al, 1997).

Metabolic disturbances – hyperglycaemia

Corticosteroids reduce the uptake of glucose by cells. This causes the plasma glucose concentration to rise which can lead to diabetes and cataract (Laskin et al, 1997). Hyperglycaemia is a particular danger in women with diabetes or if beta$_2$ agonists (for example ritodrine) have been administered.

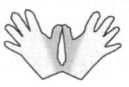 **Practice Point**

- Anyone receiving oral or parenteral steroids (including those receiving tocolytic therapy) should be monitored for hyperglycaemia.

A single course of dexamethasone is probably insufficient to cause bone demineralization (Ogueh et al, 1998).

Neonatal adrenal suppression may occur following repeated ante-natal courses of corticosteroids (see Chapter 15). Therefore the neonate should be examined for signs of weakness, cardiovascular insufficiency and hypoglycaemia.

Central nervous system side effects

Steroids may induce headache, vertigo, insomnia, mood changes or psychoses, or aggravate pre-existing mental illness (BNF, 2000). There may be euphoria or depression or mood swings which may resemble post-partum depression. Steroids lower the seizure threshold, causing restlessness or convulsions, especially with intravenous administration.

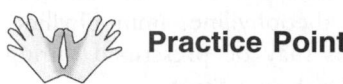 **Practice Point**

Administration to women with epilepsy requires caution.

Infection

Administration of corticosteroids increases the risk of infection in women whose membranes are ruptured (Crowley, 1999).

Effects on the fetus

The risk of intrauterine growth retardation is significant if administration of corticosteroids is prolonged or repeated. Repeated courses of steroids cause neurodevelopmental delay and poor growth in animals and possibly in humans (Brocklehurst et al, 1999; Smith et al, 2000). An observational study in humans suggested that repeated ante-natal courses of corticosteroids reduced fetal growth and head circumference (French et al, 1999).

Case Report

A paediatrician expressed concern regarding a one-year-old boy in his care, with moderate developmental delay, some spasticity in the legs and a head circumference on the third centile. The boy was born at 20 weeks' gestation following multiple doses of dexamethasone, and no complications of prematurity (Klinger & Koren, 2000).

This issue is surrounded by uncertainty, but long term follow-up of such infants is advisable.

Authorities state that no adverse outcomes have been noted in association with a single course of dexamethasone for fetal lung maturation (BNF, 2000; Crowley, 1999).

Interactions with corticosteroids

Fluid retention will be accentuated if steroid therapy is combined with high sodium intake, either orally or by intravenous infusion.

Pulmonary oedema has been associated with co-administration of dexamethasone and ritodrine (McKenry & Salerno, 1998).

Hypokalaemia is a particular danger if corticosteroids are co-administered with beta$_2$ adrenoreceptor agonists (ritodrine), theophylline, aminophylline, digitalis, or diuretics; these drug combinations may be prescribed during tocolytic therapy or management of an acute attack of asthma.

Conclusions: corticosteroids

The use of multiple courses of corticosteroids is currently widespread in the UK. It is not certain that this confers any benefit over a single course (Smith et al, 2000). However, in view of the potential side effects of prolonged administration of corticosteroids, and the data from animal studies, this practice requires further evaluation (Brocklehurst et al, 1999). The effects of antenatal corticosteroids may not be apparent until adolescence; therefore long term follow-up of these infants is required. Randomized control trials of multiple courses of corticosteroids versus a single course may not be ethically justifiable.

Further Reading

Brocklehurst, P., Gates, S., McHarg, K.M., Alfirevic, Z. & Chamberlain, G. (1999) Are we prescribing multiple courses of antenatal corticosteroids? A survey of practice in the UK. *British Journal of Obstetrics and Gynaecology*:106:977–9.

Smith, G., Kingdom, J., Penning, D. & Matthews, S. (2000) Antenatal corticosteroids: Is more better? *Lancet*:355:251–2.

Smith, P., Anthony, J. & Johanson, R. (2000) Nifidipine in pregnancy. *British Journal of Obstetrics and Gynaecology*:107:299–307.

Steer, P. & Flint, C. (1999) Preterm labour and premature rupture of membranes. *BMJ*:318:1059–62.

PART III

DISORDERED PHYSIOLOGY IN CHILDBIRTH

This part of the book discusses the management of disorders associated with, but not necessarily exclusive to, pregnancy. In some circumstances, it is the midwife who identifies these conditions and refers the woman to obstetricians. Midwives also play a crucial role in administering appropriate medications in primary, secondary and tertiary care.

CHAPTER 8

Drugs Affecting the Coagulation Process

SUE JORDAN AND MARIA ANDRADE

This chapter considers the anti-coagulants employed in the management and prophylaxis of thromboembolic disorders. Vitamin K administration, both therapeutic and prophylactic, is also discussed.

Chapter Contents

- Haemostasis

- Anti-coagulants

Aspirin is discussed briefly in Chapter 9. Of the oral anti-coagulants, only warfarin is considered, since others are seldom prescribed in the UK.

The number of maternal deaths due to pulmonary embolism increased in the last triennium (1994–6) from 30 to 46 cases. Maternal deaths represent only a very small proportion of the women who suffer pulmonary emboli (PE), deep vein thrmboses (DVT), cerebral thromboses or arterial occlusion of limbs. Consequently, professionals are urged to maintain a high index of suspicion for thromboembolic disorders, and wider use of prophylactic anti-coagulants is 'urgently recommended' (DoH, 1998:20). Also, there is increasing recognition of the need for anti-coagulant therapy in women with inherited pro-coagulant disorders who are at high risk of thromboembolic events. Therefore midwives are likely to encounter an increasing number of women prescribed anti-coagulants.

Haemostasis

When a blood vessel is damaged, the clotting mechanisms are activated to seal the vessel and minimize blood loss. Initially, the damaged vessel constricts,

Stage	Requirements	Drugs Affecting	Antidote to Drug
1. Temporary plug	platelets	aspirin, possibly heparin	none
2. Fibrin clot	clotting factors, vitamin K	warfarin, coumarin	vitamin K
	anti-clotting factors	heparin	protamine sulphate
3. Fibrinolysis	plasmin, fibrinolytic system	streptokinase, tissue plasminogen activator (tPA)	aminocaproic acid aprotinin

Figure 8.1   Summary of the three stages of haemostasis

and a temporary plug of platelets forms which is then converted into a permanent clot by the activation of fibrinogen. Normally, various anti-clotting mechanisms restrict and prevent clot formation in undamaged vessels. In due course, blood clots are broken down by the fibrinolytic process, and the vessel heals. The three stages of the coagulation process are summarized in Figure 8.1.

Normal blood flow is dependent on maintaining the delicate balance between circulating and endothelial [glossary] anti-coagulant and pro-coagulant factors. If this equilibrium is disturbed, a thrombosis [glossary] may occur. The likelihood of thrombosis can be assessed from known risk factors which include:

● increased plasma concentrations of oestrogens or progesterone;
● pregnancy (increased concentration of some clotting factors);
● childbirth, especially emergency Caesarean section, instrumental delivery and grand multiparity (para 4+);
● age >35, >30 with operative delivery;
● obesity, weight >80 kg;
● immobility, bed rest > four days, long term paralysis of lower limbs;
● trauma and surgery;
● dehydration (for example emesis or hyperemesis);
● haemorrhage;
● current infection, sepsis (especially staphylococcal toxins), inflammation;
● vessel wall compression, for example from delivery table stirrups, pressure of presenting part;
● smoking;
● stress;
● hypertension, pre-eclampsia;
● high fat, low fibre diet;
● gross varicose veins;
● thrombophilia (one of several inherited pro-coagulant disorders), anti-phospholipid syndrome, lupus anticoagulant, a family history of cardiolipin antibody;

- personal history of thromboembolism;
- diabetes;
- pre-existing disease: respiratory disorders, cardiovascular diseases, arterio-sclerosis, nephrotic syndrome, inflammatory bowel disease, cancer.
(Buckley, 1990; Toglia & Weg, 1996; DoH, 1996; 1998)

Case Report

A thorough history should be obtained from every woman to assess the risk factors for thromboembolism, including past history and family history.

An older parous woman did not declare a history of DVT at the booking clinic. (How specifically was it sought?) She was discharged home three days after a forceps delivery, but a few days later she was readmitted overnight for evacuation of retained products of conception. She suffered headaches and episodes of loss of consciousness. A week later she collapsed at home. The problem was diagnosed as a venous thrombosis in the cerebral cortex. However, the diagnosis was questioned and no anticoagulants were administered. Death occurred on the 27th day post-partum (DoH, 1991:40).

This case illustrates the importance of history taking and the potential seriousness of headaches.

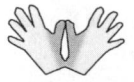 **Practice Point**

All risk factors for thrombosis should be included when the midwife takes the woman's history, so that the prophylactic use of leg stockings and/or anticoagulant therapy can be prescribed (DoH, 1998).

Any situation which leads to slow or sluggish blood flow places the woman at risk of a thromboembolic event: following Caesarean section, it is estimated that thromboembolism occurs in 1–2 per cent of women (Buckley, 1990). Management of a thromboembolic event will be divided into an acute phase of intensive treatment (usually involving heparin), followed by a later preventive phase lasting several months using either heparin or warfarin (De Swiet, 1995).

Thrombolytic drugs, such as streptokinase, and recombinant tissue plasminogen activator (rtPA) are used in some clinical situations to break down existing clots, but the use of these in pregnancy is considered hazardous (De Swiet, 1995a). For further information on thrombolytics, see McKenry and Salerno (1998).

Anti-coagulants

Neither heparin nor warfarin affect any existing clot but act to prevent the formation of further clots. Following a thromboembolic event, anti-coagulants will be prescribed to prevent further clot formation.

Case Reports

It is imperative that breathlessness, cough, 'anxiety attack' or chest pain and tachycardia are recognized as signs of pulmonary embolism. This can be difficult because shortness of breath, tachypnoea, swelling and discomfort of the legs are common in late pregnancy (Toglia & Weg, 1996).

1. An obese woman in her thirties was induced at 42 weeks, and had a normal delivery. Twelve days after delivery she was readmitted with DVT. A ten-day course of heparin plus support stockings were prescribed. Cough and breathlessness were inadequately monitored and treated. PE occurred 42 days after delivery (DoH, 1994:46).

2. A woman booked for elective Caesarean section was admitted with spontaneous rupture of the membranes. Following Caesarean section, she developed a low grade pyrexia and a week later was complaining of faintness, giddiness, and breathlessness. She died of massive PE on the tenth day. It would appear that no anti-coagulation was administered (DoH, 1994:50).

It is important to assess for all risk factors and ensure that the DoH (1996:56) guidelines are followed. For all women, this involves early mobilization and good hydration. For the highest risk women, this means support stockings (correctly worn) and heparin at least until the fifth post-operation day **and until fully mobilized**.

Anti-coagulants are also prescribed as prophylaxis for those women defined as being at high risk of a thromboembolism (De Swiet, 1995). Investigation into recurrent miscarriage has highlighted the need for heparin prophylaxis in pro-coagulant disorders such as antiphospholipid (Hughes') syndrome* (Rai et al, 1997; Khamashtra & Mackworth-Young, 1997; Lima et al, 1996). Administration of aspirin may be combined (Greaves, 1999).

* *Note: Anti-phospholipid syndrome is defined as thrombosis or recurrent miscarriage plus laboratory evidence of the presence of certain antibodies in the blood, such as lupus anti-coagulant (Greaves, 1999:1348).*

Due to the considerable risk of iatrogenic haemorrhage with anti-coagulants, treatment should be closely monitored and the midwife needs to be aware of the available antidotes (Lima et al, 1996). See Implications for Practice.

Heparin

Synthesized heparins closely resemble natural anticoagulants, which are found on the inner surfaces of capillaries. Two categories of heparin are in general use: standard or unfractionated heparin and low molecular weight heparins (such as enoxaparin, dalteparin, certoparin, tinzaparin). The differences are summarized in Figure 8.2. Standard heparins stimulate or catalyse the activity of antithrombin III, an endogenous anticoagulant which binds and inactivates several clotting factors (thrombin, Xa, IXa, XIa and XIIa), thereby preventing the formation of fibrin. However, long term use of standard heparin will deplete the supply of antithrombin III, decreasing the effectiveness of the therapy (Levy et al, 2000). Measurement of antithrombin III concentration is not usually possible in clinical settings.

	Standard/unfractionated heparins	Low molecular weight heparins
Routes of administration	iv or sc	sc
Frequency of administration	continuous ivi or sc every 12 hours	sc every 12 or 24 hours, depending on preparation
Site of action	thrombin, Xa, IXa, XIa, XIIa	only Xa (probably)
Uses	established DVT and PE prevention of DVT and PE	prevention of DVT and PE
Advantages	proven efficacy in established disorders	ease of administration reduced incidence of side effects (no studies of long term administration) reduced need for haematological monitoring

Figure 8.2 Comparison of standard and low molecular weight heparins

Low molecular weight heparins, such as enoxaprin, are now used in many UK maternity units (Khamashta & Mackworth-Young, 1997; Ellison et al, 2000). They inhibit only clotting factor Xa which may account for their increased bioavailability, predictability and safety when compared with standard/unfractionated heparins (Heaton & Pearce, 1995; Geerts et al, 1996). In normal doses, they do not inhibit thrombin. Therefore their use is not detected by most laboratory tests for coagulation. Since the rate of coagulation is limited by factor Xa, low molecular weight heparins are effective prophylaxis when the coagulation process has not been initiated (Malseed et al, 1995). They have a lower incidence of side effects than standard/unfractionated heparin and are equally effective in DVT prevention (Nelson-Piercy et al, 1997; Lensing et al, 1999), but further evaluations of their use in pregnancy are needed (De Swiet, 1995a). Where low molecular weight heparins have been used in established DVT and PE in pregnancy, this has been accompanied by monitoring concentration of factor anti-Xa (Thomson et al, 1998; Greer, 1999).

How the body handles heparin

Administration of heparin

In acute situations, heparin is given as a loading dose, followed by continuous intravenous infusion; intermittent intravenous injection is no longer recommended. For prophylaxis, heparin is given as subcutaneous injections, which may be self-administered (BNF, 2000).

Doses of standard/unfractionated heparin are prescribed in 'units' and low molecular weight heparins are prescribed in milligrams or 'units' which are not necessarily interchangeable between preparations. Different systems exist in the USA and the UK. USP (United States Pharmacopeia) units are not equivalent to international units (IU), although they are essentially very similar (Reynolds et al, 1996). Staff also need to be alert to the dangers of decimal place errors.

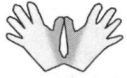 **Practice Points**

- If a loading dose is prescribed, it should never be given in less than one minute, due to the risks of hypersensitivity responses.
- Heparin flushes designed for maintaining intravenous patency are not suitable for injection.
- Subcutaneous heparins may be injected into rotated sites in the lower abdomen, using a small gauge needle.
- All subcutaneous injections should be two inches away from the umbilicus and scar tissue and a 'bunching' or Z-track technique is advised (Malseed et al, 1995).
- To avoid bruising, administration should comprise gentle needle insertion, a ten-second hold and gentle needle withdrawal. Gentle pressure should then be applied to the site for one or two minutes (McKenry & Salerno, 1998).
- The use of ice-packs pre- and post-injection reduces pain but not bruising (Ross & Soltes, 1995).
- If the subcutaneous injection is too shallow or the site is massaged following administration, bruising is intensified and the action of heparin will be shortened.
- The pain of subcutaneous injections increases with the volume injected; therefore large doses of heparin should not be given by this route (Jorgensen et al, 1996).
- Women may prefer low molecular weight heparins, because they are less painful to inject, and some forms can be given just once a day (De Swiet, 1995a).

Subcutaneous standard/unfractionated heparin takes effect within 20–60 minutes and is maximally effective two to three hours after administration (Lutomski et al, 1995; Malseed et al, 1995). Intravenous heparin takes immediate effect, therefore close observation of cannula sites may allow early detection of bleeding. Heparin infusion rates are determined from tables incorporating height and body weight (Lutomski et al, 1995).

Clearance of heparin

Heparin is bound to plasma proteins and inactivated by macrophages, the liver and activated platelets. Since standard/unfractionated heparin has a short half-life, (60–90 minutes at usual doses), intermittent infusion may be unreliable. The risk of bleeding is increased for two to six hours after an intravenous injection and 8–12 hours after a subcutaneous injection. Due to individual differences in response, and the dose dependent half-life of standard heparin, dosage is adjusted according to results of coagulation tests (Majerus et al, 1996).

The longer half-life and duration of action of low molecular weight heparins allow once daily administration for prophylaxis. The response to any given dose is more predictable, allowing fixed dose administration without laboratory monitoring in many circumstances (Ginsberg, 1996).

Heparin does not cross the placenta or enter breast milk in appreciable amounts, therefore administration during pregnancy and lactation is considered safe for the fetus and neonate (BNF, 2000). However, use of heparin in pregnancy has been associated with an increase in miscarriage and premature labour (Hall et al, 1980), but more recent reviewers dispute these findings (Toglia & Weg, 1996).

Side effects of heparin

The side effects and problems arising from short term heparin use are:

- bleeding;
- thrombocytopenia (low platetlet count);
- hypotension, due to preservative (chlorbutol) in some preparations;
- diuresis starting 36–48 hours after initiation of therapy, lasting 36–48 hours after discontinuation;
- vasospastic reaction (rare), leading to raised blood pressure, chest pain and parasthesia;
- hypersensitivity responses.

Further problems may arise with long term use of heparin; for example in any woman with a history of repeated thromboembolism:

- abnormalities of liver function tests;
- decreased renal function;
- aldosterone inhibition, leading to hyperkalaemia;
- hair loss (usually reverses on discontinuation);
- osteoporosis or osteopenia;
- abrupt withdrawal, which may cause rebound coagulation;
- heparin resistance.

Bleeding

Bleeding is problematic for 1–33 per cent of patients. The importance of this is demonstrated in several studies: Hall et al (1980) cite 14 haemorrhages and three deaths in 135 women using heparin during pregnancy; Sadler et al (2000) report anticoagulant related post-parum haemorrhage following Caesarean section in four of 14 women receiving heparin; Ellison et al (2000) report one ante-partum and four post-partum haemorrhages in 57 pregnancies where low dose heparin was administered. Haemorrhage remains a common reason for maternal admission to intensive care and hysterectomy (DoH, 1998). Bleeding is more likely with: high doses, intravenous administration, an increased activated partial thromboplastin time (aPTT) [glossary]; standard/unfractionated heparin (Majerus et al, 1996).

Case Report

Heparin administration increases the risks of bleeding, necessitating careful monitoring.

A woman with several risk factors for pulmonary embolus complained of severe chest and abdominal pains. A diagnosis of pulmonary embolism was made, and heparin was administered. Later that day she collapsed, and resuscitation was unsuccessful. A retro-peritoneal haemorrhage was found at autopsy (DoH, 1998 p.133).

The exact contribution of heparin to this death is not clear, but it probably intensified the severity of the bleeding.

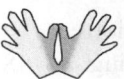 **Practice Points**

- It is important to observe for the first signs of bleeding such as bruising, petechiae, haematoma, nosebleeds, bleeding gums or cannulation sites.
- The recognition of internal bleeding is more difficult but can be identified by symptoms such as abdominal pain or distension, low backache, joint pain or swelling, headache or dizziness. Intra-adrenal haemorrhage is a rare complication.

- Practitioners should be alert to the possibility of retroplacental bleeding, which may only become apparent following a scan. Should the woman complain of severe abdominal pain and contractions or shivering and breathlessness (symptoms of a transfusion reaction), she must be immediately referred to her obstetrician.
- Checking urine and stools periodically for the presence of blood, both by laboratory tests (multistix and faecal occult blood reagent strips) and observations will give practitioners an early warning of bleeding problems. The woman should also be asked to report any increase in bleeding from the gums (Malseed et al, 1995).
- To detect any haemorrhage as early as possible, the midwife should monitor vital signs every four hours during heparin administration in hospital (McKenry & Salerno, 1998), and be aware that life-threatening haemorrhage may occur without a tachycardia and hypotension (Little et al, 1995).
- Anticoagulants will be withheld and urgently reviewed if bleeding is suspected.

Doctors may reduce or discontinue heparin 24 hours prior to delivery or during labour to minimize the risks of both bleeding and thromboembolism (Majerus et al, 1996; De Swiet, 1995, Toglia & Weg, 1996).

Box 8.1 Haematological monitoring for women receiving heparin

Use of full dose standard/unfractionated heparin entails haematological monitoring during therapy, usually aPTT [glossary] on a daily basis (McKenry & Salerno, 1998; Lensing et al, 1999) and initially every six hours (Majerus et al, 1996).

- Venous blood samples are taken from the arm not receiving any infusions, 30 minutes before the next dose is due.
- Heparin doses are adjusted in the light of laboratory findings, with the aim of maintaining aPTT 1.5–2.5 times the standard value (Majerus et al, 1996).

However, aPTT is unreliable during pregnancy: antifactor Xa concentrations, activated clotting time and plasma heparin concentrations may offer better alternatives (Greer, 1999; Lutomski et al, 1995).

At normal doses, low molecular weight heparins have no effect on haematological indices, therefore routine monitoring is not required with standard regimens (BNF, 2000).

Although heparin has a short half-life, the administration of the antidote, protamine sulphate, is occasionally necessary. This is expanded later on p. 210.

Thrombocytopenia

Early recognition of thrombocytopenia [glossary] is important because it is reversible if heparin is discontinued but causes life-threatening arterial emboli if left unattended (Majerus et al, 1996).

There are two forms of thrombocytopenia encountered with heparin administration:

- The early/mild form occurs in up to 33 per cent of recipients and resolves spontaneously.
- The delayed/severe form is rare and leads to arterial or venous thrombosis.

In the severe form of thrombocytopenia, antibodies are formed against a heparin-platelet complex. These cause the platelets to aggregate and form a thrombus which may be asymptomatic or present as venous or arterial thromboembolism. The clinical manifestations of this include: deep vein thrombosis (DVT), pulmonary embolism (PE), skin necrosis, occlusion of the circulation to limbs, thrombosis of mesenteric, coronary or cerebral arteries. The sequestration of the platelets into thrombi reduces the number in circulation, causing thrombocytopenia.

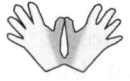 **Practice Points**

- The BNF (2000) recommends regular platelet counts for those taking heparin for longer than five days.
- If the patient has previously received heparin, thrombocytopenia may arise in less than five days, necessitating earlier platelet checks (Reynolds et al, 1996).

The risks of heparin-induced thrombocytopenia, associated thrombotic events and antibodies to heparin are reduced or delayed but not eliminated by the use of low molecular weight heparins (Warkentin et al, 1995; Nelson Piercy, 1997; Lindhoff-Last et al, 2000). Thrombocytopenia has also been reported following the use of heparin flushes for intravenous infusions (for example Hepsal®) (Reynolds et al, 1996).

Hypersensitivity responses

All heparin preparations may induce hypersensitivity responses, such as, chills, rash, pruritus, urticaria, hair loss, pyrexia, nasal congestion, bronchospasm, lacrimation, diarrhoea and even anaphylaxis. Since heparin is derived from animal products, hypersensitivity reactions are relatively common, particularly in atopic individuals [glossary].

Abrupt withdrawal

Discontinuation of heparin may lead to rebound coagulation and a rise in plasma lipid concentrations, causing hyperlipidaemia (Majerus et al, 1996). Heparin administration is usually followed by oral anti-coagulation with warfarin. This prevents rebound coagulation and the formation of DVT or pulmonary emboli.

Heparin resistance

If extensive clotting is present, heparin will be rapidly destroyed and larger doses will be required; this is termed 'heparin resistance' (Lutomski et al, 1995). Also, heparin is neutralized by activated platelets present in arteriosclerosis which reduce its effect. In very high risk women, there is considerable risk (4/14) of thromboembolic events if heparin is the sole anti-coagulant (Sadler et al, 2000).

Some individuals have a congenital excess of clotting factor VIII or heparin-binding proteins which interfere with the haematological monitoring required for heparin administration. If this occurs, heparin concentration monitoring will be necessary (Majerus et al, 1996). Heparin resistance is summarized in the Table 8.1.

Osteoporosis and osteopenia

Bone density is reduced in pregnancy, due to fetal demands for calcium and enhanced bone turnover. This may be compounded by prolonged administration of heparin. Diabetics are particularly at risk (Chapter 17).

Heparin binds to calcium ions and, with prolonged administration, this may induce osteoporosis and osteopenia. The risk is increased after 3–6 months' use (Majerus et al, 1995) and with doses over 15 000 units/day (Rubin, 1995). Doses of 10 000 units/day for 19 weeks have led to bone demineralization in pregnant women: 2.2 per cent of women receiving heparin during pregnancy and the puerperium sustained osteoporotic fractures (Dahlman,

Table 8.1   Heparin resistance

In some circumstances, heparin may not have its usual efficacy:	
Lack of antithrombin:	DIC, cirrhosis of liver, nephrotic syndrome arteriosclerosis, that is in women over 40 long term use, for example women with a previous PE
Increased clearance of heparin:	pulmonary embolus, pleurisy fever, infection, thrombophlebitis smoking tobacco extensive surgery (such as abdominal hysterectomy) myocardial infarction cancer

1993). Low molecular weight heparin (40 or 20 mg enoxaprin) has also been associated with loss of bone density in the spine and hip when compared with unmedicated controls (Dahlman et al, 1994; Barbour et al, 1994; Nelson-Piercy et al, 1997). Rai et al (1997) state that bone loss is reversible and equivalent to the loss caused by six months' lactation; however the results of long term follow-up studies are contradictory (De Swiet, 1995a).

Case Report

This case illustrates the possibility of **compression fractures** in women receiving heparin.

A woman had received heparin prophylaxis (5000 IU three times per day) during pregnancy and lactation. During the last two weeks of pregnancy, she complained of back pain. Six weeks after delivery, she sustained a compression (crush) fracture of the sixth thoracic vertebra, and general osteopenia was noted. Vitamin D concentrations were found to be low (Haram et al, 1993).

In view of these risks, women receiving heparin long term should be given dietary advice.

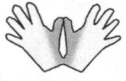 **Practice Points**

- Women receiving any form of heparin during pregnancy should be advised to enhance the calcium, vitamin D and protein contents of their diets and take calcium supplements (Ginsberg, 1996).
- Women receiving heparin for recurrent miscarriage and antiphospholipid syndrome during pregnancy should be reviewed regularly, as unduly prolonged treatment increases the risk of osteoporosis (Greaves, 1999).

Effects on the fetus

Although heparin does not cross the placenta, heparin may deprive the fetus of calcium or other nutrients by binding them in the maternal plasma. This could account for the high rates of stillbirth and prematurity in early studies of heparin in pregnancy (Hall et al, 1980). In women heparinized for the management of articifial heart valves, the fetal loss rate was 25 per cent, all within the first trimester (Sadler et al, 2000). In the USA, pregnancy safety is category C, implying that despite adverse animal studies, and a lack of controlled studies in humans, the benefits of administration are deemed to outweigh the risks. Heparin preparations containing benzyl alcohol are considered unsafe for administration during pregnancy (BNF, 2000).

Cautions and contra-indications

Heparin is contra-indicated where bleeding would be life threatening, for example in women with severe hypertension, pre-eclampsia, eclampsia and HELLP syndrome, thrombocytopenia, haemorrhagic disorders or active haemorrhage. Anticoagulants are avoided if hypertension (including pre-eclampsia or eclampsia) exists, due to the increased risk of cerebrovascular accident.

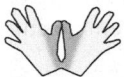 **Practice Points**

- Blood pressure should be checked before initiating heparin treatment and monitored subsequently. A sustained rise in diastolic BP of 15 mmHg may be considered significant.
- It is advisable to perform a full clotting screen and FBC before administration (McKenry & Salerno, 1998).

Regional anaesthesia in women who are concurrently receiving anti-coagulants is generally contra-indicated due to the small but definite risk of spinal haematoma. The use of low dose subcutaneous heparin remains controversial (Reynolds et al, 1996); Ellison et al (2000) experienced no problems during 22 deliveries under epidural and spinal analgesia. Toglia and Weg (1996) advise that safety is increased if aPTT is normal and heparin has not been administered for four to six hours before the anaesthesia is commenced. *The Report on Confidential Enquiries into Maternal Deaths* (DoH, 1996:59) states that on current, non-obstetric evidence subcutaneous heparin as prophylaxis is not associated with an increased risk of spinal haematoma.

Storage

Heparin should be stored in airtight containers at 15–25°C, without freezing (Reynolds et al, 1996).

Drug interactions

Non-steroidal antiinflammatory drugs such as aspirin, other salicylates, ibuprofen and diclofenac inhibit the procoagulant action of platelets. Should a woman receiving anti-coagulants require simple analgesia, for example for a headache, paracetamol is suitable, although there are isolated reports of bleeding after seven days' concurrent use (Stockley, 1999). Penicillins, cephalosporins, quinine and dextrans also interfere with coagulation, increasing the risks of bleeding, particularly from the gastro-intestinal tract. If acid-citrate dextrose converted blood is transfused, it may potentiate the action of heparin (Malseed et al, 1995). Nicotine accelerates heparin elimination; therefore smokers may require higher doses.

Most other drugs react with heparin if given via the same intravenous line; therefore this practice should be avoided. Glucose has a variable effect on heparin infusions (Reynolds et al, 1996). However, the BNF (2000) advises administration in glucose 5 per cent or sodium chloride 0.9 per cent, using a motorised pump.

Antidote to heparin – protamine sulphate

This forms an inactive complex with heparin and interacts with platelets and fibrinogen. However bleeding due to low molecular weight heparins is only partially reversed (Reynolds et al, 1996; Ginsberg, 1996). Protamine sulphate must be given by a slow intravenous infusion, since rapid administration may cause dangerous hypotension and bradycardia and the dose should never exceed 50 mg (De Swiet, 1995a). Following administration, feelings of warmth and flushing are common. Other potential problems with protamine sulphate treatment are:

- bleeding, if given in excess;
- anaphylactic reactions (particularly in diabetics and those with an allergy to fish);
- pulmonary vasoconstriction.

Protamine sulphate acts within five minutes and is active for one to two hours; however its safety in pregnancy and lactation are unknown (Malseed et al, 1995).

Conclusion

In order to minimize the potential problem of bleeding, the midwife should be in a position both to offer the woman practical advice and to ensure that appropriate monitoring is undertaken, as outlined in Implications for Practice. It is important that all those delivering care are aware that a client is receiving anti-coagulant therapy.

Implications for Practice: heparin

Potential problem	Management
Risk of haemorrhage	Observe (for example catheter sites, mouth) for signs of bleeding.
	Check vital signs every four hours, initially.
	Avoid rectal thermometers.
	Advise a medi-alert band with medication clearly written.
	Test urine and stools daily for occult bleeding.
	Ensure that coagulation and FBC are monitored regularly and that the woman understands the need to attend clinics for this.
Bleeding tendencies	Avoid vigorous nose blowing or teeth cleaning. Use a soft toothbrush.
	Avoid razors (electric razors are the least abrasive).
	Avoid going 'barefoot'.
	Avoid intramuscular injections, catheters, enemas, if possible.
Risk of recurrence of thrombosis	Avoid constrictive clothing, leg stirrups.
	Mobilize, encourage use of anti-embolic stockings.
	Measure and compare calf circumferences every eight hours.
	Avoid tobacco.
	Assist in turning, coughing and deep breathing every four hours.
	Check for dyspnoea, pulmonary oedema, cough and haemoptysis at least every four hours initially.
Thrombocytopenia	Ensure monitoring of platelets on the fifth day of therapy and regularly thereafter.
	Check for purpura or petechiae in dependent areas and under the BP cuff.
	Be wary of heparinoids for anticoagulation in women with a history of heparin-induced thrombocytopenia.
Heparin resistance	Inform physician if an infection or thrombophlebitis develops, since the dose of heparin may be increased accordingly.
Hyperkalaemia	Potassium concentrations should be monitored on commencement and seven days later.
Osteoporosis	For those on long term (one month plus) heparin, dietary calcium supplementation and review of diet to include fish and milk if possible. Advise on the need for exercise in the long term.

Warfarin

Due to the risk of fetal malformations, oral anti-coagulants are rarely pre-scribed during pregnancy but may be used post-partum, following throm-boembolic episodes. Warfarin is a more powerful anti-coagulant than heparin, and may be used if heparin has been ineffective (Toglia & Weg, 1996). Oral anti-coagulants interfere with the action of vitamin K, which is needed for formation of clotting factors II, VII, IX and X, the anti-clotting factors protein S and protein C, and bone formation in the fetus.

How the body handles warfarin

Administration and absorption of warfarin

Following oral administration, coagulation is gradually affected over several days; this is because warfarin interferes with the production of several clot-ting factors, each with its own half-life. Because thrombin has a half-life of 50–60 hours, warfarin will take two to four days to be fully effective. There-fore, heparin is used for four days or until the internal normalized ratio (INR) [glossary] has been in the therapeutic range for two consecutive days (Ginsberg, 1996).

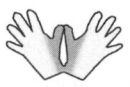 **Practice Point**

It is important that warfarin is taken at the same time each day in relation to meals, as absorp-tion is decreased by the presence of food in the gastro-intestinal tract.

Elimination of warfarin

There is considerable individual variation in the half-life of warfarin (25–60 hours). Warfarin continues to act two to five days after the last dose. Clearance is dependent on hepatic metabolism, which is influenced by age, diseases, such as heart failure and thyroid disorders, and many other drugs, including alcohol and tobacco.

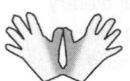 **Practice Point**

Ingestion of a high dose of alcohol (a binge) will inhibit the clearance of warfarin, and precipitate a haemorrhage.

Although warfarin does enter breast milk, breastfeeding may be possible (De Swiet, 1995a; Majerus et al, 1995). There may be an increased risk of haemorrhage in the neonate, accentuated by deficiency of vitamin K (BNF, 2000). Therefore, Malseed et al (1995) consider heparin the preferred anticoagulant if a mother wishes to breastfeed.

Side effects of warfarin

Bleeding

Approximately 10 per cent of those receiving warfarin experience an episode of bleeding; therefore a full blood count, platelets and prothrombin time should be assessed prior to initiation of therapy (McKenry & Salerno, 1998). The risk of bleeding is related to the intensity of therapy and is reduced by regular monitoring of prothrombin time (as INR). The INR may not be entirely accurate in some women with antiphospholipid syndrome (Greaves, 1999); therefore clinical tests of bleeding (see Implications for Practice) assume greater importance.

Should haemorrhage occur, vitamin K_1 (phytomenadione; see below) may be given by slow intravenous injection although this will take up to 24 hours to restore coagulation. Therefore, a concentrate of clotting factors II, VII, IX and X is needed to cover the immediate danger (BNF, 2000).

Skin necrosis

In extremities or fat rich areas this has occurred, typically three to ten days after initiation of therapy. This is attributed to widespread thrombosis of the microvasculature, caused by reduced availability of the anti-clotting factors, proteins C and S. It is important to be aware of this rare problem because lesions may spread rapidly and cause disfigurement (Majerus et al, 1996). Another rare circulatory problem is blue-tinged discolouration of feet three to eight weeks after initiation of therapy due to cholesterol emboli.

Warfarin may cause mouth ulcers, gastro-intestinal disturbances (diarrhoea and vomiting) and liver damage. Hypersensitivity responses may occur: rash, urticaria, fever, nephropathy, reduction in white blood cells, and even agranulocytosis [glossary]. Hereditary resistance to oral anticoagulants has been reported (Majerus et al, 1995).

Effects on the fetus

Risk of fetal damage is appreciable in all trimesters (Hall et al, 1980). Because subcutaneous heparin is less effective than warfarin, warfarin will occasionally be prescribed to women with pre-existing disease; in these circumstances, the midwife will need to understand the associated risks, and the need for close fetal monitoring (De Swiet, 1995a). Malformations are probably dose-related, and warfarin has been used without incident in women with artificial heart valves (n = 20). Warfarin and related drugs interfere with bone formation. This results in a high (30 per cent) incidence of cartilage and bone abnormalities, facial deformities and epiphyseal damage. Use of warfarin is also associated with: high risk of spontaneous abortion (36 per cent), low birth weight, abdominal and CNS malformations (microcephaly, subdural haemorrhage, blindness, spasticity, learning disability) and optic atrophy, possibly secondary to intracranial bleeds. Sadler et al (2000) report only 8 per cent live births in women warfarinized for management of artificial heart valves. Other authors suggest that these incidences are over-estimated by 50 per cent (Reynolds et al, 1996).

Cautions

- Use of warfarin within three weeks of delivery risks intrapartum bleeding, either retroplacental or fetal intracerebral (De Swiet, 1995a).
- Warfarin is used cautiously, if at all, in people with haemorrhagic tendencies (see heparin).
- Atopic individuals may display hypersensitivity responses. The tartrazine present in some brands of warfarin may give rise to allergies (Karch, 1990).
- Warfarin is usually withdrawn over three to four weeks, due to the risk of rebound coagulation (Malseed et al, 1995).

Interactions with warfarin

Warfarin interacts with most (approximately 300) other drugs, some foods, and alcohol. Co-administration of other drugs, such as aspirin, with anticoagulant actions increases the risk of bleeding. Other drugs increase bleeding by decreasing the availability of vitamin K: aminoglycosides, vitamin E, tetracyclines, mineral oils, colestyramine, antibiotics or other agents causing diarrhoea. The effectiveness of warfarin is influenced by the diet. Vitamin K, in cabbage, onions, caffeine or soy, opposes the action of warfarin. A high fat diet increases the absorption of vitamin K. There are reports of ice cream and avocado reducing the effects of warfarin (Stockley, 1999). Oestrogens (including the oral contraceptive pill) and tobacco antagonize the actions of anticoagulants and promote clotting.

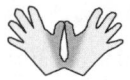 **Practice Point**

A higher dose of warfarin will be needed if the oral contraceptive pill is co-prescribed.

Co-ingestion of antacids may discolour urine (red); although harmless, this may provoke anxiety.

Storage should be in airtight containers, away from heat, light and moisture. Tablet containers should be closed securely.

Implications for Practice: warfarin

Potential Problem	Management
Bleeding	See section on heparin, above.
	Ensure prothrombin time is measured regularly.
	Avoid intramuscular injections.
	Ensure that vitamin K1 and clotting factors are available for intravenous administration.
	Warn women to report any oozing from cuts, bleeding gums, or petechiae.
Drug interactions	Advise against use of OTC medications, tobacco or alcohol and casual use of aspirin or vitamin supplements.
	Assess diet and advise on the importance of regular food intake.
Hepatitis (rare)	Report any symptoms of itching.
Agranulocytosis (rare)	Report any fever, chills, sore throat.
Teratogenicity	Advise of the risks and the need for effective contraception in women using warfarin post-partum.

Conclusion

In the UK, during the triennium 1994–6, there were 48 maternal deaths attributed to thrombosis and thromboembolism, with 46 due to pulmonary embolism and two due to cerebral thrombosis; in addition, there were two late deaths from pulmonary embolism (occurring between 42 days and one year post-partum). These deaths occurred in all stages of pregnancy and the puerperium (DoH, 1998). This represents a noticeable increase over the previous three years. The (very real) risks of osteoporosis may be deterring some doctors from prescribing heparin prophylaxis (Nelson-Piercy, 1997). To minimize the complications associated with these conditions, the midwife has an important role in informing women about the value and potential side effects of anti-coagulant therapies.

Vitamin K₁ phytomenadione

There are two groups of preparations of Vitamin K:

- Water soluble (menadiol). This is contra-indicated in neonates, infants and late pregnancy.
- Fat soluble (phytomenadione), which is discussed in this chapter.

Vitamin K is required for bone formation in the fetus and the formation of clotting factors II, VII, IX and X and anti-clotting factors protein C and protein S in the liver. Deficiency of vitamin K may lead to haemorrhage. Vitamin K is obtained from the diet (green plants, vegetable oils, eggs, cows' milk) and the gut flora. It is fat soluble, stored in the liver, and may be deficient in any malabsorptive state (for example coeliac disease). Vitamin K deficiency is associated with:

- neonates whose mothers who have received antenatal anti-epileptic drugs or anticoagulants or anti-tubercular drugs;
- neonates (particularly premature infants);
- dietary deficiency, including prolonged intravenous feeding;
- malabsorption;
- disruption to gut flora by antibiotics;
- liver disease (including alcohol related), biliary tract disease or surgery;
- oral anticoagulant therapy.

Haemorrhagic disease of the newborn (HDN)

The first report of HDN was by Townsend, in 1894, when the distinction from haemophilia was made (Lane & Hathaway, 1985). It has since been observed that haemorrhage usually begins on the second or third day of life, commonly from the gastro-intestinal tract and is normally self-limiting. Reported incidence in the UK varies widely from 1:20000 in some areas to 1:1200 in others, giving an overall prevalence of 1:10000 (McNinch et al, 1985; McNinch & Tripp, 1991). To date, research has been directed at finding a cure for HDN rather that establishing a cause; thus in most respects, the aetiology of HDN is unknown.

The disease has been sub-divided into three categories:

- **Early onset** at delivery or within 24 hours, in neonates whose mothers have received drugs affecting the metabolism of vitamin K: for example warfarin phenytoin, barbiturates, rifampicin, isoniazid.
- **Classical** during the first two to seven days of life, when bleeding is normally from the umbilicus or gastro-intestinal tract, and is usually self-limiting.

Table 8.2   Haemorrhagic Disease of the Newborn (HDN): comparison of strategies for prophylaxis

Oral vitamin K in neonates
Single dose vitamin K mm offers protection against classical HDN
Dose may not be complete due to dribbling or spitting
Single dose is not effective against late onset HDN, therefore two or three doses are recommended
Prolonged administration time (first six weeks of life) may lead to non-compliance
Is not effective prophylaxis for early onset HDN in high risk babies
More expensive

Intramuscular vitamin K in neonates
Fear and uncertainty of possible association with childhood cancers
Pain and swelling at injection site
Risk of kernicterus in premature infants
Risk of hypersensitivity response
Greater potential for errors

- **Late onset**, eight days – 12 months, predominantly in breastfed babies. This involves sudden onset of intracranial haemorrhage with serious sequelae (Nishigguchi et al, 1996). Vitamin K deficiency may be precipitated by diarrhoea or malabsorption, for example following prolonged administration of antibiotics. Other risk factors include: birth trauma, chronic diarrhoea, cystic fibrosis, malabsorption syndromes, liver disease, biliary atresia, α_{-1} anti-trypsin deficiency (Reynolds et al, 1996).

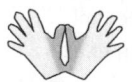 **Practice Point**

High risk infants can be identified, and their parents should receive specialist advice regarding vitamin K therapy.

The fetus acquires a store of vitamin K during the last month *in utero*; however fetal plasma concentrations are always lower than maternal concentrations since the placenta acts as a partial barrier. For the first few days after birth, until the gut flora are established, the healthy neonate has a low intake of vitamin K, particularly if breastfed. In the first few days of life, there is a transient decline in both vitamin K-dependent clotting factors and anti-clotting factors, although the coagulation balance should be maintained in healthy term neonates. Neonatal administration of vitamin K prevents the physiological decline in vitamin K-dependent clotting factors and anti-clotting factors.

Case Report

Late haemorrhagic disease of the newborn is extremely rare. A case is reported from Spain following administration of 1 mg vitamin K intramuscularly at birth.

> The baby was healthy and exclusively breastfed until four weeks of age. Umbilical bleeding then began, followed by an intracranial haemorrhage four days later. Coagulation studies indicated deficiency of vitamin K-dependent clotting factors which was corrected on administration of vitamin K (Solves et al, 1997).

The intramuscular dose in the BNF (2000) is 1 mg. This case illustrates the importance of all health care professionals and parents being alert to the potential severity of bleeding around the umbilicus.

HDN is more likely in infants who are premature, are at high risk (see above) or whose mothers use drugs which affect the metabolism of vitamin K (Marcus & Coulston, 1996). Some anticonvulsants (phenytoin, barbiturates, carbamazepine) and anti-tubercular drugs (rifampicin, isoniazid) increase the clearance of vitamin K-dependent clotting factors. If these drugs have been prescribed during late pregnancy, there is an increased risk of neonatal haemorrhage. However, the inefficiency of placental and breast milk transfer of vitamin K means that antenatal prophylaxis to raise maternal levels of vitamin K will be relatively ineffective in elevating the infant's levels.

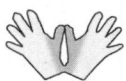 **Practice Points**

- Women taking carbamazepine, phenytoin or phenobarbital should commence oral supplementation with vitamin K four weeks before expected delivery (Nulman et al, 1999).
- Women with intrahepatic cholestasis of pregnancy should receive oral supplements of vitamin K (Campbell & Lees, 2000).
- Intramuscular vitamin K should be given to these neonates immediately following delivery and repeated if necessary (Sawle, 1995; Marcus & Coulston, 1996).

How the body handles vitamin K

Administration of vitamin K may be oral, intramuscular or intravenous. The last route is reserved for emergencies, such as haemorrhage. The route and dose of vitamin K administration to neonates has been the subject of controversy; see Table 8.2 and Implications for Practice. The licensed oral formulation, vitamin K_1 (20) mm (mixed micelle) Paediatric (Konakion ® MM), appears to offer protection from both classical and late onset HDN (Amedee-

Menasme et al, 1992; Isarangkura et al, 1994; Greer et al, 1998). The manufacturer recommends doses at birth and at four to seven days for all babies, followed by a further dose at one month for breastfed babies (*Drugs and Therapeutics Bulletin*, 1998).

Absorption of oral preparations may be too slow to prevent early onset disease in high risk neonates, who should be given intramuscular vitamin K at birth (Reynolds et al, 1996). International comparisons indicate that oral regimens are less effective than intramuscular prophylaxis (Cornelissen et al, 1997).

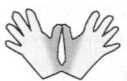 **Practice Point**

Preparations of vitamin K should not be administered by an unlicensed route unless they are so prescribed on a named patient basis, as absorption may be uncertain (*Drugs and Therapeutic Bulletin*, 1998).

Vitamin K_1 is rapidly metabolized and excreted via the liver and kidneys.

Side effects of vitamin K

Vitamin K in the newborn has been associated with haemolytic anaemia, hyperbilirubinaemia and kernicterus [glossary], particularly in premature infants and infants with congenital deficiency of glucose-6-phosphate dehydrogenase (G6PD) or vitamin E deficiency. These problems are much rarer with phytomenadione than with menadiol (Reynolds et al, 1996). Parenteral vitamin K should be administered cautiously to infants under 2.5 kg, because of the increased risk of kernicterus (BNF, 2000).

Thromboembolic disorders have occurred following vitamin K administration in adults; therefore the prothrombin time is monitored for adults receiving regular vitamin K supplementation (Reynolds et al, 1996). Heparin may be used as a 'rescue' medication in these circumstances.

Oral vitamin K is generally well tolerated but may cause nausea, headache or flushing. In liver failure, hepatic function will be further depressed (Peschman, 1992).

Intramuscular administration in adults may cause hypertension, bradycardia, chills, sweating, dyspnoea and hypersensitivity reactions. Alterations in blood viscosity and RBC aggregation have been triggered when vitamin K has been used over a period of several days, probably due to the non-ionic surfactant contained in 'Konakion'® ampoules (Roche, 1995).

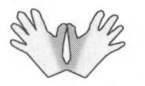 **Practice Point**

Pain and swelling at injection site are not uncommon and should be managed symptomatically.

Intravenous administration is reserved for emergencies, due to the potential severity of the side effects and hypersensitivity responses Administration may be followed by vasodilation and, rarely, cardiovascular system collapse or hypersensitivity responses from rashes to anaphylaxis. Therefore intravenous injections should always be given very slowly (BNF, 2000). Overdose of vitamin K results in anaemia and gastrointestinal tract disturbance.

Childhood malignancy

Childhood malignancy has been linked to intramuscular, but not oral, vitamin K administration in well-publicized studies (Golding et al, 1990; 1992). The possibility of association between intramuscular vitamin K administration and acute lymphoblastic leukaemia between ages one and six was confirmed by a case note retrieval study which simultaneously refuted links with the overall incidence of childhood cancer and leukaemia (Parker et al, 1998). A small additional risk of borderline statistical significance was also found by Passmore et al (1998a). However, other studies have not confirmed this association (von Kries et al, 1996; Ansell et al, 1996; Passmore et al, 1998b; McKinney et al, 1998). The potential human carcinogenicity of vitamin K remains undetermined, but no increase in childhood cancer has been reported since the introduction of vitamin K prophylaxis in the 1960s (Zipursky, 1996).

The research methods used appear to influence the findings in these studies. For example, results may depend on: whether information on route of administration is obtained from notes or inferred from hospital policies; whether matched or unmatched controls are obtained and on how many of the factors (known and unknown) causing 'clustering' of leukaemia are taken into consideration (Parker et al, 1998). It is unfortunate that vitamin K prophylaxis was introduced randomly without prospective randomized controlled trials. Until results of such trials are available, no firm conclusions can be drawn in relation to the safety of vitamin K either as a treatment or prophylaxis. Unfortunately, the follow-up period in these studies will be many years. The relatively low risk of haemorrhagic disease of the newborn (early 0.4–1.7 and late 4.4–10.5 per 100 000 births) is well documented and must be offset against any possible increase in the risk of childhood malignancy, which is a much more common condition (Zipursky, 1996).

Interactions with vitamin K

Vitamin K is rendered ineffective by oral anti-coagulants but not by heparin. These effects persist for two to three weeks after discontinuation of oral anti-coagulants. See Appendix 1 for others.

Cautions and contra-indications

Safety in pregnancy has not been established (Roche, 1995).

Storage

Intramuscular vitamin K and oral vitamin Kmm (mixed micelle) should be stored in light-resistant containers, below 25°C. Freezing must be avoided and turbid solutions should not be used (Roche, 1995). Vitamin K is an irritant; therefore skin contact with the administrator and the recipient should be avoided (Reynolds et al, 1996).

Implications for Practice: vitamin K

Due to continuing uncertainty and controversy, midwives involved in the administration of neonatal vitamin K should ensure that parents are fully informed prior to consenting to prophylactic administration.

Potential Problem	Management
Failure of oral administration	Ensure compliance. Repeat dose if medicine is extruded.
Pain at injection site	Injection should be given slowly and the area gently compressed on completion of the procedure. The site should not be rubbed as this increases bruising.
Concerns over cancer risks	Advise parents of risks and benefits. Offer to discuss the relevant information leaflets. Have current research papers available, should parents require further information. Konakion® MM paediatric oral preparation is likely to be the most effective alternative to intramuscular injection.
Parent refusal	Document refusal and monitor neonate for signs and symptoms of HDN (particularly bleeding around the umbilicus) for the first 12 months of life.

Conculsion

The neonate is born with relatively low concentrations of vitamin K. With breastfeeding, these rise slowly to adult values during the first year of life, thereby putting a small number of babies at risk of HDN.

Further research is needed to:

- determine the aetiology of HDN in order to identify those babies at risk of the disease;
- explore the possible advantages of physiological concentrations of neonatal vitamin K;
- establish the safety of vitamin K for routine prophylaxis.

Further Reading

Greer, F., Marchall, S., Severson, R., Smith, DA., Shearer, M., Pace, D. & Joubert, P. (1998) A new mixed micellar preparation for oral vitamin K prophylaxis. *Archives of Disease in Childhood*:79:4:300–5.

Majerus, P., Broze, G., Miletich, J. & Tollefsen, D. (1996) Anticoagulant, thrombolytic and anti-platelet drugs. In: Hardman, J., Limbard, L., Molinoff, P., Ruddon, R. & Goodman Gilman, A. (eds) *Goodman & Gilman's: The Pharmacological Basis of Therapeutics*. New York, McGraw-Hill, 9th edition, pp. 1341–60.

McKenry, L. & Salerno, E. (1998) *Pharmacology in Nursing*. 20th edition. St. Louis, Mosby.

CHAPTER 9

Cardiovascular Disorders in Pregnancy

SUE JORDAN

This chapter focuses on hypertensive disorders in pregnancy. Cardiac dysrhythmias and cardiac failure are considered briefly

Nifedipine is included under tocolysis, Chapter 7.

Cardiovascular disorders may arise during pregnancy or pre-date conception. The commonest cardiovascular abnormality detected in pregnancy is hypertension. This may be due to pre-existing hypertensive disorders, pregnancy-induced hypertension or pre-eclampsia. These conditions continue to impact on maternal mortality: in the last triennium (1994–6), hypertension accounted for 20 maternal deaths in the UK.

Blood pressure in pregnancy

Normally the blood pressure, systolic and diastolic, falls by 10–15 mmHg during mid-pregnancy. This reverses on delivery, causing blood pressure to peak 3–4 days post-partum. The midwife should explain that observations and any treatment will be continued during this period. For hypertensive women, monitoring for proteinuria and hypertension should continue for 6–12 weeks after delivery (Girling & De Swiet, 1996).

In pregnancy, diastolic BP* should normally be below:

- 75 mmHg in the second trimester;
- 85 mmHg in the third trimester (Badr & Brenner, 1991).

* *Note: It is important that BP measurements are standardized, with instruments that have been validated for use in pregnancy. To avoid confusion, clinicians need to standardize the diastolic measurement using either the K4 (muffled sounds) or the K5 sound (silence) or both (Girling & De Swiet, 1996; Nelson-Piercy, 1996, Helewa et al, 1997).*

Hypertension in pregnancy is defined** as:

- a diastolic BP 15 mmHg above the earliest recorded reading (MacKay & Evans, 1995) *or*
- a systolic BP 30 mmHg above the earliest recorded reading (Campbell & Lees, 2000) *or*
- a diastolic BP above 90 mmHg on two readings four hours or more apart (Gallery, 1995) *or*
- a single diastolic BP reading above 110 mmHg. (Redman & Jefferies 1988; Helewa et al, 1997).

** *Note: There is no consistency in the literature regarding a single definition of either hypertension or pre-eclampsia (Chappell et al, 1999).*

Pregnancy renders the mother's cerebral circulation vulnerable to any hypertensive episode, while, simultaneously, the uterine and placental circulations are unable to autoregulate (adjust) to compensate for hypotension and the associated reduced perfusion pressure (Williams, 1991). Management aims to steer between:

- uncontrolled hypertension, leading to cerebral ischaemia and convulsions or a cerebrovascular accident;
- hypotension, jeopardizing the blood supply to the placenta;
- possible damage to the infant from any drugs administered.

Pre-eclampsia and eclampsia

The literature offers no consensus on a definition of pre-eclampsia. Most authors use a definition of a combination of blood pressure above 140/90 mmHg plus proteinuria greater than 300 mg in 24 hours (Chappell et al, 1999) or a diastolic BP >90 mmHg on two separate days after 20 weeks' gestation plus significant proteinuria, in the absence of pre-pregnancy hypertension (MCHRC, 2000). The safest method of measuring proteinuria in hypertensive women is by estimation of total protein in 24-hour urine collections, as reliance on 'dipstick urinalysis' may fail to detect significant proteinuria (Halligan et al, 1999). Clinical signs and symptoms and other laboratory indicators, such as abnormal liver function tests, coagulopathy, raised haematocrit, raised uric acid and thrombocytopenia, are of the utmost importance (Badr & Brenner, 1991; Gallery, 1995; DoH, 1996).

Pre-eclampsia and eclampsia may occur any time between 20 weeks' gestation and six weeks post-partum. Fifteen per cent of primagravidae are affected. To date, the only effective treatment is removal of the placenta (MacKay & Evans, 1995). Risk factors for pre-eclampsia are listed in Box 9.1 and complications are listed in Box 9.2.

Box 9.1 Risk factors for pre-eclampsia

Linked to possible immune-mediated reactions
- First pregnancy
- Rhesus incompatibility
- Renal disease
- Connective tissue disease (for example rheumatoid arthritis)

Linked to genetic predisposition
- Family history
- Black race
- Age < 16 or > 40
- Prior pre-eclampsia
- Trisomy 13 of fetus

Linked to large placenta
- Multiple pregnancy
- Diabetes
- Molar pregnancy

Linked to atherosclerosis
- Adverse lipid profile
- Essential hypertension
- Obesity
- Insulin resistance
- Raised homocysteine concentrations (associated with low dietary folate)
  (Girling & De Swiet, 1996; Brown, 1997; Roberts & Hubel, 1999)

Box 9.2   Complications of pre-eclampsia

Eclampsia – seziures
Cerebral oedema
Cerebral haemorrhage
Retinal haemorrhages, cortical blindness
DIC (disseminated intravascular coagulation), usually in association with HELLP
HELLP syndrome (haemolysis, elevated liver enzymes, low platelets) in 4–12 per cent of severe cases
Fulminant hepatic failure
Hepatic infarction, subcapsular haematoma and rupture
Acute renal failure
Bilateral renal cortical necrosis
Haemolytic uraemic syndrome
Thrombocytopenia
Disseminated intravascular coagulation (DIC)
Pulmonary oedema, adult respiratory distress syndrome
Congestive cardiac failure
Intra-uterine growth retardation
Placental abruption
Fetal distress, prematurity, intrauterine death
                    (Mackay & Evans, 1995; Girling & De Swiet, 1996; Knox &
                                    Olans, 1996; Nelson-Piercy, 1996)

The **pathophysiological changes** underlying pre-eclampsia and eclampsia require further research which, at present, is hampered by the absence of an animal model for this disease. A variety of mechanisms have been proposed, some of which have led to trials of therapeutic interventions (Brown, 1997). It would appear that placentation fails, leaving the blood vessels supplying the placenta too narrow to sustain development during the second and third trimesters. The failure of the maternal spiral arteries to dilate (during second wave trophoblast invasion) impairs fetal development and induces placental ischaemia. The placenta responds by releasing cytokines [glossary] which activate platelets, promote coagulation and damage maternal endothelial cells [glossary], triggering widespread vasoconstriction (Pipkin et al, 1996). This reduces the intravascular volume, making the woman vulnerable to both fluid overload and dehydration. Eventually, deposition of fibrin on the lining of the blood vessels leads to end-organ damage, particularly in the kidneys (Knox & Olans, 1996).

Eclamptic seizures are attributed to unremitting vasospasm, raising BP beyond the autoregulatory adjustment capacity of the cerebral blood vessels. This produces oedema, ischaemia, micro-infarctions and patches of small haemorrhages in areas of cerebral cortex on the borders of the territories of major arteries, particularly in the occipital cortex. In turn, ischaemia reduces the threshold for seizure activity (Chen et al, 1995; Naidu et al, 1996). This can occur with only a moderately elevated BP.

Case Report

It is important that complaints of headache are not dismissed as trivial (Katz et al, 2000).

A patient admitted with severe pre-eclampsia of 29 weeks' gestation, complained of a headache. Junior medical staff prescribed co-proxamol over the telephone, failing to appreciate the significance of a rise in BP. Ninety minutes later, she convulsed. (DoH, 1996: 27).

Detection of pre-eclampsia traditionally depended on the triad of hypertension, proteinuria and oedema. However rapid deterioration in the presence of only one of these signs has been known (DoH, 1996). Any delay in recognition of pre-eclampsia may be fatal to both mother and baby.

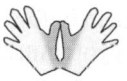 **Practice Points**

- Hypertension with proteinuria (>300 mg in 24 hours) indicates the need for urgent (same day) hospital admission (Girling and De Swiet, 1996).
- Important clinical changes include: severe headache, visual disturbance, epigastric tenderness, proteinuria, retention of uric acid or sodium, consumptive coagulopathy and hyper-reflexia leading to convulsions (Badr & Brenner, 1991). Other diagnostic indicators include: thrombocytopenia, raised uric acid levels and abnormal liver function tests (DoH, 1996).

Management of pre-eclampsia and eclampsia

While the underlying causes of pre-eclampsia and eclampsia remain unclear, management will continue to be empirically based. The goals of management remain: prevention of convulsions, control of severe hypertension and delivery of the fetus and placenta (Chen et al, 1995).

- The initial management of mild or moderate pre-eclampsia may be non-pharmacological. **Rest**, combined with **careful monitoring**, at home or in hospital may be considered. By centrally redistributing the blood flow, bed rest improves the perfusion of the placenta, kidneys, heart, brain and liver and alleviates ischaemia (MacKay and Evans, 1995). The woman should be warned that a diuresis usually follows. A left lateral position may be optimal (Kulb, 1990). When bed rest is prescribed, the risks of thromboembolic disorder should be considered.

- **Controlling blood pressure** protects the mother from the cerebral complications of hypertension but does not influence the disease process underlying pre-eclampsia. There is a danger that signs of disease progression may be masked (Girling and De Swiet, 1996).

Case Report

Anti-hypertensives may be ineffective in eclampsia.

An in-patient of 29 weeks' gestation was treated with labetolol for severe pre-eclampsia. A course of corticosteroids was commenced to hasten fetal maturity. However, after five days, BP suddenly rose, precipitating convulsions (DoH, 1996: 26).

The administration of corticosteroids to a woman whose circulation was contracted due to severe pre-eclampsia may have been the decisive factor in precipitating hypertension.

- **Close monitoring** of urine output and vital signs is essential, before, during and after pharmacological intervention. The density of proteinuria indicates the extent of renal damage. Coagulation may cause necrosis of the renal cortices which indicates a poor outlook for renal function. Renal failure may follow (Badr & Brenner, 1991).
- **Dietary supplements and aspirin** (see Box 9.3) have been suggested as prophylaxis, but larger, prospective, randomized controlled trials have not confirmed efficacy (Sibai, 1998). Calcium supplementation did not improve outcomes in hypertensive disorders in pregnancy in a large randomized controlled trial (n = 4589, Levine et al, 1997). Aspirin, fish oils and evening primrose oil alter the composition of endothelial cell membranes. However they may be metabolized to produce free radicals which damage, rather than heal, cell membranes (Pipkin et al, 1996) or increase the risk of infant brain haemorrhage (Olsen et al, 2000). Oral magnesium taurate has also been investigated (McCarthy, 1996).
- **Sedatives**, including opioids and prochlorperazine, are **avoided**, due to depressant effects on the central nervous systems of mother and fetus which interfere with monitoring (MacKay & Evans, 1995).
- **Diuretics** will **dangerously worsen** the condition. In pre-eclampsia, the circulating volume is already contracted. This is compounded by the administration of diuretics, thus jeopardizing the already precarious blood supply to the placenta (Hopkinson, 1995).

Box 9.3 Aspirin and pre-eclampsia and pregnancy

Pre-eclampsia may be characterized by increased endothelial thromboxane [glossary] activity; this would imply that aspirin could be an effective therapeutic strategy. Accordingly, aspirin has been investigated as prophylaxis in women at high risk of early onset pre-eclampsia. In a review of 42 trials, 75 mg aspirin/day from 12–20 weeks slightly reduced the risk of pre-eclampsia, pre-term delivery and neonatal death (Knight et al, 2000). However in large studies, low dose aspirin* (for example 75 mg/day controlled release) had no effects, either beneficial or deleterious (CLASP, 1994; Rotchell et al, 1998; Duley, 1999).

Further research is need to establish the safest and most effective dose of aspirin for the prevention of pre-eclampsia. The 60 mg/day dose of aspirin has been widely used, but while this is sufficient to inhibit platelet activation, it does not prevent other inflammatory processes which may be more important in pre-eclampsia. This requires a 150 mg/day dose of aspirin (Pipkin et al, 1996).

The prescription of high dose of aspirin (3 g or ten tablets per day) for various condition in pregnancy resulted in: prolonged gestation and labour; increased blood loss at delivery; higher risks of pre-eclampsia and neonatal intracranial haemorrhage (Byron, 1995). Aspirin use in the last trimester risks increasing blood loss at delivery, the incidence of minor bleeding complications in neonates (Howden, 1995) and premature closure of the ductus arteriosus, associated with neonatal lung damage (Lee & Schofield, 1994b). Even 60 mg/day in early pregnancy for pre-eclampsia has been associated with an increased risk of placental abruption, bleeding disorders and post-partum haemorrhage (Golding, 1998). Therefore use of aspirin may be reserved for women with high risk of severe disease (Reynolds et al, 1996). However occasional use of aspirin for migraine is probably not harmful (Pfaffenrath & Rehm, 1998).

* Aspirin tablets for analgesia contain a dose of 300 mg (BNF, 2000).

- **Anticonvulsant prophylaxis** in women who have not suffered a seizure remains controversial. Magnesium sulphate is currently the preferred anticonvulsant in severe pre-eclampsia (Chien et al, 1996; Duley et al, 2000). In a randomized controlled trial (n = 685) of women with severe pre-eclampsia, Coetzee et al (1998) found that magnesium prophylaxis reduced the risk of convulsions (by a ratio of 11 to 1). Some obstetricians prescribe magnesium to pre-eclamptic patients if hyper-reflexia is present (Smith and McEwan, 1997).

- **Control of convulsions** may involve either magnesium sulphate or diazepam. Since diazepam is familiar to all junior doctors in the UK, and the therapeutic range is relatively wide, it may be given by intravenous injection or rectal solution to rapidly terminate seizures. Any delay in controlling convulsions will be detrimental (Fox and Draycott, 1996).

Magnesium sulphate

This section focuses on the use of magnesium sulphate to control eclampsia. However there is ongoing debate as to the optimum management of pre-eclampsia and eclampsia.

Magnesium sulphate is currently the drug of choice to prevent further fits in established eclampsia (Eclampsia Trial Collaborative Group, 1995). In this large study (n = 1680), magnesium sulphate was demonstrated to be more effective than either diazepam or phenytoin in preventing recurrent seizures and was associated with fewer maternal deaths. Subsequently, the role of phenytoin in obstetrics has been very limited. Following publication of this trial, magnesium sulphate was widely adopted for the management of eclampsia in the UK. However the dose used varies with institution (Smith and McEwan, 1997). Analysis of the trial data indicated that the higher doses used in the intramuscular regimen were more effective in reducing seizures where laboratory monitoring facilities were limited (Graham, 1998). In the USA, magnesium has been employed as an anticonvulsant and a tocolytic since 1925 (Robson, 1996). The administration of magnesium sulphate is not without hazards (DoH, 1996), and it is therefore reserved for women who are seriously ill (see Implications for Practice).

How the body handles magnesium

Administration of magnesium

Magnesium sulphate may be administered by deep intramuscular injection (into the gluteal region) or intravenously with rapid effect. With the patient placed in the recovery position, seizures may be arrested by an intravenous bolus of magnesium sulphate, administered slowly, for example as 4 g or 16 mmol over five to ten minutes. An infusion is then administered and continued for 24 hours after the last fit at a rate of 1 g every hour (BNF, 2000), but regimens of 2 g/hour are also recommended (Robson, 1996; Graham, 1998). Bolus doses of 2 g may be given slowly, over at least five minutes, should convulsions recur (BNF, 2000). The dose of magnesium may be reduced gradually over a two to three hour period (Kulb, 1990).

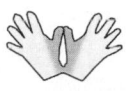 **Practice Points**

- If intravenous infusions are administered, the patient must be carefully monitored for signs of fluid overload, particularly in pre-eclampsia and eclampsia, when intravascular space is contracted.
- Absorption from intramuscular injections may be slow or unpredictable if circulation has been reduced due to pre-eclampsia or shock.
- Kulb (1990) reports the use of lignocaine to minimize the pain of intramuscular injections, which are repeated every four hours for 24 hours after the last fit.
- Local abscess formation complicates 0.5 per cent of im administrations (Eclampsia Trial Collaborative Group, 1995).

Distribution of magnesium

Magnesium crosses the placenta and affects the fetus in a manner similar to the adult. Magnesium concentrations remain elevated for 24–48 hours after birth (Kulb, 1990). The blood/brain barrier may delay the passage of magnesium into the CNS; plasma and CNS concentrations equalise in approximately three hours (Chen et al, 1995). In eclampsia (but not pre-eclampsia) the blood brain/barrier may not be intact, allowing rapid entry in the CNS.

Elimination of magnesium

The kidneys are responsible for the elimination of magnesium. The elimination half-life of magnesium is four hours in pregnancy but much longer if the glomerular filtration rate [glossary] falls (Lu & Nightingale, 2000). Therefore the rate of infusion must be in line with renal function, which may change rapidly during the course of the illness. Since pre-eclampsia and eclampsia cause renal impairment, it is important that an accurate measure of renal function (usually serum creatinine*) is available for all women likely to require magnesium sulphate in an emergency.

* Note: When interpreting laboratory results, it should be remembered that 'normal' values change during pregnancy. Both renal plasma flow and GFR (glomerular filtration rate) increase 30–50 per cent, in keeping with increased metabolic demands. Therefore, serum creatinine falls, and any value over 70 μ mol/l is indicative of renal compromise. In pre-eclampsia, the glomerular endothelial cells become vacuolated and swell. This reduces the blood flow into the glomeruli and hence the GFR, causing serum creatinine to rise to the normal level for a non-pregnant female (up to 120 μ mol/l). Failure to consider this could result in seriously abnormal laboratory tests being misinterpreted as 'normal', leading to administration of more magnesium than can be cleared by the patient's kidneys.

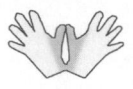 **Practice Point**

During magnesium administration, urine output is closely monitored, as a guide to renal function. Urine output must be at least 25 ml/hour or 100 ml in the four hours prior to administration of each dose (Malseed et al, 1995).

Toxic levels of magnesium can be reached very quickly if the urine output is below normal (Kulb, 1990). If urine output falls and there are no other signs of magnesium toxicity, infusion may be maintained at half the normal rate, combined with plasma magnesium concentration monitoring (Duley, 1996; Robson, 1996).

The literature offers no consensus on the need to monitor plasma magnesium concentration. Robson (1996) advises monitoring if seizure prophylaxis fails, urine output falls below 100 ml every four hours, signs of toxicity are apparent or staff are inexperienced in administering magnesium (see Table 9.2).

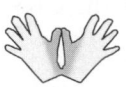 **Practice Points**

- To minimize the effect of cell leakage and obtain an accurate result, blood for magnesium monitoring should be delivered to the laboratory immediately.
- Current therapy should be noted, particularly calcium gluconate, which can interfere with laboratory tests (Byrne et al, 1986).

Actions of magnesium

Magnesium is vitally important for metabolism, smooth muscle regulation, nerve conduction and impulse transmission (Rude & Oldham, 1990). Increased concentrations of magnesium (hypermagnesaemia, see Table 9.2) depress the activity of all excitable tissue (see Box 9.4).

It is thought that magnesium treats eclampsia by relieving the spasm of cerebral blood vessels which improves cerebral perfusion (Naidu et al, 1996). Magnesium also protects the capillary endothelium from damage by free radicals [glossary], which are released in all inflammatory processes. However eclamptic fits have occurred despite magnesium phrophylaxis and concentrations within the therapeutic range (Katz et al, 2000).

Box 9.4   Actions of magnesium

Hypermagnesaemia depresses the activity of all excitable tissue by:

1. **Reduced calcium entry** into:
   (a) **Nerve cells**
   Magnesium ions compete with calcium ions for entry into presynaptic nerve terminals. This decreases neurotransmitter release at synapses. Reduced release of acetylcholine at myoneural junctions causes relaxation of skeletal muscle. Similarly, reduced release of noradrenaline (norepinephrine) from sympathetic nerves supplying vascular smooth muscle causes hypotension.
   (b) **Cardiac muscle**, causing heart block
   Hypermagnesaemia reduces entry of calcium ions into muscle cells which induces relaxation of smooth muscle and, in high concentrations, heart muscle. The competitive actions between calcium and magnesium mean that calcium is an effective short term antidote to magnesium toxicity (Rude & Oldham, 1990).
   (c) **Smooth muscle**
   Contraction of all smooth muscle, including blood vessels, uterus and gut, is inhibited.
   This reverses cerebral vasospasm but induces hypotension.
2. Reduced nerve conduction velocity, that is slowing nerve impulse transmission.
3. Blocking excitatory receptors in the CNS.

Side effects of magnesium

Magnesium sulphate is extremely potent and must be administered cautiously, as its side effects are various and hazardous, affecting all systems of the body, and combining to cause problems ranging from generalized discomfort to cardiac arrest (See Implications for Practice). Side effects may be understood in terms of depression of excitable tissue (Table 9.1) and increasing magnesium concentrates (see Table 9.2).

Cardiovascular system

Arterioles   Magnesium relaxes the smooth muscle of arterioles. This reverses the cerebral vasospasm responsible for eclamptic seizures. It also improves blood flow in the maternal uterine artery, which is responsible for some cases of preterm labour. However, smooth muscle of systemic arterioles is also relaxed, inducing flushing, sweating, hypothermia, hypotension and even cardiovascular collapse.

Table 9.1 Summary of actions and side effects of magnesium sulphate

Depressant actions of magnesium on:	Potential end point or disaster
Smooth muscle of:	
Blood vessels, especially arterioles	Cardiovascular collapse
Uterus	Tocolysis
Gut	Vomiting, paralytic ileus
Heart	Cardiac arrest
	Pulmonary oedema
Skeletal muscle	Flaccid paralysis, respiratory arrest
CNS	Somnolence, loss of consciousness
Coagulation	Bleeding
Plasma calcium concentration	Tetany

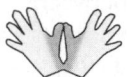 **Practice Points**

- Thirst, warmth and flushing are early signs of magnesium toxicity (Malseed et al, 1995).
- Hypothermia may mask the signs of infection (Hill, 1995).
- The anti-hypertensive effect of magnesium may not be sustained (Kulb, 1990). Therefore it is important that vital signs are monitored regularly throughout administration.

Heart

Magnesium, in high concentrations, depresses the rate and force of cardiac contractions. This results in: bradycardia, widened QRS complexes, heart block, chest pain and eventually cardiac arrest or pulmonary oedema. Cardiac toxicity intensifies with increasing magnesium concentrations, culminating in asystole; however the concentration of magnesium at which asystole occurs varies among individuals (4–15 mmol/litre). Continuous ECG monitoring may reduce the risk of serious cardiac dysrhythmias.

Case Report

A multiparous woman with signs of pre-eclampsia was admitted to hospital and a magnesium infusion was started. The fetal heart rate decreased, and the woman was transferred to theatre for an emergency Caesarean section. During transfer, the woman complained of nausea and flushing. She suddenly vomited, lost consciousness, stopped breathing and developed ventricular fibrillation. It was then discovered that, during transfer, the magnesium infusion pump had been removed, and the woman had received 1 gram of magnesium sulphate per minute for some ten minutes. After resuscitation, the woman made a full recovery in intensive care. After delivery by emergency section, the baby was initially flaccid but had an Apgar score of 7 at five minutes (Morisaki et al, 2000).

If a magnesium infusion is allowed to flow freely, cardiopulmonary arrest can occur without warning signs.

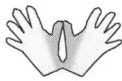 **Practice Point**

Too rapid administration of magnesium may induce serious dysrhythmia or maternal cardiac arrest (Crowther, 1990).

The fetus may demonstrate decreased heart rate variability and baseline heart rate (Hill, 1995); continuous fetal heart monitoring is essential (Robson, 1996; Kulb, 1990).

Pulmonary oedema has been associated with magnesium administration for tocolysis in around 1 per cent of patients. Pulmonary oedema is the main cause of death in severe pre-eclampsia (Walker, 2000). Excessive infusion of fluids, and the associated plasma dilution, is the commonest cause of pulmonary oedema (Hill, 1995).

Case Report

Attention to fluid balance is of vital importance. In the UK, six of the 20 deaths due to hypertensive disorders were associated with circulatory overload.

One patient with severe pre-eclampsia suffered a post-partum haemorrhage after induction of labour. She was transfused with 2.5 l of crystalloid plus 4 litres of colloid plus blood. This volume of fluid can not be accommodated in the contracted vascular compartment of eclampsia, and pulmonary oedema and adult respiratory distress syndrome ensued (DoH, 1996: 27).

Very close observation of input and output must be maintained. High risk situations include:

- decreased intravascular fluid volume, as in pre-eclampsia and eclampsia;
- fluid overload;
- administration of corticosteroids (to aid fetal lung maturation);
- fluid retention;
- decreased renal function;
- impaired cardiac function/contractility;
- tachycardia;

- infection: occult sepsis injures pulmonary capillaries;
- prolonged therapy >48 hours;
- anaemia;

Bleeding tendency

Alongside the altered coagulation of pre-eclampsia and eclampsia, magnesium sulphate also affects clotting times. Magnesium administration was associated with a higher rate of post-partum haemorrhage in a retrospective cohort study (Szal et al, 1999). Hypermagnesaemia depresses the activity of platelets, increases clotting times and reduces thrombin generation, thereby impairing coagulation (Rude & Oldham, 1990; Assaley et al, 1998). However disseminated intravascular coagulation may still occur (Crowther, 1990). Therefore venous blood samples are frequently needed for coagulation monitoring.

Skeletal muscle paralysis

Magnesium inhibits contraction of skeletal muscle, depressing deep tendon reflexes and contractility of all muscles, including the muscles of respiration. Muscle weakness and fatigue are early signs of impending toxicity. Flaccid paralysis is possible in mother, fetus or neonate.

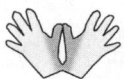 **Practice Point**

- Reflexes, such as the patellar reflex (knee jerk), are tested regularly, certainly before each dose, as this may be the first indication of magnesium toxicity. If reflexes are absent, magnesium must be withheld, because respiratory depression is likely to follow (Malseed et al, 1995; Duley, 1996).

Weakness and gastrointestinal tract stasis combine to cause nausea and anorexia. Reduced protein intake may be compounded by high renal losses.

Respiratory system

Weakness of **respiratory muscles** depresses ventilation and causes hypoxia (see Chapter 4, opioids). Regular oxygen saturation monitoring will reduce this danger (Robson, 1996). At very high concentrations, magnesium causes apnoea, in mother or neonate, due to a combination of central and peripheral actions (Rude and Oldham, 1990). Pritchard et al (1984) report one maternal death from respiratory arrest.

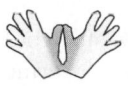 **Practice Points**

- Respiratory rate and depth are checked regularly, and a minimum value of 16 resps/minute should be recorded before each dose is administered (Malseed et al, 1995).
- It is also important to check the neonate for adequate ventilation and to guard against sudden cessation of respiratory movements (Olsen & D'Oria, 1992; Hill, 1995).

Central nervous system (CNS)

Somnolence, blurred or double vision, nausea, nystagmus [glossary] and slurred speech may be the first signs of a rising magnesium concentration, but these may not be easily detected in an eclamptic patient. Higher concentrations of magnesium lead progressively to confusion and coma (Rude & Oldham, 1990). Therefore regular assessment of conscious level is extremely important.

Kidneys

Magnesium dilates renal arterioles, which maintain urine output (Crowther, 1990). Since magnesium is osmotically active, its elimination may cause an osmotic diuresis (Hill, 1995). These factors may combine to dehydrate the patient, unless fluid balance is carefully maintained.

Uterus

Magnesium sulphate decreases the amplitude and frequency of uterine contractions; therefore it is employed as a tocolytic in the USA. Magnesium antagonizes oxytocin, making vaginal delivery more difficult (Kulb, 1990), and Caesarean section more likely (Chien et al, 1996; Khan & Chien, 1997). Women receiving magnesium require higher doses of oxytocin (Witlin et al, 1997). However duration of labour may be more closely associated with epidural anaesthesia than magnesium therapy (Chapter 4). A statistically insignificant trend towards longer labour with magnesium therapy has been reported (Szal et al, 1999).

GI tract

Nausea and vomiting are common side effects of magnesium therapy; they result from the combination of actions on the CNS and GI tract. Constipation becomes clinically significant with long term parenteral therapy. Paralytic ileus is a rare complication of magnesium therapy (Hill, 1995).

Hypocalcaemia

With long term therapy, magnesium reduces the secretion of parathyroid hormone, which is responsible for controlling calcium losses in the urine (Rude & Oldham, 1990). This results in increased urinary losses of calcium, and eventually causes bone demineralization in mother and fetus. It is reversible on discontinuation of therapy (Hill, 1995). Short term administration of magnesium increases the quantity of calcium lost in the urine, and may cause maternal or neonatal hypocalcaemia, tetany and even fits (Lu & Nightingale, 2000).

Emergency measures/'rescue' medications

The depressant actions of magnesium are competitively inhibited by calcium. Therefore, calcium gluconate is an effective **temporary** antidote in magnesium toxicity. Ten ml of 10 per cent calcium gluconate is administered intravenously over three to five minutes (Kulb, 1990). Dialysis provides a more permanent means of correcting magnesium imbalance.

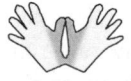 **Practice Point**

To facilitate use in an emergency, it is recommended that 10 per cent calcium gluconate (10 ml) is kept in a pre-filled syringe by the side of any patient receiving a magnesium infusion (Smith & McEwan, 1997).

Management of eclampsia, severe pre-eclampsia or preterm labour entails infusion of magnesium until the plasma concentration is above the normal physiological range; therefore the midwife should observe the patient closely for the first signs of these problems.

Neonatal side effects of magnesium

The neonate should be monitored for the side effects of magnesium, particularly respiratory depression, for the first 48 hours. If the mother is ill enough to be receiving magnesium therapy, the neonate is likely to be at high risk (see Table 9.2). Currently, there is little evidence of any association between long term problems and magnesium therapy (Idama & Lindow, 1998; Riaz et al, 1998).

Table 9.2 Clinical effects of increasing serum magnesium concentrations

Serum magnesium concentration in mmol/l	Clinical effect
0.75–1.5	Normal physiological range
1.8–3*	Therapeutic range for tocolysis and seizure control, some depression of deep tendon reflexes (for example patellar reflex)
2.5–3.5*	Target range for severe pre-eclampsia Depression of deep tendon reflexes
3.5–5	ECG shows some evidence of heart block, that is wide QRS complex and prolonged PQ interval; hypotension; somnolence; loss of deep tendon reflexes. **Warning signs of toxicity**
5	Respiratory depression. **Toxicity**
6–7.5	Respiratory paralysis; complete heart block, that is extreme bradycardia of 15–40 beats/minute and collapse
12.5 (range 4–15)	Cardiac asystole

* *Target range varies among authors*
Source: McKenry and Salerno, 1998:340; Olsen and D'Oria, 1992; Idama & Lindow, 1998; Lu & Nightingale, 2000.

Breathing

High concentrations of magnesium may cause apnoea in the neonate. The risk of neonatal respiratory depression is increased if magnesium is administered within two hours of delivery (McKenry & Salerno, 1998). In one study (n = 64), magnesium administration was associated with poor Apgar score and increased Caesarean section rate for fetal distress (Chen et al, 1995). However babies born after administration of magnesium were less likely to have a low Apgar score at one minute or to be admitted to special care baby units than those whose mothers had received either diazepam or phenytoin (Crowther, 1990; Eclampsia Trial Collaborative Group, 1995). Neonatal depression may not be easily reversed by calcium gluconate administration (Pangle, 2000), and intensive care facilities may be needed.

Unchecked, **hypocalcaemia** may result in tetany or neonatal convulsions (Malseed et al, 1995). Therefore monitoring for serum clacium concentration is undertaken and calcium gluconate administered if necessary (see Chapter 16).

Breastfeeding

If the neonate is hypermagnesaemic, this may cause drowsiness, blunted reflexes and respiratory depression (Hill, 1995). The neonate may have poor muscle tone (be 'floppy'), cry weakly or demonstrate neurobehavioural impairment (Chen et al, 1995; Riaz et al, 1998). Drowsiness, combined with decreased muscle tone, makes breastfeeding difficult. However, since magnesium will have been eliminated by 24–48 hours, extra support may be sufficient to establish breastfeeding, if the mother is well enough. Breast-feeding is considered safe 24 hours after the last dose of magnesium, as women with normal renal function will have normal plasma magnesium concentrations by that time (Idama & Lindow, 1998). Decisions will be taken in the light of post-partum magnesium and renal function measurements.

Cautions and contra-indications

Pre-existing heart block, cardiac disease, or myasthenia gravis are likely to be worsened. Caution is advised in renal, hepatic or respiratory impairment.

Interactions with magnesium sulphate

Since magnesium administered to the mother passes into the neonate, it is important that drugs administered to the neonate as well as the mother are checked for potentially dangerous interactions.

- Increased CNS depression, leading to confusion and loss of consciousness may occur if sedatives are administered: for example opioids, benzodiazepines, alcohol, phenothiazines (for example prochlorperazine/Stemetil®) and anaesthetics, including nitrous oxide.
- Magnesium potentiates and prolongs the actions of all drugs inhibiting neuromuscular transmission, including muscle relaxants, local anaesthetics (for example epidurals), calcium antagonists (such as nifedipine) and aminoglycoside antibiotics (such as gentamicin). This increases the risks of hypotension, paralytic ileus, and respiratory depression or paralysis (Malseed et al, 1995; Hill, 1995). If a Caesarean section is performed on a woman who has received magnesium sulphate, the dose of muscle relaxants will be adjusted accordingly. Intravenous calcium gluconate is always available, should it be needed to assist recovery (Stockley, 1999).

Case Reports

Drug interactions must be checked before drug administration to either neonate or mother.

A woman with pre-eclampsia had been successfully managed with magnesium sulphate. However, she was noted to have muscle weakness and a serum magnesium concentration above normal limits. When the baby girl was 12 hours old, she received ampicillin plus gentamicin for a severe infection. After the second dose of gentamicin, the baby stopped breathing; she survived, due to prompt intubation. Her condition improved when the gentamicin was discontinued (Stockley, 1999:118).

The additive effects of magnesium plus gentamicin are sufficient to induce neuromuscular blockade. The kidneys of neonates eliminate magnesium very slowly. Therefore, this drug combination is potentially hazardous, and is only safe where facilities exist for artificial ventilation. Where two drugs have the same action, they may dangerously potentiate each other (Stockley, 1999:412).

A woman of 32 weeks' gestation received nifedipine for premature uterine contractions. However, 12 hours later, contractions returned and intravenous magnesium sulphate was administered for tocolysis. The woman developed jerky movements in the extremities (tetany), difficulty in swallowing, paradoxical respirations and muscle weakness so intense that she was unable to lift her head from the pillow. Magnesium was discontinued, and the woman recovered within the next 25 minutes.

This case illustrates the hazards of drug interactions, particularly in units where certain agents are rarely needed.

- The risks of cardiovascular side effects, particularly pulmonary oedema, become unacceptably high if magnesium is combined with a β_2 agonist (such as ritodrine for tocolysis or salbutamol for asthma).

Implications for Practice: magnesium

Magnesium infusions are adjusted in accordance with the results of laboratory and clinical monitoring. The midwife should be prepared to discontinue magnesium therapy and place the patient in the recovery position should signs of toxicity develop. In the Eclampsia Trial Collaborative Group (1995) protocol, patellar reflexes and respirations were checked every 15 minutes, more frequently during the first one to two hours of an intravenous infusion and before each intramuscular dose (Duley, 1996). In many centres, blood is taken every four to six hours to monitor magnesium concentrations, in addition to close clinical observations (McKenry & Salerno, 1998).

Potential problem	Management
Hypotension	Vital signs every 15 minutes. Monitor urine output.
Muscle weakness/ flaccid paralysis	Deep tendon reflexes, for example patella reflex every 15 minutes and before each dose.
Respiratory depression and apnoea	Monitor respiratory rate and depth every 15 minutes. 16 resps/min. is the minimum acceptable rate. Pulse oximetry. Ensure oxygen is available by mask. Ensure facilities for intubation and ventilation are in place. Ensure calcium gluconate is available, for example in a pre-filled syringe at the bedside containing 10–20 mmol calcium gluconate 10 per cent for slow intravenous injection. Monitor neonate; apnoea may occur suddenly. Ensure ventilatory support is available for the neonate, if required.

Implications for Practice: magnesium (*continued*)

Potential problem	Management
Cardiac dysrhythmia and cardiac arrest	Continuous ECG to detect dysrhythmias. Calcium gluconate, and a protocol for administration, must be available to manage any magnesium toxicity (see above). Expertise to carry out emergency intubation must be available. Continuous monitoring of fetal heart rate.
Pulmonary oedema	Strict fluid balance records. Monitor heart rate. Auscultation of lung bases. Note the development of dyspnoea/breathlessness. Monitor protein loss in the urine.
CNS depression	Assessment of conscious level of patient. Special care facilities available for neonate. Support mother in breastfeeding. This may be difficult for the first 48 hours, while the neonate is eliminating magnesium.
Decreased uterine activity	Monitor uterine activity. Ensure facilities for Caesarean section are in place.
Impaired coagulation	Haematological monitoring: platelets plus clotting times. Monitor blood loss at delivery. Facilities for transfusion should be in place.
Accumulation of magnesium	Monitor urine output. Record every hour. Minimum level is 25 ml/hour. Ensure a measure of renal function, for example creatinine concentration, is available for women who may require magnesium therapy.
Nausea and vomiting	Strict fluid balance. Provide support. Monitor plasma proteins.
Paralytic ileus	Monitor appetite and intake post-partum. Monitor stool output until bowel function is restored.
Tetany, neonatal convulsions	Ensure availability of calcium gluconate.
Hypothermia	Monitor core temperature. Ensure signs of infection are not overlooked. Maintain patient comfort. Ensure neonate is well protected from the cold.
Sweating and flushing	Maintain patient comfort and check for further signs of rising magnesium concentration.
Lack of effect, seizures	Convulsions may occur before or after delivery, despite magnesium therapy. Therefore, vigilance will need to be maintained. Monitor serum calcium in mother and neonate.

Conclusion

At the time of writing, the role of magnesium therapy in pre-eclampsia remains uncertain (Khan & Chien, 1997; Thornton, 2000). The use of any anticonvulsants in pre-eclampsia, where the risk of convulsions is only 1 per cent, remains controversial (Chen et al, 1995; Robson, 1996). In South Africa, Coetzee et al (1998) demonstrated the benefit of magnesium for women with the most severe pre-eclampsia, defined as symptoms of imminent eclampsia, diastolic BP ≥110 mmHg and proteinuria; however Hall et al (2000) found that women with pre-eclampsia prior to labour derived no benefit from magnesium therapy. Unfortunately, as few as 9/53 (17 per cent) of eclamptic seizures can be predicted from the presence of pre-eclampsia, and not all of these will be prevented by administration of magnesium sulphate (Katz et al, 2000). Before the use of magnesium sulphate can be extended to lower risk women, it will be important to demonstrate conclusively that it carries no substantial risk to the neonate (Duley & Neilson, 1999). If magnesium is employed indiscriminately for pre-eclampsia, it will gain a reputation for serious adverse effects (Chen et al, 1995).

In view of the findings of the Eclampsia Trial Collaborative Group (1995), failure to use magnesium in established eclampsia can no longer be justified. Unfortunately, in some centres/units, this is likely to produce a situation where a potentially dangerous drug is used only once or twice a year, so that problems may arise due to inexperience with this potent drug (Smith & McEwan, 1997). This will strengthen the arguments for the establishment of regional centres specializing in the management of eclampsia in high dependency environments (DoH, 1996).

Pregnancy induced hypertension and hypertension in pregnancy

The clinical presentation and management of these conditions may be indistinguishable. Hypertension noted during the first trimester is likely to predate pregnancy, but pre-eclampsia* cannot be automatically excluded without thorough investigation, as this will dramatically affect clinical management. Unlike chronic essential hypertension, pregnancy induced hypertension will have resolved spontaneously by six weeks post-partum. Hypertension may be secondary to other, non-pregnancy related conditions which will require investigation such as renal disease (repeated UTI), steroid therapy, endocrine disorders, co-arctation of the aorta (Nelson-Piercy, 1996).

* *Note: Pre-eclampsia is distinguished from other forms of hypertension by the presence of proteinuria, coagulation disorders, liver dysfunction or contracted cirulatory volume (raised haematocrit) (Gallery, 1995).*

Mild, uncomplicated chronic hypertension is a relatively benign condition (Sibai, 1996). However hypertensive disorders in pregnancy have been associated with superimposed pre-eclampsia, placental abruption, IUGR, increased maternal and perinatal morbidity and mortality, and increased long term risks of renal disorders and hypertension (Nisell et al, 1995; Sibai, 1996; see Implications for Practice). Severe hypertension (>170/110 mmHg) will require pharmacological intervention to prevent maternal cerebrovascular accidents (Plouin et al, 1990; Sibai, 1996). Perinatal outcome is related to both duration and severity of hypertension (Shah & Reed, 1996). However, the effect of hypertension and antihypertensive medications on IUGR is disputed (McCowan et al, 1996; Plouin et al, 1990). Whatever drug is used, reduction in BP may be excessive, jeopardizing the blood flow to the placenta, which lacks autoregulatory capability; this may explain purported associations with IUGR and prematurity (von Dadelszein et al, 2000).

Some uncertainty remains concerning the selection and initiation of antihypertensive medications in pregnancy: some authors prescribe antihypertensives when diastolic BP is persistently above 100 mmHg (Walker, 1996) or 90 mmHg (Brown & Buddle, 1996), while other authors adopt less stringent criteria (Sibai, 1996). A variety of antihypertensive agents are used in pregnancy, including methyldopa, calcium antagonists (nifedipine), hydralazine or labetolol. Other agents are rarely used in pregnancy:

- Beta blockers (for example atenolol) may cause intra-uterine growth retardation which restricts their use to the last trimester (Magee et al, 1999; see above).
- ACE inhibitors (for example captopril, enalopril) are implicated in oligohydramnios, stillbirth and renal damage, and are therefore contra-indicated in pregnancy.
- Diuretics reduce circulating volume, thereby jeopardizing placental blood flow and fetal growth. During pregnancy, they are reserved for management of pulmonary oedema or heart failure (Hopkinson, 1995; Girling & De Swiet, 1996).

Methyldopa

Due to its long record of safety, including seven-year follow-up studies of infants, methyldopa is often considered the first choice antihypertensive in pregnancy (Hopkinson, 1995; Sibai, 1996; Nelson-Piercy, 1996; BNF, 2000). Unlike other antihypertensives, methyldopa does not impair renal function and does not reduce cardiac output in young people (Oates, 1996). However, some 60 per cent of women experience sedation or depression which makes it unpopular for long term use (Reynolds et al, 1996).

How the body handles methyldopa

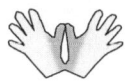 **Practice Points**

- *Methyldopa is taken one hour before or two hours after meals* to minimize the variability in oral absorption.
- *The woman may opt to take a single dose at bedtime or to divide the dose* in order to minimize dose-related side effects, particularly sedation. The long half-life of methyldopa makes this possible.
- Follow-up monitoring is essential because:
  - Maximal effects are not seen for several days, although onset of action occurs at six to eight hours (Malseed et al, 1995).
  - As tolerance develops, over the first seven days, both the adverse effects and the benefits of the drug may lessen.
  - Any impairment or deterioration in renal function (as in pre-eclampsia) prolongs half-life, necessitating a dose reduction.

Methyldopa passes into the fetus and reduces BP in neonates, but this is not known to be harmful (Hopkinson, 1995). There are occasional reports of methyldopa causing a tremor in neonates whose mothers received methyldopa (Reynolds et al, 1996). Methyldopa passes into breast milk, causing undue sedation; therefore, alternative drugs are used for nursing mothers.

Actions and side effects of methyldopa

Methyldopa acts centrally, in the brain stem, to oppose the actions of adrenaline (epinephrine) and noradrenaline (norepinephrine) and dopamine. This causes:

- Inhibition of the sympathetic nervous system, which is normally responsible for controlling BP, regulating the viscera and maintaining a state of 'alertness' (Oates, 1996). The resultant vasodilatation and bradycardia reduce BP.
- Impairment of the reticular activating system (of the brain stem). This induces sedation, weakness and a reduction in mental energy.

Methyldopa also blocks the dopamine receptors (Chapter 5).

Postural hypotension

Methyldopa impairs blood pressure regulation, particularly on standing (via the baroreceptor reflex). As the woman stands, the BP may suddenly drop, which leads to sudden dizziness and even falls.

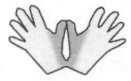 **Practice Points**

- BP should be taken in both a sitting and a standing position.
- Women should be warned to stand up slowly and carefully, particularly during the first week of therapy and in hot weather.
- Women should also be advised to avoid: prolonged standing; hot showers or baths; alcohol ingestion; strenuous exercise (McKenry & Salerno, 1995).

Oedema

Prolonged (12 weeks) use of methyldopa may lead to vasodilation with salt and water retention, causing oedema and jeopardizing blood pressure control (Oates, 1996). Women should be advised to report any new oedema to their midwife, as the possibility of pre-eclampsia will need to be investigated.

Sedation

Women prescribed methyldopa should be advised that they will (almost certainly) feel an increased need to sleep, and should be encouraged to do this. Resting will reduce hypertension by redistributing the blood flow (see pp. 227–8). The midwife could advise women to adopt the 'sick role' for the first week, while tolerance is developing, and avoid physical activity, including housework. Driving may be impaired. Sedation will be compounded by alcohol or anti-histamine medications, which are best avoided (Nelson-Piercy, 1996) (Chapter 5).

Depression

Since it is likely to cause or intensify depression, methyldopa is avoided postpartum (Nelson-Piercy, 1996) or if the woman is clinically depressed prior to therapy (BNF, 2000). The midwife should be alert for symptoms of depression in women prescribed methyldopa which will suggest the need to substitute an alternative antihypertensive.

Reduced production of saliva

Methyldopa inflames salivary glands, reducing the production of saliva. Scrupulous oral hygiene should be maintained. The tongue may become inflamed or discoloured. Irritation of the lining of the nose may cause an uncomfortable 'stuffiness'.

Nausea

Nausea is another problem which may limit the use of methyldopa in practice. Small frequent meals or taking the drug with food may help (Malseed et al, 1995).

Tremors

Posture and movement disorders, similar to Parkinson's disease, may occur in susceptible people (particularly those taking antipsychotic medication) and in neonates (Chapter 5).

Breast discomfort

The reduced activity of dopamine causes increased production of prolactin which may cause breast discomfort and reduction in libido.

Dark urine

A metabolite of methyldopa may darken urine; this is harmless, but women should be aware of this as it may cause alarm.

Liver damage

Hepatotoxicity, with impaired coagulation has been reported in pregnancy. This potentially serious situation may be avoided by monitoring liver function three weeks before and three months after initiation of methyldopa (Smith & Piercy, 1995; Oates, 1996).

Interference with blood tests

Methyldopa may induce the formation of auto-antibodies which interfere with blood cross matching (BNF, 2000). Therefore, this must be done before therapy is initiated.

Other immune-mediated side effects include: rashes; a 'flu-like syndrome; haemolytic anaemia; thrombocytopenia; myocarditis and pancreatitis (Reynolds et al, 1996). Therefore, the BNF (2000) advises monitoring FBC before and during therapy.

Cautions and contra-indications

Pre-existing depression or history of depression, liver or endocrine disease or blood dyscrasias would make methyldopa an unsuitable antihypertensive. Iron salts interact with methyldopa to reduce the antihypertensive effect. Separation of ingestion by two hours only partially reduces this interaction (Stockley, 1999).

Drugs used in hypertensive emergencies

Rapid control of hypertension may be achieved by intravenous hydralazine or labetolol or oral nifedipine (Girling & De Swiet, 1996). Hydralazine is associated with more adverse events (maternal hypotension, Caesarean section, placental abruption and low Apgar score) than either labetolol or nifedipine (Magee et al, 1999). If a nifedipine capsule is bitten (or pierced) then swallowed, blood pressure will fall within five to ten minutes (Smith et al, 2000). However, some prescribers prefer to avoid nifedipine because of its potentially dangerous interaction with magnesium (Magee et al, 1999). (Nifedipine is described further in Chapter 7.) These antihypertensives are also used antenatally, usually for women who cannot tolerate methyldopa. Unlike methyldopa, their use cannot be supported by long term follow-up studies of infants.

Hydralazine is a potent vasodilator, capable of achieving rapid reduction of BP when administered intravenously in hypertensive emergencies. Onset of action is within 10–20 minutes and peak effect within 15–30 minutes. Nitroprusside is an alternative (Reynolds et al, 1996).

Side effects of antihypertensives for emergency use, for example hydralazine

With any drugs in this situation, there is a danger that BP will fall too quickly, risking cardiovascular collapse. Maternal cardiovascular collapse has been reported with sublingual nifedipine (Girling & De Swiet, 1996).

Rapid changes in vital signs

Parenteral hydralazine rapidly lowers BP, particularly diastolic. As this happens, heart rate suddenly rises (via the baroreceptor reflex). This may cause myocardial ischaemia, palpitations or chest pain, particularly if any cardiovascular disease pre-exists, for example in women over 30 who smoke (Robertson & Robertson, 1996). If BP falls too rapidly, this endangers the blood flow to the placenta, and the oxygen supply to the fetus (Reynolds et al, 1996). The woman may sweat profusely and complain of nausea.

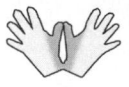 **Practice Points**

- Women receiving parenteral antihypertensives are closely monitored, including vital signs every five minutes until stabilized.
- Fetal distress may complicate administration of hydralazine, and close monitoring is undertaken (Sibai, 1996).

Changes in blood supply

Vasodilation

As blood vessels dilate, the blood supply to the brain, kidneys, and skin initially improves. All vasodilators, including hydralazine and nifedipine, cause headache, flushing, nausea, nasal congestion. Co-administration of methyldopa may prevent the complications of tachycardia (Nelson-Piercy, 1996) but not the headache and facial flushing (Hopkinson, 1995).

Ischaemia

Generalized vasodilation may divert blood to the skin and prevent an adequate circulation to the brain, retina, heart or kidney, leading to ischaemic injury, including blindness (BNF, 2000). Use in those over 40 is 'inadvisable' (Oates, 1996).

Fluid retention and pulmonary oedema

Hydralazine causes fluid retention, which reverses its hypotensive effects. (This should not be mistaken for pre-eclamptic oedema.) Muscle cramps may be associated (Reynolds et al, 1996). There is also a danger of pulmonary oedema, particularly if intravenous fluids are being administered. This is because the drugs dilate the blood vessels, allowing tissue fluid to dilute the blood. There may be an associated proteinuria.

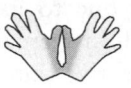 **Practice Points**

- Fluid balance should be strictly monitored, and the patient weighed at least daily to detect fluid retention (McKenry & Salerno, 1998).
- Urine monitoring and pulse oximetry are advised (Hill, 1995).

Cautions

Because of the dangers of rapid reduction in blood pressure, the intravenous route is reserved for hypertensive crises (BNF, 2000). Any abrupt reduction in BP would be dangerous in certain situations such as severe pre-eclampsia, cardiogenic shock, heart failure or aortic stenosis.

Hydralazine – maintenance therapy

Hydralazine may be given orally to control hypertension in the ante-natal period; it is usually reserved for women who have failed to tolerate methyldopa and beta blockers. Due to toxicity in animal studies, this drug is avoided in the first and second trimesters (BNF, 2000).

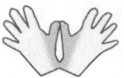 **Practice Points**

- Hydralazine should be administered with food at the same time each day.
- Women should be warned that abrupt cessation of therapy may lead to a sudden, dangerous rise in BP (McKenry & Salerno, 1998).

Prolonged (6 months plus) therapy with hydralazine has been associated with serious side effects, including peripheral neuropathy, tremor, blood disorders and lupus-like syndromes. Vitamin B_6 may minimize these side effects. Those with reduced renal function are most at risk. Hydralazine crosses the placenta, and there are reports of neonatal thrombocytopenia following maternal administration (Reynolds et al, 1996).

Beta blockers (including labetolol)

Beta blockers may be used to manage pregnancy associated hypertension. They are better tolerated than methyldopa. Beta blockers may be the treatment of choice in controlling hypertension post-partum when, due to its depressive effects, methyldopa is relatively contra-indicated (Nelson-Piercy, 1996). However beta blockers can also depress mood. Before the third trimester, some beta blockers reduce the fetal blood supply (Sibai, 1996), causing intra-uterine growth retardation (BNF, 2000), but the importance of this is disputed (Hopkinson, 1995). Beta blockers are also used to manage thyrotoxicosis, angina and cardiac dysrhythmias.

Actions of beta blockers

Beta blockers lower BP by reducing heart rate and cardiac output and depressing the renin-angiotensin system [glossary] (Massie, 1995). They act by competing with beta agonists (such as epinephrine/adrenaline) for occupation of the $beta_1$ and $beta_2$ receptors which control the heart, the liver, the pancreas and the smooth muscle and/or glands of many organs, including blood vessels, uterus, bronchioles and gut.

Side effects of beta blockers

The side effect profile of beta blockers is related to the physiology of the sympathetic nervous system.

Cardiovascular system

Cardio-depressant actions may lead to bradycardia, heart block and even heart failure, precluding use in women with cardiovascular disease. As with all anti-hypertensive medications, orthostatic hypotension is a potential problem.

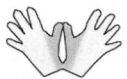 **Practice Points**

- Vital signs, including orthostatic intolerance, should be assessed regularly (see methyldopa).
- The neonate should be monitored closely for 48 hours to detect and action any transient hypotension and bradycardia (Pangle, 2000).

Beta blockers impair the peripheral circulation, making the arms and legs feel uncomfortably cold.

Asthma

Beta blockers prevent the relaxation of the smooth muscle of the bronchioles and cannot be used in women with any history of asthma.

Diabetes

Beta blockers impair the normal sympathetic response to hypoglycaemia, dangerously blocking warning signs and symptoms. They are not suitable for diabetic women.

Discomfort

Although generally well tolerated, beta blockers can cause fatigue, nightmares, gastro-intestinal upsets, dry eyes or rashes. Psoriasis may be exacerbated.

Withdrawal reaction

Abrupt withdrawal of beta blockers may lead to tremor, headache, sweating, rebound hypertension, and, in susceptible people, myocardial infarction or thyrotoxicosis (McKenry & Salerno, 1998).

Breastfeeding

Beta blockers pass into breast milk. US texts caution against use during lactation (Malseed et al, 1995), but the BNF (2000) is less proscriptive. The half-life of some agents (for example labetolol) is prolonged in the neonate, increasing the dangers of accumulation (Reynolds et al, 1996). The infant should be carefully monitored, as toxicity cannot be discounted.

Labetolol

Labetolol is a combined alpha and beta blocker. Alpha blockade induces vasodilation. This improves the blood flow to various organs, including the kidneys, and labetolol may be more effective in curtailing the development of proteinuria than methyldopa (Qarmalawi et al, 1995). However vasodilation also causes postural hypotension (see methyldopa).

Labetolol has a faster onset of action than other beta blockers, and may be administered intravenously to control severe hypertension. Hypotension is maximal within five minutes of iv administration and persists for 8–12 hours after discontinuation (Malseed et al, 1995).

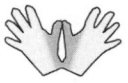 **Practice Points**

- During, and for three hours after, iv administration, the patient should not be allowed into an upright position, due to the risk of profound postural hypotension (BNF, 2000).
- Intensive BP monitoring is required, for example, every five minutes for the first 15 minutes, then every 15 minutes during iv infusion.
- Atropine, vasopressors and bronchodilators should be available during intravenous administration (McKenry & Salerno, 1998).

Administration of labetolol is also associated with nasal congestion, a sensation of scalp tingling, headache, dizziness, nightmares and depression. Raynaud's phenomenon may be worsened by labetolol. Severe liver damage has been reported with both long and short term use of labetolol (BNF, 2000).

Implications for Practice: antihypertensives

- With all anti-hypertensives, vital signs will require continuous monitoring to avoid, simultaneously, the dangers of inadequate treatment of hypertension and catastrophic hypotension.
- Unless fluid balance is accurately recorded and maintained, it will be impossible for the prescriber to avoid pulmonary oedema *and* underperfusion of the placenta and vital organs simultaneously.
- Practitioners may need to distinguish between drug side effects and symptoms of disease: for example nausea and headache may be symptoms of impending eclampsia or side effects of anti-hypertensives.
- The midwife should also offer the woman reassurance over the 'minor' (non-life-threatening) side effects of therapy, such as nasal congestion and flushing. The delivery of such informed care has the potential to make a positive impact in practice.
- Concerns over the putative link between fall in mean arterial pressure and reduction in birthweight suggest that fetal growth should be very carefully monitored in women prescribed antihypertensives.
- Where pre-eclampsia is excluded, prescribers may adopt a 'watchful vigilance' regimen in women with blood pressures below 170/110 mmHg (von Dadelszen et al, 2000; de Swiet, 2000). This will involve the midwife in regular monitoring of these 'at risk' women.

Cardiac dysrhythmias in pregnancy

Cardiac dysrhythmia may be detected during antenatal examinations. Supraventricular tachycardia (SVT) is the commonest dysrhythmia in pregnancy. While prompt medical referral is vital, it is important to consider the possible origins of any SVT:

- unaccustomed exercise;
- anxiety;
- fever/infection – always consider UTI;
- hypovolaemia/dehydration;
- evolving pulmonary embolus (even in apparently healthy women);
- use of sympathomimetics: OTC cold cures, amphetamines (including ecstasy), cocaine, asthma medications (salbutamol, terbutaline), tocolytics (ritodrine);
- anti-psychotic or anti-depressant medications;
- undetected heart valve disease;

- undetected cardiac conduction abnormalities (e.g. Wolff-Parkinson-White syndrome);
- undetected thyroid disease;
- undetected heart failure;
- hypocalcaemia (particularly diabetic women).

The management of cardiac dysrhythmia in pregnancy requires specialist input. Adenosine has been used to restore sinus rhythm safely in pregnant women. Verapamil is used in young people for prophylaxis of supraventricular tachycardias, and some specialists will continue this drug during pregnancy. Amiodarone is associated with a variety of long term side effects, including thyroid dysfunction in mother and neonate; it is regarded as a drug of 'last resort' (Hopkinson, 1995).

Heart failure in pregnancy

Cardiac output is increased during pregnancy, and further increased during labour. This is achieved by increasing stroke volume. Women with heart failure, congenital heart problems or valve disease are unable to raise stroke volume to meet the demands of pregnancy. Pregnancy carries a recognized risk for a significant number of these women. In the UK, most of these women will be receiving specialist medical care prior to pregnancy.

Digoxin

Digoxin is prescribed for atrial fibrillation and cardiac failure. From many years of experience, digoxin is known to be safe for use in pregnancy, provided digoxin concentrations remain within the therapeutic range. Due to changes in drug distribution and elimination (Chapter 1), the dose of digoxin frequently requires adjustment during pregnancy. Also, the signs of digoxin toxicity and therapeutic failure, such as nausea, may be masked by pregnancy. It is important that digitalis toxicity does not occur, as this can be fatal to the fetus (Hopkinson, 1995). Therefore, regular therapeutic drug monitoring is essential, in addition to regular clinical monitoring, including HR, BP, ECG, lung bases, renal function, electrolytes, thyroid function. The midwife should encourage a diet containing plenty of fruit, vegetables and museli to ensure adequate levels of potassium and magnesium because deficiency of these electrolytes predisposes to digoxin toxicity.

   Digoxin crosses the placenta and enters breast milk. Although the amount of digoxin entering breast milk is small, infants are unduly susceptible to digoxin, and the midwife should pay close attention to weight gain in the neonate (Malseed et al, 1995).

Conclusion

Although the midwife does not initiate the prescription of antihypertensives, in hospital practice she will be expected to manage acutely ill women receiving antihypertensive therapy. It is important that this is prioritized, and close surveillance is undertaken.

While delivering ante-natal or post-natal care to hypertensive women, the midwife will undertake client education on the need for antihypertensive therapy and the management of side effects; see Implications for Practice. A full understanding of side effects will empower the woman to minimize both the incidence and the inconvenience of such common problems as postural hypotension, nausea and sedation.

Further Reading

De Swiet, M. (2000) Maternal blood pressure and birthweight. *Lancet*:355:81–2.

Idama, T. & Lindow, S. (1998) Magnesium sulphate: a review of clinical pharmacology applied to obstetrics, *British Journal of Obstetrics and Gynaecology*:105:260–8.

Lu, J. & Nightingale, C. (2000) Magnesium sulfate in eclampsia and pre-eclampsia: pharmacokinetic principles. *Clinical Pharmacokinetics*:38:305–15.

CHAPTER 10

Rhesus Incompatibility and Anti-D Immunoglobulin (Rh$_0$)

YAMNI NIGAM

This chapter discusses Anti-D immunoglobulin administered to Rhesus negative women. An understanding of genetics and immunology will be helpful in reading this chapter.

Chapter Contents

- Introduction

- The Rhesus system

- Haemolytic diseases of the newborn

- Prevention of Rhesus sensitization

- Conclusion

Introduction

An individual's blood group is determined by inherited glycoprotein antigens on the surfaces of erythrocytes and other cells. In the early 1900s, Karl Landsteiner discovered the presence of two antigens (A and B), on the surface of red blood cells. He found that individuals possessed either one, two, or neither of these antigens on their erythrocytes, and thus provided an explanation for the fatal incompatibility seen in early blood transfusions (Landsteiner, 1900). Although discovery of the ABO system improved safety, transfusion reactions were still occurring, and it was not until some 40 years later that the Rhesus (Rh) blood groups were identified (Landsteiner & Wiener, 1940).

Several other blood group systems have also been found, although the ABO blood group system is easily the most important, since antibodies to antigen A and/or antigen B are found in virtually everyone who lacks the corresponding antigens. These antibodies cause intravascular haemolysis (the bursting or lysis of erythrocytes) when incompatible red cells are transfused.

The Rhesus system

The Rhesus system is of clinical importance because individuals without the Rhesus (Rh) antigen readily form antibodies when exposed to it. The Rhesus antibody is capable of causing haemolytic transfusion reactions, for example when it crosses the placenta, giving rise to Haemolytic Diseases of the Newborn (HDN) or *erythroblastosis foetalis*. There are six main genes coding for the Rh antigen (designated dominant genes C, D, and E and corresponding recessive genes c, d, and e), with genes D/d being the most important.

We inherit only one Rhesus gene from each parent. Gaining the combination of genes DD or Dd gives rise to the presence of the Rhesus D antigen and makes the individual Rh-positive (approximately 85 per cent of UK population is positive). Those individuals born with the genes dd lack the Rh antigen and are Rh negative. Fifteen per cent of Caucasians, 5 per cent of West Africans and less than 1 per cent of Asians are Rhesus negative.

In contrast to the ABO system, there are no preformed antibodies to antigen D present from infancy. However under certain circumstances, Rhesus negative women can form Rhesus antibodies (Anti-D). Formation of Rhesus antibodies (Anti-D) follows the exposure of an Rh negative person to Rh positive blood. This will happen if:

- Rh positive blood is transfused to a Rh negative person [about 90 per cent of Rh D negative subjects transfused with Rh D positive blood will make Anti-D, that is they will become Rh sensitized or immunized (Contreras, 1998)]; or
- an Rh negative woman is pregnant with a Rh positive fetus.

In midwifery, problems may occur when fetal Rh positive erythrocytes enter the maternal (Rh negative) circulation via the placenta. The mother will often react to them by forming Anti-D, but, since the transfer of red cells most commonly occurs during the delivery of the placenta, the first baby born to an Rh negative woman is rarely affected. However there are exceptions, for example if the mother has been previously inadvertently transfused with Rh positive blood. In circumstances where the first pregnancy (miscarriage or termination) has resulted in the sensitization of an Rh negative mother, all subsequent pregnancies may carry a considerable risk to the developing fetus.

If an Rh negative woman in her first pregnancy has an Rh positive fetus *in utero*, it is possible that fetal red cells may enter her circulation prior to the third stage of labour due to partial placental separation and an ensuing fetomaternal bleed, for example during miscarriage.

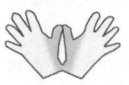 **Practice Point**

The midwife should be prepared to administer Anti-D following miscarriage/abortion and
certain obstetric manipulations which can increase the risk of a transplacental haemorrhage:
  amniocentesis;
  chorionic villus sampling;
  caesarean section;
  external cephalic versions;
  manual removal of the placenta.

Placenta praevia and choriocarcinoma are often associated with large antepartum haemorrhages, and should therefore be followed by administration of Anti-D (Contreras, 1998). Formation of Anti-D in the mother depends on several factors, including the volume of fetal erythrocytes crossing the placenta into the mother (transplacental haemorrhage). Often this is too small to induce Rh (iso) immunization. Hence, only 17 per cent of Rh negative women will become sensitized to Rh D after a pregnancy with an ABO compatible Rh positive infant (Contreras, 1998).

Haemolytic diseases of the newborn (HDN)

Once Rh antibodies (Anti-D) have developed in the maternal circulation, they are capable of agglutinating, haemolysing and destroying red blood cells carrying the D antigen and can pass to the developing fetus and continue their haemolytic activity, causing pathological responses such as anemia, hypoxia, oedema or *hydrops foetalis* in the fetus.

Rhesus antibodies generated in the mother, if present in a high enough concentration, may cause the breakdown of fetal red cells, resulting in an anaemic and hypoxic fetus. If the fetal haemoglobin level drops below (4 g/dL) heart failure leads to oedema (Chamberlain et al, 1989), which may develop into *hydrops foetalis* – the most serious form of Rh haemolytic disease: the baby at birth is grossly oedematous with an enlarged abdomen, usually stillborn and macerated.

The accelerated rate of red cell breakdown may cause the fetus to become severely jaundiced. This is due to increasing levels of bilirubin released from the damaged and destroyed erythrocytes. This becomes increasingly problematic after birth, when placental transfer and excretion by the maternal liver has ceased, and the neonatal liver cannot cope with such high concentrations of bilirubin. Residual maternal Anti-D circulates in the baby's bloodstream and continues haemolysis of red cells. If serum bilirubin levels rise above

120 µmol/litre, damage to the brain cells (kernicterus) may occur. This results in a variable degree of cerebral palsy and learning difficulties.

The volume of transplacental haemorrhage, that is the passage of red cells from the fetus to the mother, is usually measured by the acid elution technique of Kleihauer-Betke which measures the number of fetal red cells as a proportion of adult cells in a sample of maternal blood. Other immunological tests, such as immunofluorescence and microscopic rosetting techniques, may also be used to calculate the volume of red cell transfer. The frequency and magnitude of this haemorrhage depends largely on gestational age; it is usually low and small in the first two trimesters, more frequent in the third and greatest at delivery (Bowman & Pollock, 1987).

Prevention of Rh sensitization

In order to detect mothers 'at risk', the blood of every pregnant woman is examined for ABO group and Rhesus type at her first ante-natal visit.

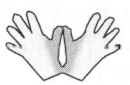 **Practice Point**

Early booking allows the blood group to be determined, so that Rh negative mothers can be appropriately treated and HDN prevented.

If the mother is Rh negative, her blood is examined for antibodies. If there are no antibodies, the test is repeated periodically during the gestation period. If Rh antibodies are found (and the baby's father is known to be Rh positive), then rapid treatment for the prevention of possible HDN is imperative.

The first study to elucidate whether serum containing Anti-D could exert a positive effect against Rh sensitization was undertaken by Stern et al (1961). It became apparent that it may be possible to destroy any fetal red cells found in the maternal circulation following delivery by means of a suitable antibody (Finn et al, 1961; Clarke and Sheppard, 1965).

In 1969, post-delivery immunoprophylaxis using Anti-D Immunoglobulin (Ig) to prevent Rhesus HDN was introduced in the United Kingdom. The initial recommendations for its use were reviewed in the 1976 Green Booklet (Standing Medical Advisory Committee, 1976a) which added the advice that Anti-D should be administered after all abortions. Further recommendations followed in 1981 (Standing Medical Advisory Committee, 1976b) which identified a number of potentially sensitizing episodes during pregnancy for which prophylaxis was recommended. Yet again, new guidelines were published in 1991 updating the use of Anti-D Immunoglobulin in pregnancy and including more detailed advice in relation to abortion (National Blood Transfusion Service Immunoglobulin Working Party, 1991).

Currently the therapeutic indications for the administration of Anti-D are:

- non-immunized Rh negative women who give birth to an Rh positive infant;
- Rh negative women who abort an Rh positive conceptus;
- Rh negative women exhibiting incidents during pregnancy that may lead to appreciable transplacental bleeding (that is amniocentesis, chorionic villus sampling, Caesarean section, external cephalic versions, manual removal of the placenta);
- Rh negative women of childbearing age who have been given blood components containing Rh positive red cells, for example in blood transfusions.

The forthcoming publication of new guidelines by the Royal College of Obstetricians and Gynaecologists will replace the current (1991) guidelines. The key expected change is the inclusion of a recommendation that Anti-D be given as routine ante-natal prophylactic treatment, that is given to all Rh negative women at weeks 28 and 34 of pregnancy, although this will increase costs (Robson et al, 1998). This recommendation is supported by the 1997 Consensus Conference on Anti-D propylatics (Urbaniak, 1998) and preliminary findings from the Cochrane Review (Crowther & Keirse, 2000).

Current doses and administration

At present, Anti-D is manufactured from venous plasma collected using a technique known as apheresis from voluntary unpaid Rh D negative donors who have been immunized against the Rhesus D antigen. Human Anti-D (Rh_0) is a liquid preparation containing immunoglobulin, mainly Immunoglobulin (Ig) G. One millilitre contains 100–180 mg human protein of which at least 90 per cent is immunoglobulin. The product is marketed in three doses – 250 International Units (IU), 500 IU and 2500 IU. This is normally a 15 per cent weight/volume protein solution for intramuscular injection. The recommended post-natal dosage is 500 IU, and should be administered as soon as possible after delivery and certainly within 72 hours.

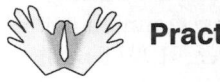 **Practice Point**

Rh negative women must not be discharged until Anti-D has been administered.

If, however, the volume of fetal red cells in the mother's circulation exceeds 4 ml, extra Anti-D (Rh$_0$) Immunoglobulin must be administered (an extra 125 IU for each 1.0 ml of red cells). Even though 500 IU (100 μg) is sufficient to cover a transplacental haemorrhage of 4 ml (99 per cent of all transplacental haemorrhages), it is mandatory to perform a screening test (such as Kleihauer-Batke which detects fetal cells in the mother's circulation) in order to assess the need for additional doses of Anti-D Immunoglobulin.

Following an incident during pregnancy such as any of those outlined previously, the recommended dose of Anti-D Ig up to 20 weeks' gestation is 250 IU per incident, and 500 IU after 20 weeks' gestation. Additionally, Anti-D Immunoglobulin should be given to all Rh D negative women with a threatened abortion after 12 weeks' gestation (250 IU before 20 weeks' gestation and 500 IU after 20 weeks' gestation). Doses should be administered at the time of the incident. Where bleeding continues intermittently, the injection should be repeated at six-week intervals. For women given blood components containing Rh positive cells, the recommended dose is 125 IU Anti-D Ig per ml of transfused Rhesus positive cells.

Storage of Anti-D

The product should be stored in the carton, at a temperature of 2°–8°C. Care should be taken not to allow the product to freeze and particular attention paid to the expiry date stated on the carton and the label.

Administration of Anti-D

Human Anti-D (Rh$_0$) must be administered by the intramuscular route as normal, and never intravenously, since the preparation may cause severe hypersensitivity reactions, including anaphylaxis, if given by this route. Extreme care must be taken to ensure that the needle does not enter a blood vessel.

This is in contrast with Anti-D Immunoglobulin used outside the UK, particularly in Canada and the USA. The Canadian product is known as Win Rh$_0$ SDF and is a sterile Anti-D polyclonal antibody which is packaged as a freeze-dried gamma globulin (Ig G). Upon reconstitution with 0.9 per cent sodium chloride, Win Rh$_0$ SDF Anti-D is administered intravenously, and not intramuscularly as is the case for Anti-D (Rh$_0$) in the UK. The mode of administration, and the fact that Win Rh$_0$ SDF provides an extra margin of human plasma product safety (in so much as solvent detergent (SD) viral inactivation and microfiltration (F) viral removal manufacturing steps have been included), are the major differences between Anti-D Ig and Win Rh$_0$ SDF Ig.

The therapeutic indications and doses remain identical, although it has recently been shown that Win Rh$_0$ SDF Anti-D is effective in the treatment of Idiopathic Thrombocytopenic Purpura (ITP), a condition characterized by a severely low platelet count (Salama et al, 1986; Andrew et al, 1992; Zimmerman et al, 1998).

Risk of infection and side effects

Solvent detergent and viral removal steps have been shown to inactivate lipid-enveloped viruses such as HIV, hepatitis B and C, although there are, to date, no known recorded cases of viral transmission from UK Anti-D (Rh$_0$); however hepatitis C infection has been reported through contaminated Anti-D in Ireland and Germany (Foster et al, 1995).

Allergic reactions to Human Anti-D (Rh$_0$) are rare, but women should be observed for at least 20 minutes following injection for signs of allergic or anaphylacticoid reaction or shock. As with all intramuscular injections, women may experience some short term discomfort at the injection site, although Anti-D (Rh$_0$) is well tolerated.

The efficacy of live attenuated virus vaccines, such as measles, oral polio, typhoid, rubella, mumps, BCG, yellow fever and varicella, may be impaired up to three months following administration of Anti-D (Rh$_0$), since Anti-D will prevent the formation of other antibodies. Such vaccinations, therefore, should only be given after an interval of three months following injection with Human Anti-D (Rh$_0$).

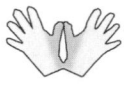 **Practice Point**

Women planning to travel abroad may need to reconsider their vaccinations following Anti-D administration.

There have been no reported ill effects of Anti-D (Rh$_0$) Immunoglobulin during pregnancy or lactation. (See Implications for Practice.) Overdosage of Anti-D is unlikely to lead to more frequent or more severe adverse reactions than the recommended dose. Anti-D is an important treatment for both acute and chronic ITP (immune thrombocytopenic purpura) and ITP developing secondary to HIV infection. There are reports of serious side effects with intravenous administration of Anti-D (Rh$_0$) Immunoglobulin in these settings (Imbach & Kuhne, 2000).

Cautions and contraindications for use of Anti-D

Use of intramuscular Human Anti-D (Rh$_0$) Ig is contra-indicated in women with clotting disorders, where intramuscular injections are inadvisable. In such cases, Anti-D (Rh$_0$) may be administered subcutaneously and careful manual pressure with a compress should be applied to the site after injection. Also, Anti-D (Rh$_0$) should not be administered to patients with severe thrombocytopenia.

Women with a weakly reacting form of Antigen-D (D^u) should not be treated with Human Anti-D, partly because most of the antibody will bind to D^u cells and not with the infants' red cells, and partly because the risk of formation of Anti-D Immunoglobulin by a D^u woman is extremely small.

Several studies indicate that the platelet count increases transiently after treatment with polyclonal Anti-D antibodies in a large proportion of Rh-D positive patients. Therefore, advice should be sought before administration to a woman with a significantly raised platelet count (Salama et al, 1986; Andrew et al, 1992; Zimmerman et al, 1998).

Implications for Practice: Anti-D Immunoglobulin

Potential Problem	Management
Development of Rhesus antibodies in Rhesus negative women	Blood group determination for all women. Administration of Anti-D Immunoglobulin injection within 72 hours of delivery, miscarriage, elective termination, antepartum haemorrhage or antenatal procedures (see p. 258) to all Rhesus negative women. Be prepared to administer additional doses of Anti-D as the results of tests indicate. Routine administration to all Rhesus negative women at 28 and 34 weeks.
Chemical instability of the injection	Regular checking of expiry date and refrigerator temperature.
Failure of live vaccines	Avoid live vaccines for three months after administration. Substitute injections for oral typhoid and polio vaccines if travelling to certain countries. It may not be possible to substitute an alternative inactivated vaccine, for example for yellow fever. In such cases, women should be aware that they are travelling with little effective immunization.
Risk of hypersensitivity response	Ensure the injection does not enter a blood vessel.

Conclusion

Despite rigorous attention to guidelines, in the UK, around 1.5 per cent of Rhesus negative women become sensitized, making their infants at risk of haemolytic disease of the newborn (Howard et al, 1997). This figure is reduced to 0.2 per cent by routine administration of Anti-D Immunoglobulin (Crowther & Keirse, 2000).

The most recent development and advance in Anti-D Ig therapy is that, as from summer 1999, the plasma used to isolate (Rh_0) Ig has been imported from USA, since there continues to be a major concern over the contamination of UK plasma with CJD (Creutzfeld-Jakob disease). It is also hoped that, in time, the product from this American plasma will be virally inactivated and thus further enhance the safety of the product.

Further Reading

Crowther, C.A. & Keirse, M. (2000) Anti-D administration for preventing Rhesus alloimmunisation (Cochrane Review) In: *The Cochrane Library*: 1, 2000. Oxford: Update Software.

PART IV

DRUGS IN PREGNANCY

This section of the book considers the agents commonly prescribed for or self-administered by women who are otherwise well. Herbal and homeopathic remedies lie outside the scope of this book. Anti-emetics are considered in Chapter 5 and over-the-counter medicines in Chapter 20.

CHAPTER 11

Nutritional Supplements in Pregnancy: Iron and Folic Acid

SUE JORDAN AND RENA MCOWATT

This chapter focuses on iron and folic acid, which are frequently prescribed as supplements. Other nutrients are mentioned briefly.

Chapter Contents

- Nutrition in pregnancy

- Iron

- Folic acid

Nutrition in pregnancy

The aim of nutrition in pregnancy is to maximize the health of the mother and enhance the development of a healthy infant or infants. There can be no guarantee of a positive outcome with optimal nutrition, but malnutrition can adversely affect the health and development of the fetus (Eastwood, 1992). Low birth weight and disease in later life are closely associated with maternal under-nutrition (Barker et al, 1990). In the UK, increased dietary intake of iron, zinc, protein and B vitamins during the last trimester proved beneficial for women attending a London teaching hospital (Haste et al, 1991). In many women, vitamin C intake may also be suboptimal (Coutts, 2000). In less privileged communities, supplements of calories, protein, iron, folic acid, vitamin A, and possibly magnesium, zinc and calcium are needed to optimize the health of women and children (Liljestrand, 1999; Makrides & Crowther, 2000).

It is important to note that the overuse of micronutrients may also prove hazardous. For example, vitamin A in daily doses > 10 000 IU was shown to increase the incidence of malformations, particularly cleft lip, cardiac defects, and central nervous system malformations (Rothman et al, 1995).

The best possible environment for the developing fetus and for its future growth is where the woman is healthy, has sensible eating habits and starts pregnancy with adequate nutrient stores. Most women who are well nourished and active have sufficient stores of minerals and vitamins to meet the increased demands of pregnancy. However, as lifestyles have become more sedentary, calorie intakes have declined. Since dietary iron intake is directly proportional to calorie intake, iron status has declined concomitantly, leaving many young women with inadequate iron stores to meet the demands of pregnancy, particularly if blood loss at delivery is high. Many women may be deficient in other essential vitamins and minerals, particularly folic acid. Those at risk include adolescents, women who have several children close together, those with chronic illness such as urinary tract or parasitic infections, pre-pregnancy menorrhagia, malabsorption or malaria, regular users of non-steroidal anti-inflammatory drugs, women who are anorexic or have a history of eating disorders and those who use appreciable quantities of recreational drugs, tobacco or alcohol. Women with very low incomes may not take in enough calories to meet the energy demands of pregnancy, let alone be able to meet the extra requirements for micro-nutrients. Therefore, some authorities recommend low dose multivitamin supplements from the preconception period. Strict vegetarians are likely to need supplements of vitamins B_{12} and D (Van Way, 1999; Coutts, 2000).

Iron

Iron is a mineral required for all biological systems in the body. It is essential for haemoglobin synthesis, catecholamine synthesis, heat production and as a component of certain enzymes needed for the production of adenosine triphosphate involved in cell respiration. Iron is stored in the liver, spleen and bone marrow. About 70 per cent of iron in the body is in haemoglobin and 3 per cent is in myoglobin (an intramuscular oxygen store). A deficiency in iron results in anaemia which reduces the maximum quantity of oxygen the blood can carry. A woman with anaemia is usually very tired, loses her appetite and feels unable to cope. Untreated, anaemia can progress to heart failure. It is important to realize that shortness of breath and tachycardia may be due to anaemia, and are not always attributable to pregnancy.

In health, the loss of iron from the body is 1–2 mg, daily. This is replaced by the average daily intake of iron which in developed countries is about 15–20 mg. Good dietary sources of iron include meats, eggs, certain vegetables (water cress) and whole grains. Most dietary iron is in the ferric (Fe^{3+}) form. Gastric secretions dissolve the dietary iron, facilitating its reduction to the ferrous (Fe^{2+}) form. This is an important physiological process as iron can only be absorbed in the ferrous form. Normally, the absorption of iron is carefully regulated so that just enough is absorbed to replace the loss. Three to ten per cent of the daily intake is absorbed. This occurs largely in the proximal duodenum, where the mucosal cells regulate the efficiency of iron absorption.

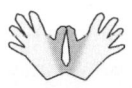 **Practice Point**

Sustained release preparations may be prescribed if other iron tablets cause side effects, but they may not release iron until the tablets have passed the duodenum, and therefore may supply no iron (Smith, 1997).

The amount of iron absorbed will depend on a number of factors such as the content of the diet, the stores of iron in the body, the rate of red cell production and whether or not iron supplements are being taken (Stables, 1999).

If body stores of iron are low, absorption increases up to 30 per cent or even 70 per cent in late pregnancy, when a larger proportion of the iron taken up by the mucosal cells is transported by a carrier mechanism into the plasma. When body stores of iron are high, the mucosal cells transport only a small amount of iron into the plasma. In the plasma, iron binds to the plasma transport protein, transferrin. Most iron is stored within the cells as ferritin. Ferritin is the tissue storage form of iron, and is found in the cells lining the gut, the liver, spleen and bone marrow. Serum ferritin measurements provide an index of tissue iron stores. To replenish iron stores, oral iron may need to be continued for several months after an improvement in haemoglobin concentrations (Smith, 1997).

Iron balance is regulated by absorption, but there is no simple mechanism regulating the elimination of iron. Iron elimination is mainly dependent on the shedding of the mucosal cells lining the gut. Therefore, overuse of iron can, in susceptible individuals, lead to iron overload (haemosiderosis/haemochromatosis). In Europe, some 12–13 per cent of women are heterozygous [glossary] and 0.3–0.5 per cent are homozygous [glossary] for the haemochromatosis gene: if these women ingest large doses of iron (as tablets), they may develop iron overload, which damages the liver and pancreas (Milman et al, 1999). Recent investigations suggest that these genes increase susceptibility to iron overload in renal failure (Fernandez, 2000).

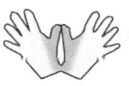 **Practice Points**

- Iron should not be continued longer than six months without medical supervision.
- A rise in haemoglobin of 2 g/dL should be seen within three weeks of starting iron.
- If there is no response to iron within three to four weeks, therapy should be reviewed by physicians.

Iron in pregnancy

Extra iron is needed in pregnancy. Iron requirements for singleton pregnancy are:

200–600 mg to meet the increase in the red cell mass;
200–370 mg for the fetus, depending on birth weight;
150–200 mg as external loss;
30–170 mg for the cord and placenta;
90–310 mg to cover blood loss at delivery.

The total iron demands of pregnancy therefore range between 580–1340 mg, of which 440–1050 mg will be lost to the mother at delivery (Hillman, 1996).

To combat these losses, pregnant women need an average of 3.5–4 mg of iron daily. The requirements increase significantly in the last trimester from an average of 2.5 mg/day in early pregnancy to 6.6 mg/day (Letsky & Warwick, 1994). The iron available from the diet ranges from 0.9 to 1.8 mg/day, depending on the adequacy of the diet. Therefore, meeting the demands of pregnancy requires mobilization of iron stores, and an increase in iron absorption. Although the absorption of iron increases considerably during pregnancy (Barrett et al, 1994), where pregnancies are close together and/or iron stores are low, sufficient iron can only be obtained by supplementation. Only in the most extreme circumstances will the baby be born iron deficient.

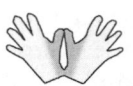 **Practice Points**

- Women with inadequate iron stores need to absorb an extra 2–5 mg of iron per day. This requires a daily supplement of 15–30 mg of iron (Hillman, 1996) or 65 mg/day from 20 weeks' gestation (Milman et al, 1999).
- A supplement of 30 mg of iron/day is sufficient for most women (Van Way, 1999). However, doses of 60–100 mg iron per day are recommended in Scandinavian countries (Milman et al, 1999).
- 15–30 mg of iron can be obtained from 50–100 mg of dried ferrous sulphate, and 65 mg iron can be obtained from 200 mg dried ferrous sulphate or equivalent (BNF, 2000) (see p. 272, Table 11.1).
- The iron content of beef is around 2 mg/100 g, of which 33–66 per cent could be absorbed. To absorb the extra 2–5 mg of iron per day, the woman would need to eat 300–1500 g of beef per day. Chicken yields less than half this amount of iron.

Lactation also increases the demands for iron; if a mother is iron depleted following delivery, her infant may require prophylactic iron. Low birth weight infants, particularly those delivered by Caesarean section, may require iron supplements. Anaemia in children has been associated with behavioural and learning difficulties (Hillman, 1996).

Anaemia in pregnancy

Although the daily requirement for iron increases in pregnancy, routine iron supplementation is not usually necessary, if the woman is active, well nourished and eating a balanced diet. However, lack of iron is the principal nutritional deficiency in the United States (Lilley et al, 1996). If there is evidence of iron deficiency, oral iron supplements may be used as there is no evidence that they cause any harm to the developing fetus in therapeutic dose. (see Implications for Practice.)

It is estimated that 40 per cent of European women have insufficient iron stores to complete pregnancy and childbirth, and half of these develop anaemia (Milman et al, 1999). Haemoglobin below 8 grams/100 ml has been associated with increased risk of neonatal encephalopathy in developing countries (Ellis et al, 2000). Low serum ferritin concentrations, particuarly in the first trimester, have been linked to increased placental vascularization and size, intrauterine growth retardation and low birth weight (Hindmarsh et al, 2000).

Diagnosis of anaemia in pregnancy is complicated by the normal changes in haematological indices:

- Synthesis of transferrin (the transport protein) increases, reducing the transferrin saturation.
- Production of ferritin (the storage form of iron) decreases. Measurements below 12 micrograms/litre are taken as indicative of iron deficiency in pregnancy (Long, 1995; Milman et al, 1999) (non-pregnant adult range 15–200 micrograms/litre). However, Barrett et al (1994) report values as low as 4 micrograms/litre in late pregnancy, without clinical evidence of anaemia.
- Haemodilution increases; circulating volume doubles, whereas red cell mass increases by 25 per cent. In late pregnancy, haemoglobin values between 9.6 and 14.5 g/100 ml are considered to be within normal limits (Milman et al, 1999). However, more stringent criteria should be adopted in women who smoke or live at high altititude (Van Way, 1999).

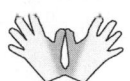 **Practice Point**

It is important to assess any tiredness, dizziness, tinnitus, anorexia, feeling cold, dry or itching skin, infections, palpitations or breathlessness which may be attributable to anaemia.

Iron tablets

Dried ferrous sulphate tablets are the most commonly prescribed treatment in the UK, as they are considered to be as effective as other products and cheaper. Ferrous fumarate tablets contain a similar proportion of iron, and may have a lower incidence of side effects. Ferrous gluconate tablets contain less iron, and, consequently, are associated with fewer gastro-intestinal side effects (Malseed et al, 1995).

Table 11.1 Comparism of iron formulations (BNF, 2000)

	Iron content %	Dose needed to obtain 60–65 mg iron in an absorbable form
Ferrous sulphate (dried)	30%	200 mg
Ferrous sulphate	20%	300 mg
Ferrous fumarate	33%	200 mg
Ferrous gluconate	11.6%	600 mg

How the body absorbs iron

Absorption of iron is increased by the presence of acid in the stomach. This can be enhanced by:

- taking with meat, veal or fish which stimulate gastric acid production;
- co-administration with ascorbic acid (vitamin C) 200 mg or orange juice;
- co-administration with alcohol (not advised in pregnancy).

Vitamin C is water soluble, and rarely accumulates in the body. However, large doses of vitamin C can cause kidney stones or precipitate a sickle cell crisis in susceptible individuals. The results of glucose testing may be obscured by large doses of vitamin C. Therefore, doses of 200 mg are recommended for concurrent use with iron tablets, up to a maximum of 500 mg/day (Spencer et al, 1993b). The relative achlorhydria [glossary] of pregnancy is not reported as an impairment to iron absorption. However, some women with iron deficiency fail to respond to oral iron. The gut is only able to absorb 40–60 mg of iron/day, even in the most severe anaemia, and higher doses may only increase gastro-intestinal side effects.

Side effects of iron therapy

Increasing iron absorption may increase the severity of side effects experienced (Smith, 1997).

Gastro-intestinal side effects

Oral iron supplements may cause nausea, vomiting, stomach cramps, heart-burn and constipation (occasionally diarrhoea). However, the degree of nausea produced by each preparation depends on the amount of elemental iron absorbed. Doses of iron above 60 mg (200 mg dried ferrous sulphate) may produce unacceptable side effects in pregnant women, leading to non-compliance (Shatrugna et al, 1999).

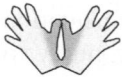 **Practice Point**

Tablets containing low doses of iron are more likely to be tolerated (and taken) than high doses. If possible, therapy should be commenced with a low dose, especially if the woman expresses concerns over gastro-intestinal symptoms. For many women, a low dose will be sufficient.

Taking iron tablets during or immediately after meals reduces the associated nausea but decreases the amount of iron absorbed. Also, many foods interact with iron, if taken within two hours (see Table 11.2).

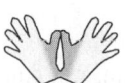 **Practice Points**

- Iron tablets may be better tolerated at bedtime (Engstrom & Sittler, 1994).
- Doses of iron should be separated by at least six to eight hours, increased to 12 or 24 hours if side effects occur (Smith, 1997).
- Vomiting and abdominal cramping are both side effects and early signs of iron toxicity. They indicate the urgent need to revise (downwards) the dosages of iron.

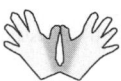 **Practice Point**

To minimize constipation, advice should be given to:
- drink two litres of fluid each day
- eat fresh fruit and vegetables
- eat plenty of fibre, two hours apart from iron tablets
- exercise regularly (see Chapter 13).

Stool and urine discolouration may occur. Women should be warned that stools may be blackened during iron therapy. This may mask any gastrointestinal bleeding.

Micro-nutrient deficiency

Absorption of zinc and calcium may be decreased by iron tablets. Zinc deficiency has been associated with anaemia, poor absorption of folates, intrauterine growth retardation, preterm delivery, low birth weight and poor wound healing (Long, 1995; Mahmood, 2000). Zinc imbalance is most likely to arise in vegetarians, smokers and heavy drinkers. However, over-supplementation of zinc leads to gastric irritation, atherosclerosis and anaemia secondary to copper deficiency (Galbraith et al, 1999).

Iron may increase the need for other micronutrients by stimulating red cell formation which also increases the body's folic acid requirements. Macrocytosis [glossary] has been reported (Barrett et al, 1994).

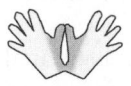 **Practice Point**

Folic acid supplements should be continued if iron is prescribed.

Iron excess

Adverse pregnancy outcomes are more likely when maternal haemoglobin falls outside the range 10.4–13.2 g/100 mL. Higher concentrations of haemoglobin increase the viscosity of the blood which may impair the blood flow to the placenta and predispose to coagulation (Long, 1995). Some 12–13 per cent of women may be vulnerable to iron overload (see above).

Table 11.2 Drugs and foods that reduce the absorption of iron

Substance	Management
Antacids	Separate ingestion by two hours.
Histamine (H2) antagonists (cimetidine, ranitidine)	Advise clients to manage nausea by adjusting food intake.
Methyldopa	Separate ingestion by two hours.
Cholestyramine	Separate ingestion by six hours.
Calcium supplements	Separate ingestion by two hours.
Tea, coffee, carbonated drinks	Separate ingestion by one hour.
Milk, eggs	Separate ingestion by two hours.
Phytates in bran, corn, beans and cereals	Separate ingestion by two hours.

Drug interactions – iron

Although foods such as orange juice, fish and alcohol help with the absorption of iron, other foods such as eggs and a number of cereal products containing phytates may impair iron absorption. Tea reduces iron absorption twice as much as coffee (Barrett et al, 1994). Black tea is particularly likely to impair iron absorption.

The antihypertensive effects of methyldopa are antagonized by iron. Administration should be separated by two hours. If blood pressure monitoring reveals the recurrence of hypertension, alternative antihypertensives should be considered.

Storage

The storage of iron tablets should be carefully considered, as they are very dangerous (even fatal) in overdose. As little as 2 g of iron (30 dried ferrous sulphate tablets of 200 mg) can be fatal to children. This typically occurs when toddlers ingest their mothers' iron tablets. Urgent referral to intensive care for administration of the antidote (desferrioxamine) can be life saving.

Other formulations of iron

Liquid iron

Liquid iron may be absorbed more readily than tablets, but can stain teeth.

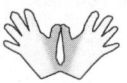 **Practice Points**

- Liquid iron should be administered to the back of the throat with an appropriate applicator or (second choice) with a straw.
- Liquid iron can be diluted with water or orange juice.
- After each dose, the mouth should be well rinsed with water.
- Stains may be removed by baking soda solution or hydrogen peroxide mouthwashes.
  (Galbraith et al, 1999; Springhouse Corporation, 1999).

Parenteral iron

Parenteral iron is occasionally used for women with gastro-intestinal disorders (e.g. ulcerative colitis), or who are unable to absorb or ingest iron for other reasons. Due to the high risks of hypersensitivity responses with these products, a test dose is mandatory (Ostrow & McCoy, 1998). Anaphylaxis may occur up to 24 hours after administration (McKenry & Salerno, 1998).

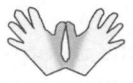 **Practice Point**

Intramuscular iron is not only painful but may cause tissue staining. Therefore, administration is into the gluteus maximus, using a Z-track technique (Ostrow & McCoy, 1998).

Conclusion

One of the aims of ante-natal care is to identify women at risk, including those at risk from anaemia. Each woman must be individually assessed, by measurement of **serum ferritin** and personal history, to differentiate the physiological changes of pregnancy from micronutrient deficiency (Engstrom & Sittler, 1994). Iron supplementation above 70 mg/day (300 mg ferrous sulphate) is rarely necessary in pregnancy, and, at this dose, side effects are less likely to be troublesome (Milman et al, 1999).

Implications for Practice: iron therapy

Potential Problems	Management
Signs and symptoms of anaemia persist despite therapy	Pre-therapy measurements of iron status and activity tolerance Administer between meals and warm drinks. Avoid sustained-release preparations. Regular evaluation of full blood count, serum iron, and ferritin. An improvement in haemoglobin should be seen after a week. Inform doctor of any decrease in white cell count which indicates an adverse reaction.
Gastro-intestinal side effects	Take in upright position, with full glass of water. Do not crush the tablets. Administer with food if nausea is a problem. Reduce the dose if necessary. Separate doses by at least six to eight hours
Dietary inadequacies	Arrange for folic acid supplements to be prescribed. Consider the diet of the whole family. Consider the possibility of micronutrient deficiencies such as zinc.
Over-medication	Careful assessment of personal and dietary history. Serum ferritin estimation. Family history of genetic disorders.
Intramuscular iron injections	Discontinue oral iron. Allow one hour between test dose and full dose administration. Advise the client to report any unusual symptoms up to 24 hours after iron injections.

Folic acid

The only supplement considered essential for all pregnant women in the UK is folic acid, which reduces the incidence of neural tube defects by 50–70 per cent (Daly et al, 1997). The administration of folic acid supplements is based on compelling evidence obtained from major studies, including randomized controlled trials (Hibbard & Smithells, 1965; Smithells et al, 1980; Laurence et al, 1981; MRC Vitamin Study Research Group, 1991; Czeizel & Dudas, 1992). The earlier studies provided convincing but not absolutely conclusive evidence of benefit of folic acid supplementation. The decision to proceed with the larger randomized studies was partly based on the difficulties with randomization in the earlier work. The Medical Research Council study recruited 1817 women whose previous pregnancies had been complicated by a neural tube defect, and randomized them to receive folic acid (4 mg), vitamin supplements, both or neither. By 1991, neural tube defects had occurred in 27 pregnancies, six in the folic acid groups and 21 in the others; this was considered to be sufficient statistical evidence to halt the trial. Czeizel & Dudas (1992) randomized over 4000 women planning a pregnancy to receive either a mineral or a folic acid supplement (0.8 mg) and found significantly lower rates of neural tube defects in those receiving folic acid (0 *versus* 6 p. = 0.029). The evidence for a protective role in other malformations, such as cleft palate and urinary tract defects is important but less compelling (Werler et al, 1999).

In humans, folic acid is essential for the production of thymidine, a component of DNA. Without folic acid, cell division is impaired which affects the embryo and the formation of blood cells. During pregnancy, folic acid requirements more than double and remain elevated during lactation (Hillman, 1996).

To help prevent the first occurrence of a neural tube defect, all women should be encouraged to take a folic acid supplement of 400 micrograms per day from the time they plan to become pregnant (at least 12 weeks preconception) until the end of the first trimester. Starting supplementation before the seventh week offers a significant advantage (Ulrich et al, 1999). Women who have not taken a supplement when they realize they are pregnant should start at once and continue at least until the 12th week (BNF, 2000) (see Implications for Practice).

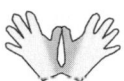 **Practice Points**

- For women who find compliance a problem, a weekly 5 mg folic acid tablet may be an alternative (Mathews et al, 1998).
- To obtain 0.4 mg folic acid from the diet, the woman would have to consume eight glasses of orange juice or ten helpings of broccoli or three helpings of brussel sprouts, lightly cooked (Wald & Bower, 1995).

Women who may become pregnant and have previously given birth to a child with a neural tube defect or have a first degree relative with this problem should be advised to take folic acid supplements at a dose of 5 mg (reduced to 4 mg if a suitable preparation becomes available) for the same period (BNF, 2000). Folic acid supplementation is associated with higher serum ferritin and haemoglobin concentrations and a reduced risk of anaemia (Hindmarsh et al, 2000).

Adverse reactions

Side effects or hypersensitivity responses associated with folic acid are extremely rare. The most common problem in midwifery is the increased risk of convulsions in women with epilepsy (see below). Such women were excluded from the major trial of folic acid (MRC, 1991). Women at high risk of developing pernicious anaemia should have serum B_{12} concentrations checked as soon as possible to exclude this potentially devastating, but treatable, condition. If given to people with pernicious anaemia, folic acid supplementation, particularly at the higher dose, masks the signs and symptoms of this progressive disorder (anaemia and glossitis), allowing the associated neurological degeneration to proceed unrecognized (BNF, 2000). This danger of masking pernicious anaemia is one of the reasons deterring the authorities from fortifying bread and cereals with folic acid. Pernicious anaemia mainly affects women in later life, but does sometimes occur in young women with a strong family history of the condition. Folic acid may cause a harmless yellow discolouration of the urine.

Drug interactions with folic acid

Folic acid absorption is decreased by oral contraceptives, isoniazid, cycloserine, glutethimide and enhanced by vitamin C.

Folic acid is antagonized by several anti-epileptics (carbamazepine, phenytoin, barbiturates, primodone). These anti-epileptics deplete the body of folates which reduces the elimination of the anti-epileptics; when folate stores are replenished, the elimination of the anti-epileptics increases, risking the return of seizures. Women taking anti-epileptic therapy should consult their doctors prior to starting folic acid therapy, as in some cases the supplement may cause serum anticonvulsant levels to fall, with possible loss of seizure control (Stockley, 1999).

Case Report

A 26-year-old woman with epilepsy, treated with carbamazepine, was planning pregnancy, and commenced a daily 0.8 mg folic acid supplement for prevention of neural tube defects.

Within the next few days, the woman experienced an increase in seizure frequency and her first grand mal fit. The authors attribute the worsening seizure frequency to folic acid supplementation (Guidolin et al, 1998).

Implications for Practice: folic acid

Potential Problems

Loss of seizure control in women with epilepsy.

Management

Ensure women with epilepsy consult with medical practitioners prior to starting folic acid.

If possible, women with epilepsy should consult their physicians prior to planning pregnancy.

Folic acid taken after conception may not be effective in preventing neural tube defects.

Folic acid should be commenced prior to conception.

Need for higher dose of folic acid in women with previous pregnancies complicated by a neural tube defect.

Identification of women at risk and preconceptual supplementation with the higher dose of folic acid (5 mg/day).

Conclusion

It has been estimated that folic acid supplementation prevents around a thousand neural tube defects every year (Wald & Bower, 1995). Pre-conceptual folic acid supplementation by tablets has been recommended for all women in the UK since 1993, as this is the most effective way to increase the availability of folic acid (Cuskelly et al, 1996). Folic acid in food may be destroyed in preparation, and universal food fortification risks masking the non-neurological signs of pernicious anaemia (Daly et al, 1997). However offering advice to women in the preconceptual period and for the first four weeks of pregnancy poses practical difficulties (Mathews et al, 1998).

During the 1980s, the incidence of neural tube defects fell from 45 per 10 000 births to 18 per 10 000 births (UK-wide). However, universal folic acid supplements were only recommended in 1993, following the Medical Research Council trial, published in 1991. It remains unclear why the recommendation of folic acid supplements has not further reduced the incidence of neural tube defects in the UK (Abramsky et al, 1999).

Further Reading

Van Way, C. (1999) *Nutrition Secrets*. Philadelphia, Hanley & Belfus.

Milman, N., Bergholt, T., Byg, K., Eriksen, L. & Grandal, N. (1999) Iron status and iron balance during pregnancy. A critical reappraisal of iron supplementation. *Acta Obstetrica Gynecoligica Scandinavia*:78:9:749–57.

CHAPTER 12

Management of Gastric Acidity in Pregnancy

SUE JORDAN

This chapter considers the available options for reducing gastric acid production, mainly H₂ antagonists and antacids. Other preparations to control gastric acidity (chelates, omeprazole) are mentioned briefly.

Chapter Contents

▨ Causes and management of heartburn in pregnancy

▨ Antacids

▨ Histamine₂ (H₂) antagonists (cimetidine, ranitidine)

▨ Chelates and complexes (sucralfate)

▨ Proton-pump inhibitors (omeprazole)

▨ Conclusion

Causes and management of heartburn in pregnancy

Acid reflux or 'heart burn' during pregnancy is a relatively common problem, affecting 45–85 per cent of women during pregnancy (Broussard & Richter, 1998). Symptoms may be managed by lifestyle adjustments or any one of a variety of medications, most of which are available over-the-counter (OTC). Gastric reflux is likely to arise for the first time in pregnancy, due to the changes occurring in the upper gastro-intestinal tract which are maximal around the 36th week. The consequences of this are:

- the lower oesophageal sphincter becomes less competent;
- reduced gastric motility and tone;
- delayed gastric emptying.

The relaxation of the gastro-intestinal tract during pregnancy is attributed to hormonal changes:

- increase in progesterone;
- decrease in motilin (a gastro-intestinal tract hormone);
- increase in enteroglucagon (a gastro-intestinal tract hormone).

These changes increase the dangers of gastric aspiration during anaesthesia. In previous triennia, aspiration of gastric contents during general anaesthesia was a major cause of avoidable maternal mortality. To lessen these dangers, some anaesthetists administer drugs to reduce gastric acidity and volume in all labouring women who are likely to require emergency surgery during labour. Prior to anaesthesia, women may receive:

- metoclopramide to minimize gastric contents (see Chapter 5);
- ranitidine;
- sodium citrate
  (Brunton, 1996; Rowe, 1997).

Women should be warned that they may experience gastric reflux during the later stages of pregnancy and be advised to minimize gastric distension by eating small frequent meals and taking fruit and fluids at different times to meals. Gastric acidity may be reduced by stopping smoking and adjusting the diet (see Box 12.1). Stooping or lying flat, peppermint and fatty foods will increase reflux.

Box 12.1   Factors which increase gastric acidity

- alcohol
- caffeine
- hypoglycaemia (missing meals)
- high calcium intake (including some antacid preparations)
- adrenaline/epinephrine (released in anger)

Disruption of gastric acid

If drugs are taken to reduce hydrochloric acid secretion or activity, the normal functions of gastric acid may be disrupted. This is particularly important if the drugs are administered long term.

- Hydrochloric acid is important in reducing the number of bacteria in food. Women using antacids should take extra care with food hygiene. Nosocomial pneumonia is more common in intensive care patients receiving H_2

antagonists for ulcer prevention: sucralfate is suggested as an alternative (Tryba & Kulka, 1993).

● Hydrochloric acid is important for protein digestion and normal flow of bile and pancreatic juice.

● Hydrochloric acid is important for the absorption of vitamin B_{12}. With long term use of drugs for peptic ulceration, vitamin B_{12} deficiency may arise.

Antacids

From long experience, most antacids are considered safe in pregnancy, particularly as they are rarely needed during the crucial phase of organogenesis (18th to 55th days of pregnancy). However, overuse can cause problems such as disruption of gastric acid production (see above). A wide variety of antacids are available OTC for symptom relief, including heartburn and non-ulcer indigestion. Examples of antacids include sodium bicarbonate, aluminium hydroxide, magnesium carbonate, sodium citrate and numerous proprietary preparations. Chewable tablets must be thoroughly masticated and followed by a drink of water. Mixing chewable tablets with water is ineffective.

Antacids provide almost immediate relief of symptoms. On an empty stomach this lasts for about 30 minutes, but the effects are prolonged by several hours if antacids are taken an hour after food. Most of these compounds (85 per cent) are eliminated in the faeces, however some constituents of antacids are absorbed and excreted by the kidneys.

Actions and side effects of antacids

Antacids decrease the acidity of the stomach which:

● neutralizes the contents of the stomach;
● reduces reflux by increasing the pressure of the lower oesophageal sphincter;
● may increase gastric acid secretion, worsening symptoms or increasing the dangers of gastric aspiration.

Magnesium carbonate and magnesium hydroxide (found in most OTC preparations including Bisodol®, Andrews Antacid®) neutralize hydrochloric acid for several hours by forming insoluble magnesium chloride. *Magnesium trisilicate* (prescribed as tablets or oral powder, Compound BP) also forms colloidal silica which adsorbs [glossary] pepsin and has a more prolonged effect. This preparation may cause kidney stones if used long term (Malseed et al, 1995). All these magnesium salts/compounds have a purgative effect (see Chapter 13, laxatives). Magnesium can accumulate in the body if renal function is poor (see Chapter 9).

Aluminium hydroxide gel (non-proprietary or as Alu-Cap ®) neutralizes hydrochloric acid and forms insoluble aluminium chloride. This inactivates pepsin by adsorption (taking it onto its surface, see glossary). Aluminium compounds cause constipation and delay gastric emptying. They are therefore not usually recommended during pregnancy or breastfeeding (Pangle, 2000). Aluminium binds to phosphates in the gut, reducing their absorption. In women at risk of malnutrition, this can contribute to osteoporosis (Brucker & Faucher, 1997).

Sodium bicarbonate (sodium biacarbonate compound BP and in proprietary products such as Bisodol ®, Gaviscon tablets ®) acts rapidly to neutralize hydrochloric acid, with the liberation of carbon dioxide. This stimulates gastrin production, which in turn increases gastric acid production and worsens symptoms. Carbon dioxide distends the stomach, promoting belching and worsening reflux (Brunton, 1996).

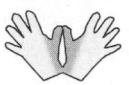 **Practice Point**

Women should be warned that these preparations may worsen, rather than alleviate, symptoms.

Sodium bicarbonate is absorbed, and is normally excreted by the kidneys. In high doses, sodium bicarbonate can cause a metabolic alkalosis [glossary] and the formation of kidney stones. Sodium bicarbonate may impede the absorption of B vitamins. Sodium intake from antacids should be limited to 0.2 mmol sodium per day (Malseed et al, 1995).

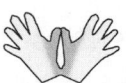 **Practice Points**

- The sodium content of antacids can be sufficient to raise blood pressure or worsen oedema. If this occurs, antacids without sodium should be substituted, for example magnesium trisilicate tablets, BP.
- Women with borderline pre-eclampsia or at risk of pre-eclampsia should be advised to discontinue antacid prepartaions.

Sodium citrate is sometimes employed prior to anaesthesia to reduce gastric acidity, to reduce the dangers of gastric aspiration. This has the disadvantage that it increases the volume of the gastric contents and reduces the efficacy of metoclopramide (Kennedy & Longnecker, 1996). Citrate ions are metabolized to bicarbonate ions, which affect the pH of the blood. In a small (n = 86) randomized placebo controlled trial to examine the effect of sodium citrate prior to elective Caesarean section, sodium citrate made no difference to either the pH or volume of vomitus, the incidence of nausea or the fluctuations in blood pressure. Despite treatment with sodium citrate, the vomitus was sufficiently acidic to have caused pulmonary damage had it been aspirated (Palmer et al, 1991).

Calcium salts are present in some OTC antacids, such as liquid Gaviscon®, Bisodol® and Settlers®. They are likely to stimulate gastric acid production and worsen symptoms. Prolonged use of calcium containing antacids can lead to the milk-alkali syndrome, kidney damage or renal stones. Potts (1991) reports that susceptible individuals may develop symptoms of weakness and irritability within days of beginning calcium and antacid ingestion. It would appear that susceptible individuals absorb a high percentage of ingested calcium, which is deposited in the kidneys, causing long term damage. The bicarbonate ions ingested with the antacid cannot then be excreted and accumulate, causing weakness, including respiratory depression.

Alginates (contained in Algicon® and Gaviscon®) and dimethicone are frequently incorporated into antacids. These reduce flatulence by forming a viscous barrier, which increases the adhesion of gastric contents to the mucosa. Dimeticone (for example as Infacol®) is sometimes used for infantile colic, but it is no longer recommended (BNF, 2000).

Many *compound preparations* are available. For example, magnesium trisilicate mixture BP also contains sodium bicarbonate, and Gaviscon ® tablets contain alginic acid, aluminium hydroxide 100 mg, magnesium trisilicate 25 mg and sodium bicarbonate 2 mmol.

Compounds containing both magnesium and aluminium are frequently used because:

- the constipating and gastric slowing effects of aluminium are countered by magnesium;
- magnesium provides immediate symptom relief, whereas the effects of aluminium are more sustained.

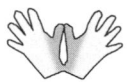 **Practice Point**

All labels of OTC products should be read carefully. It is prudent to avoid preparations containing sodium and calcium salts.

Interactions with antacids

Absorption of most drugs, including the oral contraceptive pill, is impaired by antacids and enteric coatings are destroyed (Brucker & Faucher, 1997).

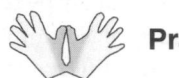 **Practice Point**

Administration of other drugs should be separated from antacids by two hours (Stockley, 1999).

Cautions

● Long term use of any antacids may cause the formation of kidney stones.
● If any degree of renal insufficiency is present (as in pre-eclampsia, or if there is evidence of repeated UTI), antacids are best avoided, as they may accumulate and cause toxicity.
● More than three months' use of antacids may be associated with birth defects (Van Way, 1999).

Storage in the refrigerator may make antacids more palatable. It is important to check expiry dates, as antacids loose their efficacy if stored too long. Liquid formulations must be shaken vigorously before administration.

Histamine$_2$ (H$_2$) antagonists

These drugs (cimetidine, ranitidine, famotidine, nizatidine) are widely used prior to obstetric anaesthesia to minimize any lung damage caused by aspiration of gastric contents. Long term use during pregnancy and lactation is unusual, as animal studies offer little reassurance on safety (BNF, 2000). (US FDA category B, except nizatidine.) They are generally reserved for use in the second and third trimesters where lifestyle changes, antacids and sucralfate have failed (Cappell & Garcia, 1998; Katz & Castell, 1998). A recent study (Ruigomez et al, 1999) found a very slightly increased risk of malformation with cimetidine and ranitidine (also omeprazole), although the confidence limits [glossary] included one in all cases, indicating that the increases could be chance findings.

How the body handles H$_2$ antagonists

These drugs are well absorbed orally. They take effect within one hour of administration, with maximum activity between one and three hours. Duration of action varies from 4–13 hours, depending on whether the drug is administered with food (McKenry and Salerno, 1998). H$_2$ antagonists are eliminated by the liver and kidneys, and are unsuitable for anyone with severe renal or hepatic disease.

The half-life of ranitidine is 2–2.5 hours; therefore if ranitidine is administered at the onset of labour, it is likely to be eliminated from the mother's body before breastfeeding is commenced.

Actions and side effects of H₂ antagonists

Histamine, via H_2 receptors, promotes secretion of gastrin, which controls gastric motility and secretion. H_2 antagonists reduce basal and nocturnal acid output, but have less effect on prandial acid output at standard doses. H_2 antagonists are effective and generally well tolerated; with long term use, the incidence of side effects is about 3 per cent (Brunton, 1996). The side effects are as follows:

Central nervous system

These drugs can cause dizziness, somnolence and fatigue, which impair the ability to drive. They may also cause headache, hallucinations, confusion and delirium. It is possible that these side effects could be mistakenly attributed to an anaesthetic.

Cardiovascular system

H_2 antagonists administered intravenously can lower or raise heart rate or cause heart block. Therefore, intravenous administration is by infusion or slow injection (BNF, 2000).

Gastro-intestinal disturbances

Nausea, stomach cramps, constipation or diarrhoea may result from administration of H_2 antagonists.

Anti-androgen actions

In long term use, *cimetidine* and, to a lesser extent, ranitidine, have anti-androgen effects, including breast discomfort and loss of libido which are reversible on withdrawal. These actions are attributed to an increase in prolactin secretion. Therefore cimetidine is not advised during lactation (Brucker & Faucher, 1997).

Rare side effects include rash, hair loss, hyperthermia, bronchospasm, interstitial nephritis, liver and bone marrow damage.

Interactions with H₂ antagonists

- H₂ antagonists are not well absorbed in the presence of antacids or meto-clopramide, and these drugs should be administered two hours apart.
- Blood alcohol concentrations may be raised by concomitant administration of H₂ antagonists due to enhanced absorption of alcohol. This exacerbates any problems with driving.
- Smoking reduces ulcer healing and increases the breakdown of H₂ antagonists.

Cimetidine, more than other H₂ antagonists, inhibits hepatic metabolism of many drugs. This is the source of numerous drug interactions. Drugs, normally eliminated by metabolism, will accumulate if taken concurrently with cimetidine. Examples include: opioids (pethidine), anti-psychotics (prochlor-perazine), warfarin, caffeine, theophylline, many benzodiazepines, nifedipine, tricyclic antidepressants, propranolol, phenytoin, carbamazepine, metronida-zole, antiarrhythmics, quinine, cyclosporin.

Chelates and complexes (sucralfate)

These bind to the base of the ulcer in the lining of the gastrointestinal tract and provide physical protection. This allows the natural secretion of bicarbonate to re-establish the normal pH gradient across the gut wall. These drugs must be taken on an empty stomach or they will combine with the protein in food, rather than the gut wall. They should be taken 30 minutes to one hour before or two hours after food. Both liquid and tablet preparations should be administered with water.

Sucralfate is widely used for reflux disorders in pregnancy in the USA, but not in the UK (Broussard & Richter, 1998). It consists of sulphated sucrose plus aluminium hydroxide. Sucralfate is only effective if the stomach contents are acid. It is not absorbed, and has few side effects, but indigestion, nausea, diarrhoea or constipation, dry mouth, back pain, rash, pruritus, dizziness and sleepiness have been reported. It is contra-indicated in renal failure. Like other antacids, it interferes with the absorption of other drugs, and administration should be separated by two hours.

Bismuth chelate (De-nol®) is not used in pregnancy since there is a risk of absorption.

Proton-pump inhibitors (omeprazole)

Omeprazole (Losec®) is rarely used in pregnancy due to reported terato-genicity in animal studies (BNF, 2000) and concerns in human studies (Ruigomez et al, 1999). It is not discussed further here.

Implications for Practice: antacids and H₂ antagonists

Potential Problem	Management
ANTACIDS	
Worsening of symptoms with administration of antacid.	Ask clients to monitor frequency of antacid ingestion.
	Avoid antacids containing sodium.
	If symptoms increase, suggest non-pharmacological management and seek medical advice.
Drug interactions	Separate ingestion/administration by two hours.
Stool discolouration (whitening)	Women should be advised of this possibility.
Kidney stones	Avoid long term use of antacids.
Alkalosis	Minimize use of antacids containing bicarbonate or citrate ions.
Unpalatable taste	Chill before taking.
H₂ ANTAGONISTS	
Cardiac conduction disturbances	Observe heart rate changes during intravenous infusion.
	Administer intravenous infusions slowly, never above the manufacturer's recommended rate.
Tiredness and confusion	Reassure women that with single doses, these effects will pass within a few hours.
Drug interactions with cimetidine	It is probably more prudent to use ranitidine if any other drugs need to be administered.

Conclusion

Ideally, gastric acidity will be managed by non-pharmacological interventions, particularly as uncertainty surrounds the administration of several of the widely used preparations. See Implications for Practice.

Further Reading

Malseed, R.T., Goldstein, F.J. & Balkon, N. (1995) *Pharmacology: Drug Therapy and Nursing Considerations*, 4th edition. Philadelphia, Lippincott.

CHAPTER 13

Laxatives in Pregnancy and Childbirth

SUE JORDAN AND BRONWYN HEGARTY

This chapter considers the management of constipation associated with pregnancy and childbirth.

Chapter Contents

▧ Constipation

▧ Laxatives

▧ Types of laxatives

▧ Conclusion

Constipation

Constipation may be defined as a delay in the passage of food residue, due to the accumulation of hard, dry stool, associated with painful defaecation, abdominal distension and a palpable mass. Constipation may lead to further symptoms such as headache, abdominal pain and appetite impairment. The normal frequency of bowel movements ranges from three per day to one in three days (Ganong, 1999).

Delays in colonic motility may be a problem at various stages of pregnancy and childbirth. During the antenatal period many women experience problems with constipation, and if this is not resolved it may affect the normal progress of labour by obstructing the birth canal (Bennett & Brown, 1993). Following the physiological evacuation of the bowel during labour, defaeca-

Table 13.1 Drugs causing constipation

opioids (pethidine, codeine)
iron tablets
anti-muscarinics [glossary], sedatives
sympathomimetics [glossary]
• amphetamines (including ecstasy), cocaine
• 'cold cures' OTC (Sudafed ®)
• salbutamol, ritrodine
anti-hypertensives: beta blockers, calcium blockers

drugs causing dehydration:
• diuretics
• alcohol
• some laxatives, for example lactulose

aluminium-containing antacids
sucralfate
anti-diarrhoeal agents
stimulant laxatives causing atonic colon (over use of)
NSAIDs (not aspirin)
muscle relaxants given for general anaesthesia

tion is usually delayed for several days. Progesterone concentrations usually remain elevated for several days post-partum which decreases colonic motility. If perineal trauma has been sustained, a combination of dehydration, pain, fear and anxiety and loss of sensation may also impede defaecation.

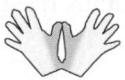 **Practice Point**

In some cases, dietary intervention (increasing fibre and water intake) and lifestyle changes (increasing exercise, heeding sensations of fullness in the rectum immediately) are not sufficient, and pharmacological agents will help in the short term. All laxatives/aperients are given only for short term use, with the primary aim of adjusting the diet when the constipation is resolved.

Pharmacological agents are useful for acute constipation, but their use should be restricted to one to two weeks (Malseed et al, 1995). The management of chronic constipation should follow physiological principles. If these are not explained to the woman ante-natally, there is a danger that she may resort to inappropriate over-the-counter (OTC) laxatives.

The midwife should consider the possibility that various pharmacological agents, such as iron tablets, (see Table 13.1) may contribute to constipation. Women who use codeine for analgesia or cough suppression are likely to find opioid-induced constipation intolerable in pregnancy (Malseed et al, 1995).

In some circumstances, clients taking drugs for recreational purposes, such as amphetamines or opioids, will complain of constipation. Occasionally, constipation may be a symptom of a serious illness and further investigation will be needed, (see Table 13.2.)

Table 13.2   Constipation may be a symptom of serious pathology

- Dehydration, debility or fever
- Hypokalaemia
- Hypocalcaemia
- Hypothyroidism – *more likely in the post-natal period*
- Gastro-intestinal disease (diverticulitis or neoplasm)
- Gastro-intestinal obstruction or post-operative ileus
- Lesions causing pain on defaecation (perineal damage during parturition, haemorrhoids)
- Scleroderma
- Muscle disease/wasting (malnutrition, hyperemesis gravidarum)
- CNS disease (multiple sclerosis, depression, anorexia)
- Autonomic nervous system disease (diabetes)
- Liver/gall bladder disease e.g. intrahepatic cholestasis of pregnancy
- Laxative abuse and eating disorders

The physiology of colonic motility

The smooth muscle of the colon undergoes peristalsis, segmentation and mass action; all gut movements are controlled by several systems, including the enteric nervous system. The factors affecting colonic motility are summarized in Table 13.3.

Table 13.3   Factors affecting colonic motility

- The autonomic nervous system
  * The sympathetic nervous system slows the gut and contracts the sphincters, for example in times of stress or anxiety, or if privacy is lacking.
  * The parasympathetic nervous system hastens the gut and relaxes the sphincters, for example when the individual is relaxed or extremely fearful.
- Higher centres (the defaecation centre in medulla) which are influenced by stress.
- Spinal and local reflexes (mainly parasympathetic nervous system).
- Mobility: colonic motility decreases if people become less mobile for any reason.
- Gastro-intestinal hormones co-ordinate the whole gut. For example eating triggers the gastro-colic reflex.
- Stretch of the gastro-intestinal tract. Bulky, high-fibre meals encourage colonic activity.
- Hydration: dehydration hardens the faeces and hinders their movement.
- Irritation of the gastro-intestinal tract, for example by caffeine, toxins or stimulant laxatives.
- Circadian rhythm. Colonic motility is maximal in the morning, after breakfast. This is upset by any change in routine or inability to heed the 'call to stool'.
- Circulating hormones such as progesterone, oestrogen and thyroid hormones.

Some of these factors can be modified by including 20–60 g of fibre/day in the diet (Brunton, 1996) and drinking one or two glasses of fluid with each meal (McQuaid, 1995). It should also be remembered that stress and tension, for example due to a strange environment such as hospital, can be responsible for constipation. Colonic inertia is more common among women with a history of sexual abuse or psychosocial problems (McQuaid, 1995). The gastro-colic reflex is most likely to be active after a high fibre breakfast (including some caffeine) in a relaxed environment.

Constipation and pregnancy

Pregnancy predisposes to constipation, due to:

- direct pressure of the uterus and fetus on the bowel;
- reduction or change in food and fluid intake;
- reduction in exercise taken;
- hormone-induced relaxation of the smooth muscle of the gut caused by
  - an increase in progesterone,
  - a decrease in motilin, which is produced by the gut wall,
  - an increase in enteroglucagon, which is produced by the gut wall.
- Faecal impaction is more likely during pregnancy because greater quantities of water and salts are absorbed from the colon due to:
  - the increased transit time, due to relaxation of the intestinal smooth muscle;
  - the actions of prolactin;
  - activation of the renin-angiotensin-aldosterone axis [glossary] in pregnancy and increased absorption of salt and water (Rutishauser, 1994; Garland, 1985).

Laxatives

A laxative is an agent that facilitates evacuation of the bowel (Malseed et al, 1995). Certain foods and drugs have laxative properties which may be useful under some circumstances.

Laxatives are used:

- when straining may be harmful, following perineal suturing or trauma, Caesarean section, abdominal surgery, or if the woman has haemorrhoids or cardiac disease;
- with opioids, if use is to continue longer than four to five days;
- during immobility from any cause.

Laxatives may be administered orally, as enemas or suppositories. Although less effective than enemas, suppositories are more acceptable to women. Current evidence does not suggest that routine administration of enemas during labour confers any benefit (Cuervo et al, 2000). While the occasional use of laxatives is considered safe, long term use is associated with complications and bowel damage (Shafik, 1993). Laxatives are contra-indicated if the gastro-intestinal tract is obstructed (BNF, 2000).

Side effects common to all laxatives

All laxatives may cause side effects by disrupting: the normal functioning of the fluid and electrolyte balance; the colonic flora; gut motility. See Implications for Practice.

Disruption of fluid and electrolyte balance

The colon plays an important part in the homeostasis of body fluids. Each day, it receives 1–2 litres of isotonic fluid from the ileum, of which it reabsorbs 90 per cent. The colon is capable of absorbing considerable quantities of water and drugs rapidly, although it does this erratically. *Tap water given by enema may be absorbed and cause water intoxication* (Ganong, 1999). Several mechanisms control the movement of ions and water across the wall of the colon. If these mechanisms are disrupted by diarrhoea or by laxatives, there is a potential for loss of important fluid and electrolytes. Thus all laxatives:

- reduce the absorption of sodium by inhibiting the Na+/K+ pump, and can cause hyponatraemia [glossary];
- reduce the absorption of water, causing dehydration, which is dangerous in volume depleted or severely anaemic people (McKenry & Salerno, 1998);
- increase the loss of potassium by increasing the rate and volume of fluid flowing through the colon. Hypokalaemia is an important side effect of laxative use, overuse and abuse; it is also a cause of constipation. (Hypokalaemia may arise in association with tocolytic therapy; see Chapter 7.)
- increase the loss of magnesium (Nichols, 1993).

These electrolyte changes may be particularly dangerous in pregnancy: any fluid and electrolyte imbalance can alter the distribution of body fluids which may compromise placental blood flow and fetal well-being (McKenry & Salerno, 1998).

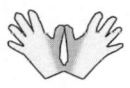 **Practice Points**

- A woman who is complaining of tiredness and constipation may be potassium depleted.
- A venous blood sample to measure the concentrations of electrolytes is helpful in assessing the disturbances caused by regular use of laxatives.
- Dehydration may lead to a fall in blood pressure on standing.

Change in colonic flora

The intestinal flora are established early in life and while these commensal bacteria use some nutrients (vitamin C, choline) they are important sources of vitamin K, some B vitamins and folic acid. Excessive use of laxatives will destroy the resident intestinal flora and recolonization by other micro-organisms may produce flatulence and discomfort.

If the colonic mucosa is damaged by overuse of laxatives, the commensal bacteria enter the circulation in sufficient numbers to overwhelm the hepatic detoxification mechanisms, and cause serious disease, including gram negative septicaemia. This is a particular danger if the blood supply to the colon is jeopardized, as in hypovolaemic shock.

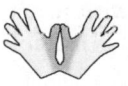 **Practice Point**

Laxatives would not be administered to women who are fluid deficient.

Increased intestinal motility

Laxatives stimulate the contractions of the intestines; this may cause abdominal cramps, diarrhoea, flatulence and discomfort.

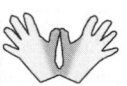 **Practice Points**

- If a laxative (even a single dose) has been effective in evacuating the colon, the woman should be advised not to expect further motions for several days (Brunton, 1996).
- Habitual use of stimulant laxatives may destroy the enteric nerve plexuses, producing an atonic or spastic colon.

Types of laxatives

Laxatives can be divided into four groups (Rang et al, 1999):

- **Bulk laxatives**
  bran, methylcellulose, ispaghula husk (Fybogel®), sterculia (Normacol®)
- **Osmotic laxatives**
  lactulose, magnesium sulphate (Epsom salts), magnesium hydroxide, phosphate enemas (Carbalax ®), sodium citrate enema (Micolette micro-enema®)
- **Faecal softeners**
  liquid paraffin, docusate, mineral oils, arachis oil enema
- **Stimulant laxatives or purgatives**
  senna, figs, prunes, rhubarb, castor oil, bisacodyl, glycerol, danthron, docusate, sodium picosylphate, phenolphthalein

The timing of various laxative actions is summarized in Box 13.1.

Bulk laxatives

Bulk laxatives are polysaccharides which are not digested. They attract water by osmosis [glossary], which increases their volume and therefore stimulates peristalsis. The more effective bulk laxatives (bran) also work by acting as a substrate for colonic bacteria; these multiply and increase faecal bulk. Bulk laxatives are a substitute for dietary fibre, and useful for patients with haemorrhoids, colostomy or ileostomy, anal fissure, diverticular disease, irritable bowel syndrome or ulcerative colitis.

Bulk laxatives are considered safer than other laxatives in pregnancy (McKenry & Salerno, 1998). However, an increase in dietary fibre to 20–

Box 13.1   Usual timing of action of laxatives

Colon evacuation usually takes:

1–3 DAYS	6–8 HOURS	1–3 HOURS
BULKING AGENTS	SENNA	MgSO₄, Cream of Magnesia
LACTULOSE	BISACODYL	SALINE CATHARTICS
	CASCARA PHENOLPHTHALEIN	CASTOR OIL

60 g/day intake is preferable to the use of laxatives. Dietary fibres, particularly pectin and lignin, have the added advantage of binding to bile acids, thereby reducing plasma cholesterol. Claims that laxatives act as appetite suppressants are exaggerated (Brunton, 1996).

Disadvantages of bulk laxatives

- Bulk laxatives take several days to work and may be ineffective. Failure of bulk laxatives is usually associated with weak pelvic floor muscles and the inability to co-ordinate the pelvic floor muscles (Po & Po, 1992).
- Flatulence is a common complaint which may subside with continued use.
- Bran and other fibres containing phytates form complexes with zinc, calcium, iron, magnesium and copper from the diet. This reduces the absorption of micronutrients which is important if the diet is marginal.
- Bulk laxatives may coalesce into a hard mass, which will then obstruct the GI tract.

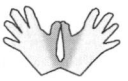 **Practice Point**

It is essential to ensure an adequate fluid intake. Bulk laxatives should be taken with at least two glasses of water (Malseed et al, 1995).

Other constituents of the laxative preparation are important to some women:

- *Some laxatives (barley malt extract, Regulan powder®) contain available carbohydrate, which will affect diabetics.*
- *Bran contains gluten and must be avoided in women with coeliac disease.*
- *Some laxatives (such as Fybogel®) contain sodium, which predisposes to fluid retention and oedema.*

Interactions: Bulk laxatives may bind to other drugs (anti-coagulants, salicylates, digitalis, tetracyclines) and minerals, so impairing absorption.

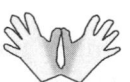 **Practice Point**

Laxatives should be administered two hours apart from food and other drugs.

Osmotic laxatives

A number of laxatives are osmotically active, retaining water by osmosis, thus increasing the volume in the gut, and stimulating stretch reflexes. The movement of water into the GI tract may deplete the extracellular fluid volume, leading to dehydration.

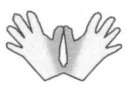 **Practice Point**

These laxatives should be taken with a full glass of water and may be added to food.

Osmotic laxatives differ in their potency, speed and site of action. Most will act in the upper GI tract, but lactulose acts only in the colon which delays and reduces its potency.

Magnesium salts

A variety of magnesium salts is on sale over the counter: for example magnesium sulphate (Epsom salts, Andrews Liver salts®); magnesium hydroxide mixture BP (Cream of magnesia®); magnesium citrate (Citramag®). They are suitable only for occasional or short term use. Liquid preparations are more potent than tablets. Chilling and flavouring improves taste.

Magnesium salts are incompletely absorbed. Their osmotic action distends and stretches the stomach, causing discomfort, abdominal cramps, even triggering the gastro-colic reflex. Flatulence and abdominal cramps may limit use. Passage of a hypertonic solution [glossary] into the duodenum may trigger vomiting, particularly if taken on an empty stomach. Magnesium salts can act rapidly, within one to three hours if taken when the stomach is empty, although lower doses may take six to eight hours to work. Some magnesium is absorbed from laxatives which is dangerous in renal and liver failure (see Chapter 9, magnesium).

Phosphate compounds (as enemas)

These can reduce the plasma calcium concentration and may irritate the colonic mucosa and Shafik (1993) suggests that warm saline provides a safer enema.

Sodium salts

Sodium salts will worsen fluid retention and heart failure and saline purgatives are not recommended due to the risk of salt retention (BNF, 2000).

Lactulose

Lactulose is used post-partum both as a treatment and a prophylactic when perineal trauma or haemorrhoids are present. Lactulose is metabolized by colonic bacteria to galactose and fructose, thence to lactic and acetic acids and formate. These attract water into the gut by osmosis, which increases faecal bulk.

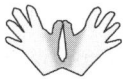 **Practice Point**

Some women may find lactulose unpleasantly sweet (McCartney, 1995).

Lactulose acts within two to three days. Tolerance to action and side effects develops; thus uncomfortable side effects such as cramps and flatulence may dissipate within a few days.

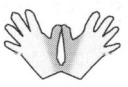 **Practice Point**

Lactulose can cause nausea, vomiting or loss of fluid and electrolytes (Brunton, 1996).

Lactulose should be used with caution in some circumstances:

- Diabetics. The sugars in lactulose may cause hyperglycaemia, so careful monitoring is required.
- Seriously ill or malnourished women may not withstand the loss of extracellular fluid and potassium ions.
- Galactosaemia (a rare hereditary condition). Galactose is extremely detrimental in galactosaemia and lactulose should be avoided.

Interactions with laxatives

Diarrhoea, including that induced by laxatives, may prevent the absorption of other drugs. Lactulose is less effective if given with antibiotics which destroy the colonic flora (McKenry & Salerno, 1998).

Faecal softeners

These are useful if haemorrhoids, anal sphincter damage and anal fissures are present.

- **Docusate**   Acts as a detergent and as a stimulant; it takes several days to work.
- **Liquid paraffin**   Interferes with the absorption of fat-soluble vitamins and some drugs.

  The oil may leak through the anus, form 'paraffinomas' in the lymph ducts or produce an aspiration pneumonia. It is usually combined with phenolphthalein (Delax®) or methylcellulose (as emulsion).

Liquid paraffin is very rarely used, because of its effect on the absorption of fat soluble vitamins.

Stimulant and irritant purgatives

These potent laxatives (for example senna) are widely available. Their role (if any) in childbirth should be restricted to use as suppositories post-partum. Suppositories may cause local irritation of the rectum. Stimulant laxatives increase smooth muscle contractions in the gut and uterus by stretch and irritation.

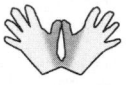 **Practice Point**

Avoid stimulant laxatives in pregnancy, due to the risk of uterine contractions and premature labour.

All stimulant laxatives reduce the absorption of fluid and electrolytes from the colon, and can cause diarrhoea, abdominal cramps, malabsorption and loss of fluids. With long term use, atonic colon, protein loss and hypokalaemia are potential problems. Damage to the gut lining may induce protein-losing enteropathy, steatorrhoea and malabsorption of calcium; therefore the use of stimulant laxatives is restricted to one week (McKenry & Salerno, 1998).

These laxatives act within 6–12 hours and they are often taken at bedtime. There is marked individual variation in response. Phenolphthalein, senna, danthron, cascara, aloe, rhubarb are passed into breast milk, causing diarrhoea in the infant and should be avoided during breastfeeding (Po & Po, 1992).

- **Glycerol** suppositories act as a mild localized irritant and stimulate the rectum, producing a bowel evacuation within 30 minutes of insertion (Shafik, 1993).

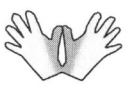 **Practice Point**

Glycerol suppositories should be stored in the refrigerator and not handled. If held at body temperature, they will begin to release their contents, and work less effectively (Spencer, 1993a).

- **Castor oil** This is a powerful laxative which acts in three to six hours. It is broken down by pancreatic lipase to form ricinoleic acid, which is an irritant to both gut and uterus. It should, therefore, be avoided in pregnancy, including topical applications (Malseed et al, 1995).
- **Senna, aloe and cascara** These contain derivatives of anthracene, which are liberated by colonic bacteria and irritate the colon. The ensuing abdominal pain and discomfort are not well tolerated. Anthracene derivatives pass into the blood stream and appear in urine, saliva and breast milk; therefore, they should be avoided during breastfeeding.
- **Bisacodyl** This causes rectal irritation; the use of suppositories may cause a burning sensation. If continued over weeks, proctitis and sloughing of the epithelium may result. Bisacodyl is sometimes given as a single dose in pregnancy and the puerperium.
- **Soap** This is a severe irritant, which inflames the rectal mucosa if given as an enema. Soap enemas should be avoided, particularly in pregnancy (BNF, 2000).

Interactions with stimulant laxatives

Biscodyl enteric coating is removed by antacids, milk or H_2 antagonists which causes excessive gastric motility/cramps. To prevent this, administration should be two hours apart and chipped tablets avoided.

Laxative abuse

Dependence on laxatives may arise from desire to lose weight or concern with bowel movements. After using stimulant laxatives or purgatives, no faeces may be passed for several days which encourages reuse of laxatives. Fluid and electrolyte imbalance may be severe; see above.

Implications for Practice: laxatives

- A single dose of a laxative is considered safe after delivery. If a laxative is needed, glycerol suppositories may be given (Silverton, 1993).
- If a laxative is indicated for medical reasons or perineal trauma, use is limited to one week. Bulking agents are preferred and liquid paraffin and stimulant laxatives must be avoided (Hibbard, 1988). If laxatives are used, the midwife should be alert to potential problems associated with their use.

Potential problem	management
Dehydration	Take with water, especially bulk laxatives.
Intestinal obstruction	
Electrolyte disturbance	Monitor. Limit use to one to two weeks. Ask the woman to report cramps, weakness, dizziness.
Discolouration of urine	Inform woman.
Laxative dependence	One to two week use maximum.
Passage to breastfed baby	Avoid stimulant laxatives during lactation.
Uterine contractions	Avoid stimulants laxatives in pregnancy.

Conclusion

Constipation is common in pregnancy and childbirth, due to the structural and physiological changes in the woman's body. Unresolved constipation can interfere with the normal progress of labour and may cause problems in the puerperium. Constipation may also be due to a variety of illnesses, or fever; therefore, serious pathology should be excluded. In ante-natal care and in the puerperium, it is also necessary to check for pyrexia and urinary tract infection. The possibility of hypothyroidism should not be overlooked in the postnatal period. Constipation is commonly cased by poor diet, lack of exercise, stress, dehydration and other drugs. Advice about the prevention and/or alleviation of constipation should be given to all women at ante-natal and postnatal visits. Additionally, a record of bowel movements can raise awareness of the problem and may prevent complications, such as faecal impaction, and reduce the need to administer laxatives.

Further Reading

Cuervo, L., Rodreguez, M. & Delgado, M. (2000) Enemas during labor. *Cochrane Database Systematic Review*: (issue 2) Update software, Oxford.

CHAPTER 14

Antimicrobial Agents

MIKE TAIT

This chapter outlines the actions and side effects of antimicrobial agents. It also considers the reasons why some courses of antimicrobials are ineffective.

Chapter Contents

▪ Pathogenic and beneficial micro-organisms

▪ Antibacterials and their actions

▪ Antifungals and their actions

▪ Antivirals and their actions

▪ Reasons for failure of antimicrobial therapy

▪ How the body handles antimicrobials

▪ Adverse effects of antimicrobials

▪ Conclusion: the future of antimicrobial therapy

An antimicrobial agent is any substance that inhibits the growth of, or kills, a micro-organism. This broad definition includes a range of chemicals that have varying degrees of toxicity to humans. Disinfectants such as chlorine and ethylene oxide are strong antimicrobial agents that are toxic to humans but can be used, for example, to prevent growth of bacteria such as *Legionella* in air-conditioning systems (chlorine) or to sterilize heat-sensitive medical equipment (ethylene oxide). Antiseptics such as chlorhexidine and silver nitrate are less toxic to humans and can be used, for example, to inhibit microbial growth on human skin (chlorhexidine) or to prevent blindness in newborn babies caused by *Neisseria gonorrhoeae* infections (silver nitrate). For use *inside* the body, however, the antimicrobials used must be selectively toxic against micro-organisms with as low a toxicity to humans as possible. This chapter focuses on this last group of antimicrobials, the *chemotherapeutic* agents. These include *antibiotics* such as penicillin, *antifungals* such as nystatin and flu-conazole and *antivirals* such as aciclovir.

Pathogenic and beneficial micro-organisms

Micro-organisms are usually divided into five groups: bacteria, fungi, algae, protozoa and viruses. Most infectious diseases are caused by bacteria, fungi or viruses, although some protozoa can cause diseases such as malaria and amoebic dysentery. Micro-organisms that cause disease are called *pathogens.*

Although there are numerous pathogenic micro-organisms, it is important to realize that there are also large numbers of micro-organisms living in association with humans that are either harmless or beneficial to us. For example, the gut is filled with bacteria that aid digestion, produce vitamins and protect against pathogens. *Escherichia coli*, for example, is a normal gut inhabitant that produces vitamin K. Other vitamins produced by gut bacteria include thiamine (vitamin B_1), riboflavin (vitamin B_2), and vitamin B_{12}. Haemorrhagic disease of the newborn, due to vitamin K deficiency, occasionally occurs in breastfed babies (see Chapter 8).

The mixture of micro-organisms in the gut – the *microflora* – is not constant. It changes as we grow older or if our diet changes. Neonates have sterile guts and acquire their intestinal microflora soon after birth. The types of bacteria present depend on whether they are breastfed or bottle fed. As diet changes from milk to solids, the microflora also changes.

Pathogenic micro-organisms spread from person to person in a number of ways, both direct and indirect: influenza and tuberculosis are spread mainly via contaminated air droplets; *Staphylococcus aureus* can be spread by direct physical contact or indirectly via contaminated bedding or surgical instruments; sexually transmitted diseases are normally spread by direct sexual contact but can be spread by other means. For example, neonates born to mothers with *Neisseria gonorrhoeae* or *Chlamydia* infections can develop acute conjunctivitis caused by contamination of their eyes with these bacteria during birth.

Case Report

Pregnant women should take all possible care to avoid exposure to infection.

A pregnant woman had been in contact with a child with chickenpox. She went to the GP with the typical rash, but was only offered symptom relief for the itching. Two days later, she was taken to hospital very ill, with varicella pneumonia. She died, despite antiviral therapy in hospital (DoH, 1998: 120).

Should infection occur, it must be recognized and treated promptly. Prescription of aciclovir would probably have saved this woman's life.

Pathogens affect the human body in several ways. The barrier defences and the immune system can usually cope with microbial invaders. For example, we all have transient bacterial infections in our blood – *bacteraemias* – caused by small cuts, and the body normally deals with these without help. Some microbial invaders, however, can evade the body's defences and grow to harmful numbers, or produce toxins that damage body tissues. In this situation, antimicrobials can help to reduce the number of invading cells and allow the body's defence mechanisms to regain control. If, however, there is no appropriate antimicrobial agent, then the body must rely on its own defences.

Antimicrobials in pregnancy

Infection is a major cause of preterm birth. Although antibiotic prophylaxis has not proved useful, prescription of antibiotics to women with preterm prelabour rupture of membranes can delay delivery and may reduce the incidence of infection (Lamont et al, 2001).

Pregnancy will influence the selection of antibiotic. Penicillins and cephalosporins are generally regarded as the agents of first choice in pregnancy, as most other drugs have been associated with increased risks of fetal malformation. For some drugs, such as erythromycin, the risk is low, and sometimes any risks to the fetus are outweighed by the seriousness of the infection in the mother. For many newer drugs, such as vancomycin, little information is available, and the manufacturers therefore advise against use by pregnant and lactating women (Box 14.1). Breastfeeding may allow drugs to be passed to the neonate, although topical preparations are generally considered safe.

Antibacterials and their actions

Since the first antibiotics were all antibacterial in their action, the term *antibiotic* is often restricted to antibacterial agents such as penicillin or gentamicin.

Antibiotics are natural products synthesized by certain species of bacteria or fungi. The best known antibiotic is probably penicillin, which is produced by some strains of a mould called *Penicillium*. Most antibiotics are produced by microbial fermentation, although some, the *semisynthetic antibiotics*, are chemically modified versions of fermentation products. Some species of bacteria are becoming resistant to the antibiotics that are currently available. Scientists are continuously searching for new natural antibiotics and for ways of creating new synthetic antibiotics, for example by genetic engineering of antibiotic producing micro-organisms.

Box 14.1 Antimicrobial agents in pregnancy: some problems and precautions

Drug	Potential problem	Comments
Chloramphenicol	Circulatory collapse of the neonate	Avoid in third trimester, when breastfeeding and for neonates.
Chloroquine and proguanil for malaria prophylaxis	Risks of teratogenesis are reduced by folate supplements	This is generally considered the safest regimen for areas where drug resistance is low.
Erythromycin	Possible liver damage to mother. Risk of gastrointestinal upsets	May be the only realistic option if the mother has a history of penicillin hypersensitivity.
Gentamicin	Risk of hearing loss (mother and neonate)	Avoid if possible. In severe illness, there may be no suitable alternative. Must be monitored.
Griseofulvin	Teratogenesis	Avoid. Potential fathers should avoid this drug for six months prior to conception.
Iodine, povidone iodine	neonatal goitre, hypothyroidism	Avoid, including topical preparations, if pregnant or breastfeeding. See nurse prescribing formulary (BNF, 2000).
Metronidazole	Considered unsafe in high doses. Low doses considered safe in second and third trimesters	Avoid high doses in pregnancy and lactation. Significant amounts in milk.
Nitrofurantoin	Haemolysis and jaundice likely at term	Avoid in third trimester and lactation.
Nystatin	Teratogenesis	Absorption from the skin or gastro-intestinal tract is considered too low to present a problem.

Box 14.1 (*Continued*)

Drug	Potential problem	Comments
Organophosphates (for example Lindane, now discontinued)	Known to be teratogenic in animals	Avoid if possibly pregnant. Absorption through the skin is possible. If the woman cannot avoid handling organophosphates, wear gloves. See malathion, Chapter 20.
Penicillins Cephalosporins	Hypersensitivity	Widely used. Generally considered safe. Manufacturer advises avoiding coamoxiclav.
Rifampicin	Teratogenesis	May be the only realistic option for TB.
	Neonatal bleeding	Monitor fetus. Extra vitamin K must be given to neonates.
Sulphonamides Dapsone	Risk of methaemoglobinaemia [glossary], haemolysis and jaundice	Avoid in third trimester and breastfeeding Dapsone requires folate supplementation.
Tetracyclines	Damage to growing bones and teeth Possible liver damage to mother	Avoid in pregnancy and lactation.
Trimethoprim	Risk of teratogenesis	Avoid in first trimester.

Antibiotics are often referred to as being either broad or narrow spectrum. Broad-spectrum antibiotics are effective against both gram-positive (*Staphylococcus*, *Streptococcus*, *Bacillus* and *Clostridium*) and gram-negative (*Escherichia*, *Salmonella*, *Neisseria* and *Pseudomonas*) bacteria [glossary], whereas narrow-spectrum antibiotics are effective against fewer species. Gram-positive and gram-negative bacteria are two major groupings of bacteria that have different cell structures and therefore different antibiotic sensitivities [glossary]. For example, penicillin is more effective against gram-positive bacteria, while gentamicin is more effective against gram-negative bacteria.

Although thousands of antibiotics have been discovered, only around a hundred are used clinically. These can be classified in a number of ways, based on their chemical structures or their targets in the bacterial cell (Table 14.1).

Table 14.1 Some antibiotics and their modes of action

Target in bacterial cell	Chemical group	Mode of action	Examples	Activity
Cell wall	β-lactams	Inhibit cross-linking of peptidoglycan backbone	Penicillin G	Effective against gram-positive* bacteria only
			Ampicillin	Effective against some gram-negative** bacteria
			Methicillin	Resistant to β-lactamases
			Oxacillin	Resistant to β-lactamases
			Cephalosporin	Broad spectrum
			Clavulanic acid	Inhibits β-lactamases
	Peptide	Inhibits cell wall synthesis	Bacitracin	Effective against gram-positive bacteria
	Glycopeptide	Inhibits cell wall synthesis	Vancomycin	Effective against gram-positive bacteria
Protein synthesis	Aminoglycosides	Bind to the smaller subunit of 70S bacterial ribosomes	Streptomycin	Effective against gram-negative bacteria, serious side-effects
			Neomycin	Effective against gram-negative bacteria
			Gentamicin	Effective against gram-negative bacteria
			Kanamycin	Effective against gram-negative bacteria
	Tetracyclines	Bind to the smaller subunit of 70S bacterial ribosomes	Tetracycline	Broad spectrum
			Doxycycline	Broad spectrum
	Macrolides	Bind to the larger subunit of 70S bacterial ribosomes	Erythromycin	Effective against gram-positive bacteria
			Clarithromycin	
	Nitroaromatics	Bind to the larger subunit of 70S bacterial ribosomes	Chloramphenicol	No longer widely used. Toxic to fast-growing human cells
	Lincosamines	Inhibit protein synthesis	Lincomycin	
			Clindamycin	
DNA synthesis	Quinolones	Inhibit DNA gyrase	Nalidixic acid	Effective against gram-negative bacteria
			Ciprofloxacin	
RNA synthesis	Ansamycins	Inhibit RNA polymerase enzyme	Rifamycins	Used against tuberculosis infections
			Rifampicin /Rifampin	
Plasma membrane	Polymyxins	Increase permeability of plasma membrane, allowing essential metabolites to leak out	Polymyxin B	Toxic but effective against gram-negative bacteria, e.g. *Pseudomonas aeruginosa*

* Gram-positive bacteria include: *Staphylococcus, Streptococcus, Bacillus, Clostridium.* ** Gram-negative bacteria include: *Escherichia, Salmonella, Neisseria, Pseudomonas.*

Cell wall inhibitors

The cell wall of most bacterial cells is formed from a polymer called peptido-glycan. This polymer is unique to bacteria and protects the cell from lysis (bursting), making it a good target for antibiotics. The most important group of cell wall inhibitors are the β-lactam antibiotics; other antibiotics affecting the cell wall include bacitracin and vancomycin, which are reserved for serious infections.

The β-**lactam antibiotics** include the penicillins, cephalosporins and clavu-lanic acid, all of which have a β-lactam ring in their chemical structures. These antibiotics block a key cross-linking reaction in the formation of peptidogly-can. This weakens the wall, causing the cell to lyse (burst) and die. Since these antibiotics only affect newly formed bacterial cell walls, they are only effec-tive against growing bacteria. Penicillin G (benzyl penicillin) is only active against gram-positive bacteria, although newer semisynthetic penicillins such as ampicillin have a broader spectrum of activity which includes some gram-negative bacteria. Other semisynthetic penicillins, such as flucloxacillin, are resistant to penicillin-degrading enzymes (β-lactamases) produced by some bacteria. Augmentin is a combination of amoxicillin with clavulanic acid.

Protein synthesis inhibitors

The **macrolide antibiotics** include erythromycin and structurally related antibiotics such as clarithromycin. They are effective against *Staphylococcus* and other gram-positive bacteria. They inhibit protein synthesis. Erythromycin is commonly used clinically where patients are allergic to penicillin or other β-lactam antibiotics. It is also used in eye ointments to prevent neonatal acute conjunctivitis caused by *Neisseria* and *Chlamydia*.

The **aminoglycoside antibiotics** include gentamicin and structurally related antibiotics such as neomycin. They are effective against gram-negative bacteria which are associated with serious infections such as septicaemia. They act by blocking protein synthesis. This action is fairly specific to bacterial cells. Since semisynthetic penicillins and tetracyclines are also available for treating gram-negative infections, the aminoglycosides are now used mainly as reserve antibiotics when the alternatives are ineffective.

The **tetracyclines**, like the aminoglycosides, block protein synthesis. They are broad spectrum antibiotics, inhibiting almost all gram-positive and gram-negative bacteria. However they are not prescribed in pregnancy and lactation.

The **nitroaromatic antibiotics** include chloramphenicol and, like the macrolide antibiotics, act by blocking protein formation. Chloramphenicol is toxic to fast-growing human cells such as those in bone marrow, and it is now only used when no alternatives are available. Its main use is for eye infections, but it is never prescribed in the third trimester (BNF, 2000).

DNA inhibitors

The **nitroimidazole** antimicrobials include metronidazole. Metronidazole is effective against protozoal infections, such as giardiasis, and bacterial vaginosis related micro-organisms such as *Chlostridium spp.* (including *Chlostridium difficile*) and *Bacteroides spp.* (Lamont, 2001). Metronidazole acts by destroying the structure of DNA, but only in a hypoxic environment. Recent reports, based on cohort studies, conclude that normal doses are probably safe in the second and third trimesters of pregnancy (Donders, 2000), although earlier work in bacteria and rodents, and three case reports of facial defects in infants, raised concerns (Thapa et al, 1998; Alef, 1999). US category B. There are no reports of adverse effects in breast fed infants, although a significant amount of metronidazole (20 per cent) passes into breast milk (Einarson et al, 2000).

Growth factor analogues

The sulphonamides were the first antibacterial drugs to be used clinically. They are called growth-factor analogues as they have a structure similar to a growth factor that is required by bacterial cells. When bacteria are exposed to a growth-factor analogue such as sulphanilimide, they cannot synthesize folic acid, which is a precursor of DNA (deoxyribonucleic acid). The sulphonamides, including cotrimoxazole (Septrin ®), have a broad spectrum of activity. They are selectively toxic to bacterial cells; human cells do not synthesize their own folic acid and use dietary folic acid instead. Trimethoprim also inhibits folic acid synthesis; it is used for urinary tract and chest infections.

Antifungals and their actions

Fungal diseases are less common than bacterial and viral diseases, but are often difficult to control because of the lack of suitable drugs. Because of the similarities in cell structure, any agent which inhibits fungal cells is likely to also affect human cells. Some antifungals and their modes of action are shown in Table 14.2.

Fungal pathogens are often opportunistic, growing normally on the surface of the body and affecting the host only when the immune system has been suppressed. AIDS, transplantation, long term treatment with broad-spectrum antibacterials or corticosteroids and possibly pregnancy, all increase the likelihood of fungal diseases. The infection can be systemic, affecting the whole body, or superficial, as in ringworm and athlete's foot. *Candida albicans*, for example, is a normal constituent of the body microflora that becomes an opportunistic pathogen under adverse conditions, causing oral and vaginal

Table 14.2 Some antifungals and their modes of action

Target in fungal cell	Chemical group	Mode of action	Examples	Activity
Plasma membrane	Polyenes	Bind to ergosterols, increasing membrane permeability and allowing essential metabolites to leak out	Amphotericin B	Broad spectrum; widely used against systemic infections; harmful side effects
			Nystatin	Used topically against *Candida* infections; less specific than amphotericin
	Azoles	Inhibit ergosterol synthesis by binding to cytochrome P_{450}	Fluconazole	Broad spectrum; used against systemic infections and cryptococcal meningitis
			Itraconazole	Used to treat systemic and skin infections
			Ketoconazole	Used to treat systemic and skin infections
			Clotrimazole	
	Allylamines	Block ergosterol synthesis by inhibiting the enzyme squalene epoxidase	Terbinafine	Used to treat ringworm
	Thiocarbamates	Block ergosterol synthesis by inhibiting the enzyme squalene epoxidase	Tolnaftate	Used to treat skin infections, for example *Tinea*
Cell division	Aromatic	Inhibits mitosis by binding to growing microtubules	Griseofulvin	Used to treat skin infections
Nucleic acid synthesis	Fluorinated pyrimidine	Converted inside cell to 5-fluorouracil which inhibits DNA and RNA synthesis	5-fluorocytosine	Used to treat *Candida* and *Cryptococcus* infections
Protein synthesis	Glutarimides	Bind to the larger subunit of 80S eukaryotic ribosomes	Cycloheximide	

thrush (candidiasis) and also systemic infections. *Candida* infections often worsen in pregnancy, due to changes in the pH of vaginal secretions.

Amphotericin and nystatin

One class of antifungals that has some selectivity for fungal cells is the **polyenes**. This group includes amphotericin B and nystatin. Their selectivity is thought to be due to their strong binding to ergosterol, which is the principal sterol in fungal plasma membranes. Amphotericin B has been used widely against systemic infections, but it has serious side effects, including renal damage. Newer formulations, combining amphotericin with cholesterol or other lipids, are less toxic. Nystatin is less selective and more toxic than amphotericin; it is therefore only used topically, mainly for vaginal and oral thrush.

Fluconazole and ketoconazole

The **azole** antifungals such as fluconazole, iatraconazole and ketoconazole are less toxic than amphotericin. They are very important in the management of patients with HIV infection. They act by inhibiting the synthesis of ergosterol. The loss of ergosterol destabilizes the fungal plasma membrane and the cell stops growing. They have also been used to treat fungal septicaemia in neonates and oral thrush in immunocompromised children. Triazoles, such as fluconazole and itraconazole, are much more selective than imidazoles such as ketoconazole and clotrimazole. Ketoconazole causes liver toxicity, possibly because it also inhibits sterol synthesis in liver cells. Resistance often develops after long term treatment with fluconazole. For example, it is estimated that 30 per cent of AIDS patients in the UK have fluconazole-resistant *Candida albicans*. This group of antifungals interacts with many other drugs, including nifedipine and ergometrine.

Terbinafine

Terbinafine (an **allylamine**) and tolnaftate (a **thiocarbamate**) also act by damaging the plasma membrane of fungal cells. Tolnaftate is used in ointments for dermatophytic fungal infections such as athlete's foot and ringworm.

Griseofulvin

Griseofulvin inhibits cell division. It is used against skin infections, but is given orally and migrates through the bloodstream to the skin. Because of its side effects, it is not used for dermatophytic infections that can be treated with topical antifungals. It is a known teratogen.

Antivirals and their actions

Viruses are responsible for a range of human diseases, ranging from the common cold and flu to more serious diseases such as AIDS. Unlike bacteria and fungi, viruses are not ceullular; they are infectious particles that enter a host cell, use it to synthesize copies of themselves, and then release these copies to infect more host cells. So far, vaccines have been the most successful way of preventing viral diseases. However these cannot be used after a person has been infected with a virus, and vaccines are not available for all viral diseases. There are far fewer effective antiviral agents than there are antibiotics. One reason for this is that it is difficult to inhibit the virus without affecting the human host. Also, viruses replicate rapidly and can reach such high numbers by the time symptoms appear that antiviral drugs may have little effect. Some antivirals that are currently in use or are being tested for use are shown in Table 14.3.

One of the best known antiviral drugs is aciclovir, which is effective against Herpes simplex and zoster, varicella (chickenpox) and Epstein-Barr viruses (glandular fever). Aciclovir is activated only within virus-infected cells, where it inhibits the formation of DNA by blocking the enzyme DNA polymerase. This reduces the replication of the virus but cannot prevent its later reactivation. Topical, oral and intravenous preparations are available. Aciclovir cream (Zovirax®) is suitable for cold sores, labial and genital *Herpes simplex*, but vaginal infections require oral preparations. Aciclovir passes into breast milk.

Table 14.3 Some antivirals and their modes of action

Target in virus	Examples	Mode of action	Activity
Penetration of the host cell	Amantadine Rimantadine	May prevent the virus from penetrating host cells	Active against influenza A virus
Nucleic acid synthesis	Zidovudine (AZT)	Blocks DNA synthesis by inhibiting the reverse transcriptase enzyme	Inhibits some retroviruses including HIV
	Acyclovir	Blocks DNA synthesis by inhibiting DNA polymerase	Used against herpes viruses
Assembly and maturation of virus particles	Saquinavir, ritonavir, indinavir, nelfinavir	Inhibit the protease enzymes that aid assembly and maturation	Used against HIV
Release of viral particles	Zanamivir GS4104	Inhibit neuraminidase	Active against influenza A and B viruses

The manufacturers advise caution in pregnancy and breastfeeding, but the amounts absorbed through the skin are likely to be small. Oral administration carries the risk of side effects, such as rashes, gastro-intestinal disturbance, headache, dizziness and potential upsets to liver, kidney or bone marrow. The intravenous infusion is reserved for severe infections.

Zidovudine (AZT) is one of several antivirals used to inhibit retroviruses such as HIV. Zidovudine slows the progression or decreases the severity of AIDS, but does not cure it. Intensive combination treatment of mothers and infants is used to reduce HIV infection in babies born to HIV-positive mothers. Zidovudine is more effective against HIV when used in combination with newer antivirals agents such as the protease inhibitors, saquinavir and ritonavir. These act by inhibiting the production of a protease enzyme that is essential for the proper assembly and maturation of new virus particles. Protease inhibitors have many side effects and no information is available on use in pregnancy (BNF, 2000).

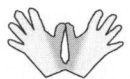 **Practice Points**

After antimicrobial therapy begins, the midwife should maintain a 'watchful vigilance' and look for signs of:
- 'drug fever' which is a form of hypersensitivity response that should not be confused with recurrent infection (Shuster, 1995; Chambers & Sande, 1996)
- failure of therapy which can have a number of causes.

Reasons for failure of antimicrobial therapy

- Wrong drug, dose or route;
- drug resistance/tolerance;
- inadequate dosage or poor compliance;
- drug not reaching the micro-organism, for example intracellular organisms.
- Superinfection.
- Undetected micro-organisms.
- Administration problems, for example incompatibilities in intravenous infusions or taking antibiotics with food.
- Foreign body, for example catheters, prostheses, such as artificial heart valves.
- Pus or haematoma or abscess formation.

How the body handles antimicrobials

Absorption

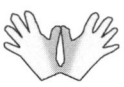 **Practice Point**

Absorption of antimicrobials is influenced by the motility of the gastrointestinal tract or the presence of food or antacids in the stomach (Stockley, 1999). If these potential problems are not considered, the infection may not be eradicated. See Box 14.2.

Case Report

Pyrexia may lead to miscarriage. Therefore, it is important that all infections are treated effectively.

A young primagravida developed a urinary tract infection, for which her GP prescribed erythromycin 500 mg every six hours. However, the patient took the tablets at 8.00 am., with breakfast, 1.00 pm., with lunch, at 6.00 pm. with dinner and at 10.00 pm. with supper. Although her symptoms subsided, some signs of infection remained. Three days later, she was admitted to hospital in premature labour and miscarried.

Had the woman assiduously taken her antibiotics two hours away from food, and without a ten-hour dosage interval, it is quite possible that the treatment would have been effective and she would not have miscarried. Therapeutic failure, due to poor compliance with medication, may occur more often than is commonly realized. Effective patient teaching could have influenced the outcome in this case.

After oral administration, the plasma concentration of an antibiotic peaks after one to four hours, depending on the drug used. When a more rapid response is required, intramuscular or intravenous injections are administered. Some antibiotics are not absorbed from the gut and are therefore given by injection, for example gentamicin, or applied directly to the infected area, for example neomycin.

Distribution

Antibiotics are widely distributed to most tissues after entering the body. Where the blood supply to an area is poor, antibiotic therapy may not penetrate to the infected tissue. This may occur where an abscess has formed, for

---

Box 14.2. Factors affecting the absorption of antimicrobials

Antibiotic	Problem	Precaution
Tetracyclines	Absorption impaired by iron, zinc, calcium or antacids in the stomach	Taken either one hour before or two hours after ingesting tablets containing these minerals or dairy products.
Doxycycline Minocycline	Can cause oesophageal or gastric irritation	Take with food and a full glass of water.
Ampicillin Erythromycin Rifampicin	Absorption reduced by food in the stomach	Taken one hour before or two hours after meals.
Amoxicillin	Absorption reduced by high fibre diets, for example bran or methylcellulose	Dose adjustments may be required.
Isoniazid	Histamine-rich foods cause histamine release and unpleasant flushing	Advise client to avoid fish and mature cheese if this reaction is suspected.
Most antibiotics	Absorption impaired by antacids, particularly those containing magnesium and aluminium	Take one hour before or two hours after antacids.
Ketoconazole	Only absorbed if the stomach contents are acid	Ketoconazole *must* be taken with food and separated by two hours from any antacid medications.

---

example following an episiotomy. It may then be necessary to drain the abscess and apply topical preparations.

Elimination

The route of elimination varies with each drug. Erythromycin, for example, is excreted into the bile, and penicillins and gentamicin are excreted into the urine.

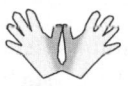 **Practice Point**

Taking a full glass of water with oral medications is very important with certain drugs, which can damage the renal tubules if they are allowed to crystallize. Patients taking sulphonamides, including cotrimoxazole (Septrin®), should therefore drink at least two litres of fluid each day.

A blood test to check renal function is necessary before certain antibiotics eliminated by the kidney are administered. These include tetracyclines (not doxycycline), gentamicin, cotrimoxazole, polymyxins and vancomycin. Some of these drugs can damage the kidneys, leading to further accumulation and a 'vicious circle'. For example, there is a danger of accumulation of gentamicin if any degree of renal impairment is present or if dehydration occurs. This may lead to dose-related side effects such as hearing loss and kidney damage.

Dosage schedules

The recommended dosage schedule varies with each individual drug and is different even for very similar drugs. Ampicillin, for example, should be administered every six hours, away from mealtimes, whereas amoxicillin should be administered every eight hours, but mealtimes are less important.

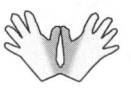 **Practice Points**

- Women should understand that 'four times a day' means every six hours, not any four convenient times. If this rule is not observed, the concentration of the drug in the tissues may fluctuate excessively throughout the 24 hours, causing therapeutic failure. (See Chapter 1, Figure 1.1.)
- Dosage schedules which require administration every six hours, away from mealtimes (ampicillin, erythromycin), must be carefully planned, as they require patients to adjust their normal routines and interrupt sleep. This is not always practicable in the community and sometimes it may be prudent to seek an alternative prescription (Bootman & Milne, 1996).

Therapeutic range

The therapeutic range of a drug is the difference between the minimum effective plasma concentration and the toxic concentration. For some drugs, such as the penicillins, this range is wide and dose-related side effects are unusual. For other drugs, such as gentamicin and vancomycin, the therapeutic range is narrow. To ensure the effectiveness and minimize the side effects of such antibiotics, venous blood samples are taken at regular intervals to measure the concentration of these drugs in the plasma.

Adverse effects of Antimicrobials

Some antimicrobials that are effective in the laboratory cannot be used clinically, because they are too toxic or are rapidly inactivated. Even when an antimicrobial is approved for clinical use, care must be taken to balance the likely benefits with the possible adverse reactions. Normally, the antimicrobial with the least severe side effects will be used, but if the microorganism is resistant to this, then a potentially more harmful alternative may have to be used.

The adverse effects of antimicrobial agents can be grouped:

- Allergic and hypersensitivity responses
- Direct toxicity of the drugs
- Superinfection
- Resistance.

The potential side effects of some antimicrobials are summarized in Table 14.5, (p. 323) and the Implications for Practice are tabulated below.

Allergy and hypersensitivity

These responses may be delayed or immediate, occurring with the first dose or on subsequent exposures. Penicillins and sulphonamides frequently cause hypersensitivity: 5–10 per cent of patients develop a rash with penicillin (Breathnach, 1993). Hypersensitivity reactions range from a skin rash and itching to fatal anaphylaxis. Reactions are more likely with intravenous administration and if the drug is given rapidly. For this reason, intravenous gentamicin should be administered over a minimum of three minutes (BNF, 2000). Cross-allergy is known to occur between similar drugs. For example, 5–15 per cent of people allergic to penicillins are also allergic to cephalosporins (Malseed et al, 1995) (see Chapter 1).

Table 14.4 Some mechanisms of resistance to antimicrobials

Mechanism	Example/target	Antibiotic affected	Organism
No uptake into cell	Cell surface	Penicillins	*Pseudomonas aeruginosa*
Removal from cell	Plasma membrane	Tetracyclines	Enteric bacteria*
Inactivation of antibiotic	β-lactamase	Penicillins	Enteric bacteria *Staphylococcus aureus* *Neisseria gonorrhoeae*
	Acetylation, phosphorylation and adenylylation	Aminoglycosides Chloramphenicol	Enteric bacteria *Staphylococcus aureus*
Modification of target	Ribosome	Streptomycin Erythromycin	Enteric bacteria *Staphylococcus aureus*
	RNA polymerase	Rifamycin	Enteric bacteria
Absence of target	Cell wall	Cell wall inhibitors	*Mycoplasma pneumoniae*
Development of resistant pathway	–	Sulphonamides	Enteric bacteria *Staphylococcus aureus*

* The enteric bacteria include *Escherichia*, *Salmonella*, *Shigella* and *Proteus*.

Direct toxicity of the drug

Several antibiotics carry an appreciable risk of organ damage (See Box 14.3). Some of the most serious problems with antimicrobials are the effects on the fetus. Trimethoprim, for example, is potentially teratogenic and may interfere with folic acid metabolism in pregnant women. Most antibiotics can cause gastrointestinal upsets, either due to the irritant actions of the drugs or interference with the normal flora of the gastrointestinal tract.

Box 14.3 Potential toxicity of some antimicrobials and appropriate precautions

Site of toxicity	Antibiotic	Precaution
Brain	Penicillins Cephalosporins	Avoid intrathecal administration. Exercise caution in administering to patients with a history of convulsions and renal failure.

Box 14.3 (*Continued*)

Site of toxicity	Antibiotic	Precaution
Inner ear (hearing and balance)	Gentamicin Vancomycin Erythromycin (rarely)	Avoid use with other drugs affecting the ear, for example furosemide/frusemide. Ensure the patient can hear and balance is not affected. Ask about tinnitus and report to prescriber.
Growing bones and teeth	Tetracyclines	Avoid in pregnant women and children.
Liver	Erythromycin Rifampicin Tetracyclines Cephalosporins (rarely)	Perform liver function tests if use prolonged. Avoid in people with a history of alcohol misuse or fatty liver in pregnancy. The liver is particularly vulnerable in pregnancy.
Pancreas	Cotrimoxazole	Be alert for severe vomiting and pain radiating to the back. Glucose estimations may be helpful.
Kidney	Gentamicin Cotrimoxazole Vancomycin Cephalosporins (rarely) Penicillins Tetracyclines	Perform blood tests to assess renal function or seek alternative drug if poor renal function is suspected, for example in a woman with a history of UTI.
Skin (photosensitivity)	Tetracyclines Aciclovir	Do not expose skin to sunlight; use sunscreen.
Bone marrow	Chloramphenicol Cotrimoxazole Cephalosporins (rarely) Aciclovir	Avoid in patients with a family history of bone marrow problems or taking other drugs (for example carbimazole) which are potentially toxic to the marrow. Perform full blood counts.

Superinfection

Superinfection occurs when antibiotics kill off the normal microflora of the skin or in the gastro-intestinal tract, allowing resistant and more harmful micro-organisms to take their place. Fungi such as *Candida albicans* are normally harmless constituents of the skin and gut microflora but can develop into pathogenic forms that cause thrush after antibiotic therapy has weakened their bacterial neighbours, leading to diarrhoea or skin infections. Superinfection is more likely to occur after administration of broad spectrum agents, prolonged therapy, low doses, or in immunosuppressed patients.

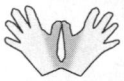 **Practice Points**

The midwife can help to minimize the problem of superinfection by:
- specifically enquiring after any diarrhoea and vomiting (which may lead to fluid and electrolyte imbalance, particularly in neonates).
- asking women to report any oral or vaginal thrush.

Pseudomembranous colitis occurs after superinfection of the gastrointestinal tract with the bacterium, *Clostridium difficile*. It can occur with almost any antibiotic, but is particularly associated with ampicillin (see Alef, 1999).

Long term use of antibiotics may cause nutrient deficiency by inhibiting the vitamin-producing bacteria in the gut. For example, the availability of vitamin K is reduced by gentamicin, tetracyclines, and possibly other antibiotics (see chapter 8). Care is also needed when drugs are prescribed long term for tuberculosis, as isoniazid may cause vitamin B deficiency (Spencer, 1993b).

Resistance

Some micro-organisms are inherently resistant to certain antimicrobials because of their structure or metabolism. Other micro-organisms can *acquire* resistance, often after exposure to the antibiotic (Jordan & Tait, 1999).

Some staphylococci produce penicillinase enzymes that break down penicillins and cephalosporins. Infections with penicillinase-producing bacteria can, however, be treated with flucloxacillin, which is less susceptible to attack by the enzymes, or by augmentin which is a combination of two antibiotics, amoxicillin and clavulanic acid.

Resistant mutants can arise spontaneously, often after long term exposure to an antimicrobial. Bacteria can also acquire resistance by transferring genetic material and information between cells or by absorbing fragments of DNA from ruptured cells. By these methods, resistance can be passed rapidly from cell to cell, making an entire population of bacteria resistant to a range of antibiotics.

Bacteria found in the gastro-intestinal tract, *Staphylococcus aureus* and *Pseudomonas aeruginosa*, can all become resistant by the spread of R (resistance) factors. Methicillin-resistant *Staphylococcus aureus* (MRSA), a common source of infection in hospitals all over the world, contains R-factors that make it resistant to a large number of antibiotics. Until recently, vancomycin and teicoplanin were the only antibiotics effective against all MRSA, but resistant strains have now appeared. (see Table 14.4, p. 319)

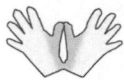 **Practice Points**

The likelihood of resistant strains arising can be reduced by:
- using short courses of treatment: a maximum of five days, where possible (BNF, 2000);
- ensuring that patients comply and complete courses of treatment;
- using high doses to reduce the numbers of bacteria before resistant strains can appear;
- using two unrelated antibiotics in the expectation that doubly-resistant mutants are unlikely to arise, particularly where prolonged therapy is necessary, as for tuberculosis or leprosy;
- reducing the overall usage of antibiotics (Dever et al, 1998);
- complying with infection control measures (Dennesen et al, 1998);
- obtaining prompt culture and sensitivity reports if resistance is suspected.

Interactions with other drugs

Antibiotics interact with a wide variety of other drugs and chemicals including alcohol, nutrients, oral contraceptives and anticoagulants.

Alcohol is a gastric irritant and is likely to exacerbate any gastrointestinal upset caused by other drugs. Some people may suffer an 'antabuse reaction' if they take even a small amount of alcohol with certain antibiotics such as metronidazole and cefamandole. This causes the peripheral blood vessels to dilate, leading to flushing, severe headache and a fall in blood pressure. Fainting, falls and even cardiovascular collapse may follow.

Where two or more drugs with the same side effects are co-prescribed, the risks are increased. For example, if two drugs with the potential to damage the inner ear are used together, such as, gentamicin and furosemide/frusemide, the chances of tinnitus, hearing loss and vertigo are high (Table 14.5).

Table 14.5 Some adverse affects of antimicrobials

Type	Antimicrobial	Reported adverse affects*		
		General	Pregnant/lactating women	Neonates/children
Antibacterial	Penicillin	Allergy (10%)*	–	Rash and diarrhoea in neonates
	Amoxicillin	Gastrointestinal upset** (5–10%) Skin rash (5–10%) Allergic reactions (2%)	–	Diarrhoea in neonates
	Cephalosporin	Allergic reactions (1–4%)	–	Gastrointestinal upset (5–20%)**
	Streptomycin	Ear toxicity; deafness Kidney toxicity Gastrointestinal upset	Crosses placenta Inner ear toxicity	Diarrhoea after breastfeeding
	Doxycycline	Gastrointestinal upset (3–4%) Allergic skin reactions (2%) Staining of teeth	Affects fetal tooth and bone development Liver toxicity	May affect bone growth
	Erythromycin, clarithromycin	Gastrointestinal upset Anaphylaxis (rare) Reversible hearing loss (rare)	–	Gastrointestinal upset (6–7%) Rash (3%) Headache (2%)
	Chloramphenicol	Anaemia	[Contraindicated if breastfeeding]	Bone marrow suppression
	Ciprofloxacin	–	[Contraindicated if breastfeeding]	–

Table 14.5 *(continued)*

Type	Antimicrobial	Reported adverse affects*		
		General	*Pregnant/lactating women*	*Neonates/children*
	Rifampicin	Gastrointestinal upset Discoloration of urine/body fluids Hepatitis. Flu-like reaction	–	–
	Trimethoprim- sulphamethoxazole	Nephrotoxicity Gastrointestinal upset Skin rashes (3–4%)	Teratogenic risk May interfere with folic acid metabolism	Mild toxic erythema (1–4%)
Antifungal	Amphotericin B	Acute kidney toxicity	–	–
	Nystatin	Gastrointestinal upset Skin/vaginal irritation	–	–
	Fluconazole	Gastrointestinal upset (3–4%) Headache (2%) Rash (2%) Hepatic toxicity (rare)	Teratogenic effects	–
	5-fluorocytosine	–	Possible teratogen	–
Antivirals	Zidovudine (AZT)	Seizures, headaches, weakness Gastrointestinal upset. Anaemia	–	–
	Acyclovir	Gastrointestinal upset. Skin rash	–	–

* Figures in brackets are reported percentages of patients affected.
** e.g. abdominal pain, nausea, vomiting and diarrhoea.

The efficacy of the oral contraceptive pill is reduced by some antimicrobials. A few drugs, such as rifampicin, rifabutin, isoniazid and griseofulvin, render all oral contraceptives ineffective; alternative methods of contraception should be used during treatment and for four to eight weeks after stopping the drug. Broad spectrum antibiotics, such as ampicillin, penicillin V, tetracycline, neomycin, sulphonamides, nitrofurantoin and chloramphenicol, interact with combined oral contraceptives and increase the risk of 'pill failure'. By eliminating the normal gastro-intestinal tract flora, antibiotics hinder the normal entero-hepatic recycling [glossary] of oestrogens, increasing their loss in the faeces and reducing their absorption. Women should be advised to use other methods of contraception during therapy and for seven days after it ends. If these seven days extend beyond the end of the pill packet, a new packet of oral contraceptives should be started immediately without a break (BNF, 2000).

Some drugs alter the absorption of antimicrobials from the gut, speed up their breakdown or alter their activity in other ways. For example, zidovudine (AZT) concentrations are decreased by clarithromycin and zidovudine toxicity may be increased when fluconazole or aciclovir are co-administered.

Many antibiotics are incompatible with other drugs when co-administered in intravenous infusions. For example, if gentamicin is combined with heparin, its antibiotic activity will be lost.

Cautions and contra-indications

With all drugs, it is important to ask patients if they have suffered previous allergies or hypersensitivity responses. People with a history of atopic or hypersensitivity disorders are particularly at risk. Some antimicrobials, such as gentamicin, depend on the liver or kidney for elimination, and any degree of organ failure, as in pre-eclampsia, may prevent this.

Implications for Practice: antimicrobials

Potential Problem	Management
Therapeutic failure	Culture and sensitivity, preferably prior to administration of antimicrobial therapy.
	Check drug administration and compliance (Box 14.2)
	Check for foreign bodies and abscesses.
	Monitor for signs of infection, for example temperature at 6.00 pm, particularly if the patient is immunocompromised.

Implications for Practice (*continued*)

Potential Problem	Management
Teratogenicity	Use penicillins and cephalosporins where possible.
	Assess and discuss relative risks and benefits.
	Use topical preparations if possible.
	Avoid certain drugs, see Box 14.1.
	Do not apply iodine if pregnant.
	Minimize infection risks; for example discontinue contact lens use during pregnancy and the puerperium.
Drug toxicity	Check renal function if there is any risk of impairment.
	Administer medication with a full glass of water.
	Ensure venous samples for therapeutic drug monitoring are taken immediately prior to administration of gentamicin or vancomycin.
	Monitor for signs of organ damage; see Box 14.3.
Gastro-intestinal upset	Monitor fluid and electrolyte balance. A venous blood sample may be necessary to check for dehydration or potassium depletion.
	Consider nutritional and vitamin deficiencies, particularly if pregnancy-induced vomiting has occurred.
	Extra caution is needed in women with diabetes or epilepsy.
Hypersensitivity responses	Obtain a history of all previous hypersensitivity responses. Check for cross-allergies, particularly before administering cephalosporins, penicillins or sulphonamides.
	Ensure protocols and equipment are in place for management of anaphylaxis.
	Administer all injections slowly.
Resistance	Culture and sensitivity.
	Ensure compliance with the full dose.
	Maintain strict asepsis, particularly in hospitals.
	Scrupulous attention to hand washing.

Conclusion: the future of antimicrobial therapy

With the recent appearance of vancomycin-resistant strains of *Staphylococcus aureus*, this bacterium has now joined *Pseudomonas aeruginosa*, *Mycobacterium tuberculosis* and *Enterococcus faecalis* in having strains that are resistant to all of the 100-plus antibiotics available to the clinician. Perhaps too late, the problem of increasing antibiotic resistance has finally been recognized and serious effort is now being put into minimizing non-essential use of antibacterials. However, despite changes in practice and continuing attempts to find and develop new antibiotics, it is likely that more strains of pathogenic bacteria, resistant to all known antibiotics, will appear. Already, scientists are investigating an interesting, and potentially very useful, alternative to antibiotics: phage therapy. Phages are viruses that specifically attack bacteria, and they may prove to be the antibiotics of the future.

Further Reading

Jordan, S. & Tait, M. (1999) Antibiotic therapy. *Nursing Standard.*13:45:49–54.

Levy, S.B. (1998) The challenge of antibiotic resistance. *Scientific American.* 278:3:46–53.

Lilley, L., Aucker, R. & Albanese, J. (1996) *Pharmacology and the Nursing Process.* St. Louis, Mosby.

PART V

PREGNANCY IN WOMEN WITH PRE-EXISTING DISEASE

This section of the book describes the medications administered to women with long term health needs who become pregnant. In the author's opinion, these topics represent the most difficult subjects in medicine. The practitioner needs to be familiar with the disease; how the disease is influenced by pregnancy; how the disease affects the outcome of pregnancy; how the drugs influence the disease; how the drugs influence the outcome of pregnancy and breastfeeding; and how pregnancy affects the actions of the drugs. As if all this were not enough, practitioners need to consider the interactions between the disease, the drugs for the disease and the drugs commonly used in labour. The following chapters are only a guide, and midwives are urged to consult specialists in tertiary referral centres.

We assume that all women affected by a disease prior to conception will be under the care of an obstetrician, and probably also a physician. However midwives can often play an important role in recognizing and referring disease arising in pregnancy. Also, we hope that the outlines provided will help midwives when advising women in pregnancy, labour and the puerperium.

For most of the drugs described, there is little or no evidence from randomized controlled clinical trials in pregnant and breastfeeding women. Evidence of safety and 'best practice' is largely based on ecological studies, often without long term follow-up. In general, the manufacturers' literature is cautious, stressing that use of medication in pregnancy and breastfeeding is based on clinical risk/benefit calculations, rather than 'scientific' evidence.

The scope of this book only allows consideration of the commonest diseases in women of child-bearing age.

US categories of drugs used in pregnancy are listed in Appendix 2.

Further Reading for Part 5

Campbell, S. & Lees, C. (eds) (2000) Medical diseases complicating pregnancy In: *Obstetrics by Ten Teachers*, 17th edition. London, Arnold.

CHAPTER 15

Asthma in Pregnancy

SUE JORDAN

This chapter describes asthma in pregnancy and the drugs commonly used in the management of asthma. This condition is so common in young people that not all women will be receiving care from a specialist in respiratory medicine. Little information is available on the use of the newest agents, the leukotriene receptor antagonists, in pregnancy.

Chapter Contents

- Asthma

- Management of asthma

- Drugs used in asthma

- Conclusion

Asthma

Asthma may affect up to 10 per cent of the population in industrialized countries, including 5 per cent of pregnant women (Serafin, 1996). Asthma is an inflammatory disease affecting the small airways. It is not always reversible, and can be fatal (McFadden, 1991). Bronchoconstriction leads to dyspnoea (breathlessness) on expiration and (sometimes) wheezing and cough. Asthma is characterized by inflammation, oedema, eosinophil infiltration and remodelling of the bronchioles. Mucus is produced in excessive amounts, and may form plugs which block the airways. The lining of the bronchioles is shed, also blocking the airways. These changes become permanent in long standing disease. Narrowing of the airways is intensified at night, following the natural circadian rhythms of hormone secretion (Holgate, 1997).

Defined allergens (such as the house dust mite) are associated with

331

worsening of symptoms. Strategies for the prevention of asthma include aller-
gen avoidance (including cigarette smoke) in pregnancy and early life, and
early treatment with anti-inflammatory agents (Holgate, 1997).

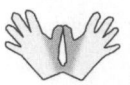 **Practice Point**

Regular, systematic monitoring of lung function and symptoms forms an important aspect
of care for asthmatic women. This will detect any changes which may occur as a result of
pregnancy or parturition, and assist compliance.

Complications of asthma

Deteriorating asthma is frequently caused by non-compliance, which may be
due to misplaced concerns that medications are teratogenic. For women with
severe asthma, there is a risk that the symptoms of asthma will intensify in late
pregnancy or post-partum. Mild or moderate asthma may improve during
pregnancy but worsen following delivery (Nelson-Piercy & Moore-Gillon,
1995; see Implications for Practice).

Hypoxia

Severe, uncontrolled asthma causes chronic or intermittent hypoxia, which
adversely affects both mother and baby. Maternal oxygen saturation should
never be allowed to fall below 95 per cent, even in an acute attack (Ebden
& Evans, 1996). Hypoxia impairs fetal development, causing intrauterine
growth retardation, fetal distress and, occasionally, death. It is important
to remember that a woman who is hypoxic may appear agitated and
confused.

Carbon dioxide retention

In a severe asthma attack, carbon dioxide is retained and the work of breathing will be so increased that a build-up of lactic acid occurs.

Acute asthma attack

These episodes may be life-threatening to mother and fetus. Nebulised
bronchodilators, oxygen, intravenous corticosteroids and, if necessary, amino-

phylline are administered as in the non-pregnant woman. (Protocols are out-lined in the BNF.) An acute attack of asthma is rare during labour; however should this occur, opioids and ergometrine should be withheld as they will intensify bronchoconstriction (Nelson-Piercy & Moore-Gillon, 1995). In rare instances, local anaesthetics can cause problems.

Case Report

Bronchospasm can complicate labour.

A 26-year-old primipara presented with premature rupture of membranes and breech pre-sentation at 36 weeks, and underwent emergency Caesarean section. No history of asthma was obtained, but examination revealed evidence of atopic dermatitis. Spinal anaesthesia was induced using 2 ml of 0.4 per cent tetracaine (a local anaesthetic) in 10 per cent dextrose. Sensory loss extended to T3. The woman began to cough and wheeze and became short of breath. This was treated as an acute attack of asthma. Both mother and baby did well post-operatively.

It would appear that spinal anaesthesia triggered an asthmatic attack by anaesthetizing the autonomic nervous system supplying the bronchioles rather than by a hypersensitivity response (Kawabata, 1996). Health care professionals need to be aware of the possibility of spinal anaesthesia precipitating respiratory difficulties in women with a history of atopic con-ditions (such as asthma, atopic dermatitis/eczema). However spinal analgesia is probably safer than opioids for women with asthma (Beischer et al, 1997).

Maternal asthma may increase the likelihood of pneumonia, hypertension, pre-term delivery, admission to neonatal intensive care, congenital malforma-tions and low birth weight, but the risks are low and related to the control of the disease (Kramer et al, 1995; Nelson-Piercy & Moore-Gillon, 1995; Schatz, 1999; Munn et al, 1999).

Management of asthma

The management goal is to control symptoms and avoid complications at all times of the day and night, in both pregnant and non-pregnant individuals. This is achieved by:

- avoidance of trigger factors (including drugs) as far as possible (see Table 15.1);
- monitoring and record keeping (see Table 15.2);
- Pharmacotherapeutic interventions.

The risks from poorly controlled asthma far outweigh any possible teratogenic effects of standard therapies.

Table 15.1 Trigger factors for asthma

An asthma attack may be *precipitated by:*

- changes in environmental temperature or humidity
- exercise
- worry, stress, or fatigue
- pollens, fungal spores, the house dust mite, animals
- smoke and environmental pollutants, for example sulphur dioxide
- infections
- hypoxia
- menstruation
- thyrotoxicosis
- industrial irritants for example laundry detergents, dusty flour or grain
- certain foods such as eggs, nuts, chocolate or fish (mainly in children)

DRUGS CAUSING or EXACERBATING ASTHMA:

- hypersensitivity response or anaphylactoid reaction to any drug
- beta blockers, for example as anti-hypertensives or as eye drops for glaucoma
- Non-steroidal anti-inflammatory drugs (NSAIDs) such as aspirin, salicylates, diclofenac
- oestrogens
- benzodiazepines
- tobacco, cannabis
- opioids, (fentanyl is possibly the least problematic)
- ergometrine (Syntometrine® rarely causes problems)
- prostaglandins (carboprost, dinoprostone)
- anti-psychotics
- tricyclic antidepressants
- atracurium muscle relaxant (use vecuronium)
- lignocaine
- angiotensin converting enzyme (ACE) inhibitors can cause cough and angioedema which may be mistaken for asthma
- hypotonic or hypertonic solutions [glossary] when in contact with the airways, for example in nebulisers; therefore normal saline is used as dilutent in nebulisers
- preservatives in inhaled drugs, for example lactose
- tartrazine for example in fruit squash, coloured fizzy drinks, curry powder, pickles
- 'sulphiting agents' for example some wines, shellfish, preservatives on fresh fruit, dried fruits, pickles

Sources: Cochrane and Rees, 1989; McFadden, 1991; Jordan and White, 2001.

Table 15.2 Always monitor airways because:

- Regular measurements of peak expiratory flow rates (PEFR) are more reliable indicators of disease than subjective symptoms.
- Some causes of exacerbations of disease (for example non-compliance, exposure to dust, menstruation, diet) only become obvious with an asthma diary.
- A change or fall in the PEFR will warn of any change in response to therapy and warn of impending 'disasters'.
- 'Nocturnal dips' will indicate loss of control of the disease.
- Inhaler technique needs checking and reinforcing.

Peak expiratory flow rates (PEFR), lung volumes and ideally FEV_1/FCV ratios (forced expiratory volume in one second/forced vital capacity) are monitored.

Source: Jordan and White, 2001.

Aerosol delivery

Asthma medication is best delivered by inhalation of aerosols, and more than 90 per cent of people treated for asthma have no need for other forms of drug delivery. Aerosols reduce the amount of drug in the systemic circulation, and therefore reduce both the maternal side effects and the drug exposure of the fetus and breastfed infant.

Even with optimal inhaler technique, only 2–10 per cent of aerosolized drug reaches the lungs, and the rest is swallowed. This is improved by the use of spacer devices, which reduce the need for co-ordination. The type of inhaler device may affect the absorption of drug by 100 per cent; therefore careful monitoring is necessary if the type of inhaler is changed. It is important that inhaler technique is checked and discussed (see Govoni & Hayes, 1990).

Drugs used in asthma

The drugs prescribed will depend on the severity of the disease. The main classes of drugs used in asthma are:

Bronchodilators
- beta adrenoreceptor agonists, for example salbutamol, terbutaline
- anti-muscarinic agents, for example ipratropium (rarely used in young adults)
- methylxanthines, for example theophylline

Anti-inflammatories
- chromones, for example cromoglycate, nedocromil
- corticosteroids, glucocorticoids, for example beclomethasone, prednisolone
- leukotriene receptor antagonists (not recommended in pregnancy)

Extensive clinical experience indicates that inhaled cromoglycate, beta$_2$ adrenoreceptor agonists and corticosteroids are safe in pregnancy (Serafin, 1996). However larger studies are needed to assess the risk of congenital malformations associated with currently prescribed therapies (Jadad et al, 2000). An underpowered [glossary] study has linked the use of beta$_2$ adrenoreceptor agonists in the first trimester with an increased risk of polydactyly in the neonate (Pangle, 2000).

Bronchodilators

The diameter of the airways is controlled by several factors (see Table 15.3). Bronchodilators relax the smooth muscle of the bronchioles and provide effective 'rescue' medication. In young people, the beta$_2$ adrenoreceptor

Table 15.3   Control of the airways

1. Normally the smooth muscle of the bronchioles is relaxed by epinephrine (adrenaline) acting on the beta$_2$ receptors – hence the use of beta$_2$ agonists, for example salbutamol.
2. Some of the airways are constricted by acetylcholine – hence the use of anti-cholinergic drugs, for example ipratropium (Atrovent®).
3. There is a third system of nerves not related to the autonomic nervous system which may be affected by cromoglycate.
4. Circadian rhythms: asthma is worst between 2.00 am and dawn.

agonists are the most widely used bronchodilators. However, asthma is a chronic inflammatory disease, involving a variety of white cells, platelets and cytokines, and therefore only mild forms of asthma are managed by bronchodilators alone. *If a pregnant woman is using 'rescue' inhalations regularly, more than once a day, her asthma is probably poorly controlled, causing hypoxaemia and compromising the fetus.* Use of more than one 200-dose inhaler per month is associated with an increased asthma mortality rate (*Drugs and Therapy Perspectives*, 1997).

Beta$_2$ adrenoreceptor agonists (for example salbutamol)

These drugs act, like adrenaline/epinephrine, by stimulating the beta$_2$ receptors which are present in the liver, the smooth muscle and glands of many organs, including uterus, lungs and gut. Aerosol salbutamol or terbutaline is the initial treatment of choice in asthma in pregnancy, provided symptoms can be controlled by inhalation less than once per day. Oral forms of these drugs are very rarely used in pregnancy. The pharmacology of the beta adrenoreceptor agonists is discussed in the chapter on tocolytics (ritodrine) and summarized in Appendix 1.

There is no evidence that inhaled beta$_2$ adrenoreceptor agonists are harmful to either the fetus or the breastfed neonate. Some fetal abnormalities have been demonstrated in animals using very high doses of these drugs. Oral or intravenous therapy may induce fetal or neonatal tachycardia, neonatal hypoglycaemia and tremor (Serafin, 1996), but this is more likely with the higher doses used for tocolysis.

Uses of beta$_2$ adrenoreceptor agonists

- rescue asthma medication;
- exercise prophylaxis;
- prevention of asthma symptoms in patients also receiving anti-inflammatory prophylaxis (usually salmeterol);
- chronic airways disease (for example cystic fibrosis): relief of pulmonary oedema;
- tocolysis (Chapter 7)

Use of inhaled salbutamol or terbutaline to treat symptoms during labour does not prolong labour or delay onset of labour, probably due to low systemic absorption (Nelson-Piercy & Moore-Gillon, 1995).

An inhaled dose of salbutamol or terbutaline acts within minutes and lasts three to five hours. Long acting preparations, for example salmeterol, fenoterol, last for 12 hours but are not effective 'rescue' medication. Tolerance to beta$_2$ adrenoreceptor agonists may develop with repeated exposure, and regular use of beta agonists may worsen disease control (Hoffman & Lefkowitz, 1996). Administration of corticosteroids may reverse tolerance and restore the effectiveness of beta$_2$ adrenoreceptor agonists (Lipworth, 1997).

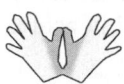 **Practice Point**

Sudden withdrawal of therapy causes rebound symptoms. Therefore it is important that asthma therapy is not discontinued (or left behind) should someone suddenly be admitted to hospital.

Methylxanthines

Theophylline is not recommended during pregnancy. It is someimtes used to stimulate breathing movements in the neonate.

Anti-inflammatory agents

Inflammation causes narrowing of the airways in asthma, both during and between exacerbations/attacks. Many inflammatory mediators, (such as histamine) are involved, therefore effective therapy is directed at the inflammatory processes rather than any single mediator. Anti-inflammatory agents are prescribed to prevent, rather than treat, asthma attacks. Cromoglycate has been widely used in pregnancy without adverse effects; there is less experience with nedocromil (Nelson-Piercy & Moore-Gillon, 1995).

Cromoglycate

Although only about 33 per cent of asthmatics respond, this is a useful drug with few side effects. Cromoglycate is administered by inhalation, as a preventative therapy, either on a regular basis or prior to exercise. Its mechanism of action is uncertain, but it probably prevents stimulation of irritant receptors and inhibits the inflammatory response. Cromoglycate is not transferred across the placenta and does not enter breast milk. Inhalation of the dry powder may cause coughing and bronchospasm. Hypersensitivity responses are very rare.

Corticosteroids

Steroids have saved lives and revolutionized the management of severe illnesses such as asthma, rheumatoid arthritis, exfoliative dermatitis and Addison's disease. Regular use of inhaled beclomethasone reduces the frequency of severe episodes of asthma in pregnancy (Wendel et al, 1996). Due to side effects, long term oral administration is avoided if possible and maintenance doses are kept to a minimum (BNF, 2000; see Implictions for Practice). However oral steroids, such as prednisolone, are essential in acute, severe asthma.

How the body handles corticosteroids

Topical or inhalational administration reduces, but does not necessarily abolish, systemic side effects (CSM, 1998). Inhaled corticosteroids will lead to oral infection such as thrush unless strict oral hygiene is maintained.

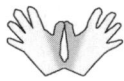 **Practice Point**

Gargling with water following corticosteroid inhalation reduces the risk of oral thrush.

Systemic side effects may occur with inhaled beclomethasone doses of 800 micrograms/day.

Steroids are dependent on liver enzymes for elimination. This gives rise to several drug interactions. Steroids cross the placenta to a variable extent. For example, over 80 per cent of prednisolone is inactivated by the placenta. The risk of intrauterine growth retardation is significant if administration of corticosteroids is prolonged or repeated (BNF, 2000; see p. 193). Prednisolone (administered orally) passes into breast milk. Doses above 40 mg per day may cause side effects in neonates, who should be carefully monitored (CSM, 1998).

Actions and side effects of corticosteroids

Side effects of corticosteroids can be summarized as:
Side effects likely to arise immediately:

- cardiovascular problems;
- central nervous system problems;
- metabolic disturbances – hyperglycaemia.

Side effects likely to arise in the longer term:

- anti-inflammatory actions;
- metabolic disturbances – growth, tissue viability and fat metabolism;
- adrenal suppression (see also Implications for Practice and Appendix 1).

This chapter will only detail problems likely to be more relevant to long term administration of corticosteroids. Short term side effects are discussed in Chapter 7, tocolysis and topical corticosteroids in Chapter 20, OTC drugs. However the potential side effects of corticosteroids may be encountered in any situation where they are prescribed.

Anti-inflammatory actions

All types and stages of the inflammatory response, both appropriate and inappropriate, are depressed, reducing redness, pain, swelling, healing and tissue repair by:

- reduced production and release of inflammatory mediators;
- failure of white cells to migrate to site of infection, increasing the risk of infections, including neonatal sepsis (Steer & Flint, 1999b);
- failure to activate macrophages, giving an increased risk of reactivation of TB (tuberculosis);
- suppression of cell-mediated immune response and reduced response to antigens. Infections are more severe, and the response to immunizations is decreased; see Box 15.1;
- reduced proliferation of fibroblasts and collagen formation. This allows rapid spread of infection without signs and symptoms and impedes healing.

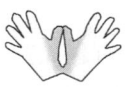 **Practice Points**

- There is a **risk of severe chickenpox,** possibly with minimal rash (BNF, 2000).
- During pregnancy, the risk of infection is higher, and extra vigilance is required to prevent and detect infections (Minerbi-Codish et al, 1998).
- After childbirth, extra vigilance will be needed to ensure that the perineum heals without infection.
- If the woman is able to breastfeed, she should be particularly vigilant for signs of mastitis.

Box 15.1   Immunizations

Live vaccines* should not be administered to anyone with impaired immunity, including those receiving high dose steroid treatment and within at least three months of discontinuation of such therapy (BNF, 2000). Live vaccines must not be administered if contacts are receiving immunosuppressive medications such as oral steroids. For example, polio may be contracted by changing the nappies of an infant who has received oral polio vaccine. Inactivated forms of polio and typhoid vaccines can be obtained for injection.

* MMR (mumps, measles, rubella), oral polio, rubella, BCG, yellow fever and oral typhoid are live vaccines.

Metabolic disturbances

Corticosteroids enhance tissue breakdown and redistribute carbohydrate, fat and protein reserves. The trunk becomes fat, while the limbs become thin. Fats are released into the circulation, and plasma lipids may rise; fat embolus is a rare complication.

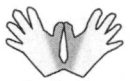 **Practice Points**

- Hyperglycaemia may occur; it is essential that anyone receiving oral steroids, or over 800 micrograms inhaled steroids per day, is monitored for this.
- Corticosteroids encourage the breakdown of glycogen and protein into glucose, and increase appetite and weight. Foods rich in salt or sugar should be avoided to reduce the risks of hypertension and dental caries.

Protein catabolism (breakdown) reduces the collagen content of all tissues, including skin and bones. Long term use may lead to osteoporosis, muscle wasting, and mineral or vitamin deficiencies (particularly B_6, C, D, K and folates). Inhaled corticosteroids has been associated with osteoporosis (Wong et al, 2000). Prolonged treatment with oral steroids has been associated with low birthweight (intrauterine growth retardation), reduced head circumference in humans and cleft palate and impaired development in rats (Serefin, 1996; CSM, 1998; Steer & Flint, 1999); increased risk of prematurity (Laskin et al, 1997).

Thinning of the gut lining may induce peptic ulceration or gastric bleeding, particularly if aspirin, NSAIDs or alcohol are also taken. Problems have occurred in neonates.

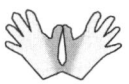 **Practice Point**

Oral steroids are taken with food to reduce gastric irritation.

Dermatological problems, such as acne, sweating, thinning of skin, facial erythema, petechiae, bruising and hirsuitism, may be caused by long term systemic steroids (Govoni & Hayes, 1990). On withdrawal of steroids, a rebound of dermatological conditions may occur; this is a particular danger in psoriasis.

Corticosteroids cause retention of sodium ions and loss of potassium ions. The associated changes in BP and fluid balance are considered in relation to tocolysis.

Adrenal suppression

Two weeks of systemic steroid therapy (including repeated courses of steroids for fetal lung maturation) is sufficient to disrupt the pituitary/adrenal axis. After two weeks' administration, abrupt discontinuation of steroids may cause symptoms and signs of adrenal insufficiency: weakness, depression, fever, muscle and joint pains, runny nose, red eyes, painful, itchy skin nodules, hypoglycaemia, electrolyte imbalance, anorexia and weight loss. In severe cases, BP falls rapidly and fatalities have occurred.

For patients taking oral steroids, labour, severe illness, fever, surgery or trauma may precipitate symptoms of adrenal insufficiency because endogenous steroid production cannot rise to meet the (tenfold) extra demands. This danger may continue for up to a year after cessation of steroid therapy. Steroid administration is increased or reintroduced for these emergencies. One hundred mg hydrocortisone is administered intravenously every eight hours during labour (Ebden & Evans, 1996).

Adrenal suppression shows individual variation but occurs with inhaled doses of 1000–2000 micrograms/day of beclomethasone (Clark & Lipworth, 1997). Fetal and neonatal adrenal suppression may arise if the mother is receiving >10 mg prednisolone per day or equivalent (Ebden & Evans, 1996). In practice, this is rarely a problem, but close observation is advisable. Breast-fed infants whose mothers are taking more than 40 mg prednisolone per day may show signs of adrenal suppression (BNF, 2000).

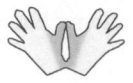 **Practice Points**

- To facilitate emergency admissions, it is important that 'steroid cards' are given to anyone receiving steroids for more than three weeks (CSM, 1998).
- The risk of adrenal suppression is least when oral steroids are given in the morning, as a single dose, before 9.00 am. This reduces the disruption to the body's circadian cycle of ACTH (adrenocorticotropic hormone) and corticosteroid secretion.

Interactions with corticosteroids

Corticosteroids antagonize the actions of many drugs (hypoglycaemic agents, anticoagulants, antihypertensives, diuretics, growth hormone) and intensify the actions of others (oestrogens).

Implications for Practice: asthma in pregnancy

Potential Problem

Undiagnosed asthma causing hypoxia and intrauterine growth retardation

Poor control of asthma, causing waking during the night with coughing and even hypoxia

Management

Inquiry to all women in antenatal clinic of a history of asthma or breathing difficulties, particularly at night. Refer to doctors for lung function tests to distinguish from 'dyspnoea of pregnancy'.

Records of PEFR or FEV_1 should be checked; any decline in function or 'nocturnal dips' should be referred to the prescriber.* Any changes in prescription or inhaler device should be noted.

Record the numbers and types of inhalations used daily and report to prescriber if > one inhalation of salbutamol or terbutaline is being taken per day.

Compliance should be discussed and monitored.

Maintain monitoring during the puerperium and for six months after delivery.

Implications for Practice (*continued*)

Potential Problem	Management
Rebound symptoms on withdrawal of therapy	Ensure the woman has a spare inhaler, particularly during the puerperium. Ensure inhalers are always available.
Intrauterine growth retardation, fetal distress	Monitor growth of fetus by serial ultrasound. Use a pulse oximeter to ensure oxygen saturation remains >95 per cent, including during delivery.
Management of labour	Ensure inhalations are maintained. Avoid carboprost and dinoprost. Use nitrous oxide as needed. Discuss the potential risks of opioids in relation to benefits during labour. Avoid general anaesthesia if possible. Be aware of case reports of asthma triggered by spinal anaesthesia (see case report). Substitute oxytocin for ergometrine as prophylaxis for the third stage.
Advice on breastfeeding	Prolonged breastfeeding may confer some protection against asthma. With the exception of methylxanthines (for example theophylline), asthma medications are no barrier to breastfeeding at normal doses.

* The predicted values for peak expiratory flow rate (PEFR) measurements are not altered by pregnancy (Brancazio et al, 1997).

Implications for Practice: steroids in pregnancy

Potential Problem	Management
Increased risk of oral thrush with inhaled steroids	Use a spacer device. Gargle with water after inhalation. Attention to oral hygiene.
Exposure to chickenpox	Obtain a history of chickenpox, if possible. If exposed to chickenpox,

Implications for Practice (*continued*)

Potential Problem	Management
	refer to physicians for prophylactic immunoglobulins. The risks are much greater if the woman is taking oral steroid therapy.
	Avoid contact with measles, chickenpox or shingles.
Chest infections exacerbating asthma	With oral steroids, a daily temperature at 5–6 pm should provide early indication of infection. Refer to doctors if antibiotics may be necessary.
Adrenal suppression if oral steroids are used for longer than two weeks	Carry 'steroid cards' in case of emergency admission.
	Intravenous steroids may be administered to cover the stress of labour.
	Check glucose and electrolytes in neonate.
	Observe neonate for appetite, weakness, lethargy, fever.
Steroid side effects	Check electrolytes, BP and fluid balance.
	Monitor weight and advise on diet.
	Check plasma glucose, and advise on diet.
	Foot care.
	Mobilize to reduce risks of DVT.
	Monitor fetal growth.
	Observe neonate for signs of sepsis.

Conclusion

Careful monitoring of airways by the multidisciplinary team is essential to prevent exacerbation of asthma, particularly in the third trimester and in the puerperium. Women with asthma should be reassured as to the likely outcome of pregnancy, so long as compliance is maintained. However larger studies are needed before this assurance can claim to be evidence-based (Jadad et al, 2000). Use of steroids must be accompanied by close monitoring of mother and fetus during pregnancy, labour and the puerperium. It is essential that help and surveillance are continued after the birth. This may be the most difficult time for asthmatics. Disturbed sleep and hormonal changes exacerbate asthma, waking the mother and intensifying sleep deprivation.

Further Reading

Serafin, W. (1996) Drugs used in the treatment of asthma. In: Hardman, J., Limbard, L., Molinoff, P., Ruddon, R. & Goodman Gilman, A. (eds) *Goodman & Gilman's: The Pharmacological Basis of Therapeutics*, 9th edition. New York, McGraw-Hill:659–82.

Jordan, S. & White, J. (2001) Bronchodilators: implications for nursing practice, *Nursing Standard 15:45–52.*

CHAPTER 16

Drugs Prescribed for Mental Illness

BILLY HARDY AND SUE JORDAN

This chapter will discuss the commonest medications prescribed to young women, the SSRIs, and brifely describe other anti-depressant and anti-psychotic medication. Many of the side effects of anti-psychotic medication are described with prochlorperazine, under anti-emetics, Chapter 5.

Chapter Contents

▨ Childbirth and mental health problems/mental illness

▨ The management of mental health problems and mental illness

▨ Drugs in mental illness

▨ Conclusion

Childbirth and mental health problems/mental illness

Midwives will encounter women with enduring mental health problems and women whose illnesses appear in the puerperium. The definitions and diagnoses of mental illness remain symptom-based, dependent, to some extent, on the clinical skills of practitioners (Bell, 1996). Some authorities consider that the aetiology of mental health problems has a neurobiological basis and that this justifies a pharmacotherapeutic approach (see Coverdale et al, 1996; Baldessarini, 1996 for a discussion).

The post-natal period is a time when the incidence of mental health problems increases sharply (Kendell et al, 1987; O'Hara & Swain, 1996). In the puerperium, women may be offered services via the primary health care team, the community mental health team or specialist psychiatric services, as described by the Royal College of Psychiatrists (1996). One treatment modality is psychiatric medications. Compliance with pharmacotherapy will be enhanced by offering detailed information regarding the relevant medications. It is at this time that the midwife's knowledge and her relationship with her clients can be used effectively, in collaboration with other professionals. The understanding of pharmacological considerations can be explained to clients and their families, possibly increasing their compliance. Discontinuation of prescribed mental health medication was associated with more than one death between 1994 and 1996 (DoH, 1998).

While there is growing evidence in support for psychological interventions for depressive episodes following childbirth (Elliot et al, 1994), it is likely that midwives will see women who are prescribed anti-depressants or medications associated with other more serious mental health problems such as schizophrenia and manic depression.

The management of mental health problems and mental illness

Harris (1996) suggests that childbirth is associated with two distinct forms of mental illness: puerperal psychosis and post-natal depression. The most devastating mental disorder associated with childbirth is puerperal psychosis, which occurs in around two per thousand births. The risk of recurrence in subsequent deliveries is 50 per cent. This psychosis, like many other forms, is characterized by florid and bizarre features and may present the professional with some very difficult decisions with regard to safety of the mother and the child (Brennan, 1991). The mother's temporary loss of reality will, in many cases, require the intervention of psychiatric services or, if available, specialist peri-natal psychiatric services offering a complete mother and baby service. It is likely that the full range of treatment options will be considered in the most disturbed women, including antipsychotics and electro-convulsive therapy.

Post-natal depression is the most common mental health problem following childbirth, affecting around 10–13 per cent of women, while a further 26 per cent of women experience a self-limiting depressive episode (Loudon, 1995; O'Hara & Swain, 1996). These conditions must be distinguished from 'the blues', episodes of tearfulness and anxiety arising around day five and continuing episodically for several weeks, particularly when the mother is tired. Prolonged post-natal depression is typically associated with adverse social circumstances; these women will benefit from post-partum screening and psychotherapeutic interventions and social support (Campbell & Lees, 2000). While the aetiological debates continue (see Elliot et al, 1994; Nicolson, 1998; Littlewood and McHugh, 1997), the most likely medical intervention in primary or secondary care will remain the prescription of anti-depressants.

Drugs in mental illness

Several drugs are used in mental illness. These are summarized in Table 16.1.

Table 16.1   Drugs used in mental illness: summary and examples

Anti-depressants	Selective Serotonin Reuptake Inhibitors (SSRIs)
	    for example fluoxetine, sertraline, paroxetine
	Tricyclic antidepressants (TCAs)
	    for example imipramine, amitriptyline, dothiepin, doxepin
	Mono-amino oxidase inhibitors (MAOIs)
	    for example moclobemide, tranylcypromine
	    (not recommended in pregnancy and breastfeeding)
	Others, such as tryptophan; see BNF for details

Antipsychotics	Typical antipsychotics
	    Oral medications
	        for example chlorpromazine, haloperidol, trifluoperazine, prochlorperazine
	    Depot medications (intramuscular injections)
	        for example fluphenzine, haloperidol (Haldol®),
	        zuclopenthixol (Clopixol®), flupenthixol (Depixol®)
	    Atypical antipsychotics (administered orally)
	        for example risperidone, olanzapine, clozapine

Anxiolytics	Benzodiazepines, such as diazepam, temazepam Buspirone (contra-indicated in pregnancy and breastfeeding)
Anti-manic agents	Lithium compounds Carbamazepine, sodium valproate (see anticonvulsants, Chapter 19)

The anti-depressants

Selective serotonin reuptake inhibitors (SSRIs)

While it can be argued that the quality and type of post-natal depression is different from other forms of clinical depression (Pitt, 1991), the anti-depressants most likely to be prescribed during this period are those generally used in primary care, the selective serotonin reuptake inhibitors [SSRIs]. These include fluoxetine (Prozac®), paroxetine (Seroxat®), sertraline (Lustral®), fluvoxamine, citalopram and related drugs, such as venlafaxine (Effexor®). SSRIs are also used in the treatment of obsessive compulsive disorders, anxiety, eating disorders and panic disorders.

Over the last decade, the SSRIs have, in part, superseded both the older anti-depressants (tricyclics) and the anxiolytics such as benzodiazepines

(Medawar, 1997). Their introduction was facilitated by concerns over the side effects of the older anti-depressants such as tricyclics, (amitriptyline, dothiepin (Prothiaden®) and imipramine). These drugs are still prescribed by some doctors, because they are viewed as been relatively safe in pregnancy and breastfeeding, with the exception of doxepin (Haberg & Mathson, 1997).

How the body handles SSRIs

SSRIs cross the placenta and enter breast milk which gives rise to safety considerations (see p. 353). Unlike the other SSRIs, fluoxetine and its metabolites have long half-lives (approximately seven to nine days). This means that fluoxetine has the potential to accumulate in the body, and will not be eliminated for three to five weeks after the last dose (see Chapter 1). It is also slower to take effect than other SSRIs, which have shorter half-lives. Therefore other SSRIs, such as sertraline, may be better choices when rapid symptom relief is needed, as in post-partum depression (Edwards & Anderson, 1999).

Actions of SSRIs

The use of this drug group depends on the specific nature of their effects on one particular neurotransmitter, serotonin (5HT, 5-hydroxytryptamine), which influences mood. SSRIs are designed to block the reuptake of serotonin in the brain, allowing higher levels to accumulate, thereby altering mood.

Side effects of SSRIs

Serotonin is important regulator of the:

- gastro-intestinal tract;
- central nervous system;
- cardiovascular system;
- platelets.

Overall, commonly reported adverse reactions are nausea, usually soon after starting treatment, feelings of nervousness, panic and insomnia. Serious adverse drug reactions occur in 1.5 per cent of inpatients receiving SSRIs, mainly psychotic and neurological disturbances, which is slightly lower than the figure for tricyclics (TCAs) (1.7 per cent) (Grohmann et al, 1999). The side effect profile of SSRIs differs from TCAs, and, in general, they are better tolerated (see Implications for Practice).

Gastro-intestinal disturbances Serotonin is important in controlling gastro-intestinal motility and secretions. Some 18–26 per cent of people taking SSRIs experience gastro-intestinal disturbances, including, *anorexia, nausea, diarrhoea, constipation and indigestion.* Weight loss commonly occurs, but this may be viewed positively by the woman. Maternal weight gain and mean birth weight may be reduced in women taking fluoxetine during the third trimester (Chambers et al, 1996); however depressive illness can also be the cause of poor weight gain and premature delivery (Wisner, 1999). In contrast, citalopram, like tricyclic anti-depressants, can cause weight gain. In diabetics, fluoxetine can alter plasma glucose concentrations.

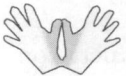 **Practice Points**

- Troublesome nocturnal gastro-intestinal symptoms may cause non-compliance with medication.
- Regular recording of weight will facilitate assessment and reduce the risks of serious weight changes.
- Fluoxetine necessitates regular glucose monitoring in diabetics.

SSRIs may cause hypersalivation or dry mouth, nasal congestion, cough, rhinitis, fever or a flu-like syndrome.

Central nervous system   By blocking the reuptake of serotonin into presynaptic neurones, SSRIs increase the availability of bioamines in the synapses of the central nervous system. While this elevates mood, it is also responsible for feelings of agitation, anxiety or even hypomania. This effect may be most pronounced with fluoxetine. Central nervous system disturbances may also lead to insomnia, amnesia, hallucinations, tremor. There are anecdotal reports linking fluoxetine to aggressive, violent behaviour and suicide (Boseley, 1999). Sensory disturbances are possible, including: pins and needles, tinnitus, visual disturbances, taste disturbance and headache. Migraine may be worsened or occur for the first time. All anti-depressants increase the likelihood of seizures in women with a history of convulsions and prolong the convulsions and amnesia induced by electro-convulsive therapy (ECT).

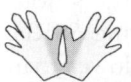 **Practice Points**

- Midwives should be particularly vigilant in observing women who are already agitated, as fluoxetine may worsen their condition.
- Anti-depressants may impair driving skills, and women should be warned of this (BNF, 2000).
- Neonates exposed to fluoxetine in the third trimester may experience poor neonatal adaption (Chambers et al, 1996). Therefore, extra help may be needed with breastfeeding.

SSRIs, particularly paroxetine, are dopamine antagonists. Therefore with prolonged administration, they share the posture and movement side effects of anti-psychotics and increase production of prolactin (see below). This may be the mechanism underlying the sexual dysfunction and loss of libido, which are frequently reported side effects, particularly with paroxetine. Frequency of micturition may be increased.

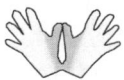 **Practice Points**

When women are prescribed SSRIs, especially paroxetine, professionals should carefully observe for signs of tremor, restlessness, abnormal movements and stiffness.

Cardiovascular system   Although SSRIs are less cardiotoxic than other antidepressants, they may cause dysrhythmias, palpitations or alterations in heart rate. SSRIs antagonize the α (alpha) receptors of the sympathetic nervous system which are responsible for maintaining blood pressure. This may lead to postural hypotension, particularly with sertraline or paroxetine. Hypotension may compromise placental blood flow and intrauterine growth, without being detectable using standard measurement techniques.

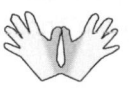 **Practice Points**

- Measuring BP in sitting and standing positions will assess the degree of postural hypotension.
- Regular monitoring of fetal growth is essential.

SSRIs may lead to increased sweating, acne, *Herpes simplex* and 'hot flushes'.

Platelets   Serotonin is important in regulating the activity of platelets. Bleeding, bruising or purpura may arise as a result of *platelet dysfunction*. This may present as haemoptysis, gastro-intestinal bleeds or even a stroke.

Hypersensitivity responses   Like all drugs, SSRIs can cause hypersensitivity responses in susceptible individuals. These are particularly common with fluoxetine. Rashes occur in 5–15 per cent of clients. In a few cases, vasculitis and blood vessel necrosis have developed, jeopardizing the blood supply of the limb.

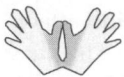 **Practice Point**

Other hypersensitivity responses include:

- alopecia (hair loss);
- joint and muscle pains;
- angioedema;
- liver function disturbances;
- pancreatitis;
- bone marrow damage – aplastic anaemia, haemolytic anaemia;
- pulmonary fibrosis. This is rare. *Dyspnoea is a warning* sign which is easily overlooked.

SSRI withdrawal syndrome

Withdrawal from treatment should be gradually phased over several weeks. Abrupt discontinuation often causes headache, nausea, pins and needles, sensory disturbance, tremor, anxiety, confusion, dizziness, fatigue, insomnia and (fluoxetine only) bleeding. These problems can persist for about three weeks.

Drug interactions with SSRIs

SSRIs inhibit key liver enzymes, reducing the elimination and causing the accumulation of several drugs, including phenothiazines (for example prochlorperazine (Stemetil®)) and anti-depressants. Similarly, the use of fluoxetine with diazepam should be treated with caution as it increases the half-life of diazepam, increasing sedation. Alcohol should be avoided.

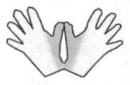 **Practice Point**

SSRIs may intensify the hypotension and sedation associated with analgesics and anti-emetics commonly used in labour.

The serotonin syndrome

The serotonin syndrome was first reported in the 1950s. It occurs in genetically susceptible people who combine SSRIs with other drugs which may increase serotonin levels in the central nervous system (for example MAOIs, tricyclic anti-depressants, alcohol, diet pills, cold cures, amphetamines, cocaine) (Nolan & Scoggin, 1999). The problem has also arisen in association with meperidine (pethidine) administration (Bowdle, 1998). The serotonin syndrome results in uncontrollable hyperthermia (and occasionally death) associated with:

- *mental state changes:* anxiety, hypomania, agitation;
- *cardiovascular problems:* tachycardia, blood pressure fluctuations;
- *gastrointestinal problems:* nausea, salivation;
- *motor abnormalities:* muscle rigidity, tremor, ataxia, shivering, nystagmus.

SSRIs and pregnancy

There is little evidence from long term studies to inform practitioners on outcomes for infants exposed to SSRIs *in utero* or via breast milk (Harris, 1996; Gupta, 1998). The safety of SSRIs in pregnancy awaits further investigation. The manufacturers advise against use in pregnancy (BNF, 2000). A US study (n = 228) found that, in comparison with controls, women taking fluoxetine during the last trimester gained less weight and delivered smaller babies. There was also an increase in minor abnormalities (club feet, hydrocoele, congenital hip dislocation, lacrminal stenosis) and evidence of poor neonatal adaptation, including jitteriness, respiratory disturbance and poor feeding (Chambers et al, 1996). A longer term study of pre-school children exposed to anti-depressants *in utero* found no performance deficits; this study included 55 children exposed to fluoxetine and 84 children exposed to a tricyclic (Nulman et al, 1997). Bhatia and Bhatia (1999) have suggested that there is little indication in the research literature that there is a substantial risk to pregnant women taking SSRIs.

Breastfeeding

SSRIs pass into breast milk and the manufacturers advise against breastfeeding (BNF, 2000). In a comprehensive review, Yoshida et al (1999) found few cases where neonates had suffered adverse effects due to SSRIs in breast milk: these included a baby with gastro-intestinal problems and another with irritability. Preterm infants and those with compromised hepatic or renal function are at increased risk. Chambers et al (1999) found that infants (n = 26) breastfed by mothers taking fluoxetine gained significantly less weight than comparators (392 grams over six months), although no infants showed signs or symptoms of either side effects or malnutrition.

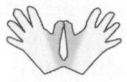 **Practice Points**

Should a mother taking a SSRI decide to breastfeed (probably against medical advice):
- A blood sample should be obtained from the neonate to ensure that renal and hepatic function are normal before exposure (Yoshida et al, 1999).
- The neonate should be monitored for signs of colic, vomiting and irritability, which may necessitate a change in feeding.
- Weight gain of the infant should be carefully monitored.
- A baby is most vulnerable in its first few days of life. Exposure to drugs via breast milk is less likely to be harmful when the infant is several months old (Suri et al, 1998).

Tricyclic anti-depressants

The use of the older tricyclics, such as amitriptyline, imipramine and doth- iepin, is declining and the SSRIs now dominate primary care. Tricyclic anti- depressants are considerably more dangerous than SSRIs in overdose, with the possible exception of citalopram: they were the immediate cause of death in two cases in the last triennium (DoH, 1998).

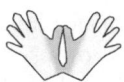 **Practice Point**

Midwives need to ensure that families are aware of the dangers of many of these medica- tions (particularly tricyclic anti-depressants and lithium) in overdose, and ensure that tablets are stored securely away from young children.

For women established on tricyclic anti-depressants, the dose may need to be increased during pregnancy to maintain the clinical response; however as mood often lifts in the third trimester, it may be possible to reduce the dose to minimize neonatal withdrawal reactions (see p. 355). Following delivery, the dose should be returned to pre-pregnancy values, and close observation maintained for emergent side effects (Wisner et al, 1999). The side effect profile of tricyclic anti-depressants is similar in many ways to the phenoth- iazines. The anti-muscarinic, cardiovascular and central nervous system side effects are described in Chapter 5, anti-emetics. Posture and movement disorders are associated with high doses. Tricyclics are also associated with agitation or even hypomania, particularly when treatment is initiated.

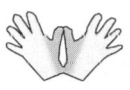 **Practice Point**

The risk of suicide is increased during the first few weeks of therapy, and particular vigilance is required during this time (Baldessarini, 1996).

If anti-depressants, like phenothiazines, are abruptly discontinued, a withdrawal syndrome may be observed: irritability, restlessness, insomnia, fever, abdominal cramps, nausea and vomiting. These problems, together with feeding difficulties, seizures, tachypnoea, gastrointestinal stasis and bladder retention, have been observed in neonates born to mothers taking these drugs during the last trimester (Loudon, 1995; Wisner et al, 1999). However tricyclics are not regarded as teratogenic (BNF, 2000), although, they may be associated with the same risks as SSRIs (Austin & Mitchell, 1998). Manufacturers advise avoiding tricyclics during breastfeeding (BNF, 2000), but, with the exception of doxepin, there is little evidence of harm (Yoshida et al, 1999).

Anti-psychotic medication

Anti-psychotics may be prescribed:

- for an acute episode of puerperal psychosis;
- as a component of the ongoing management of women with enduring mental illness, often as intra-muscular 'depot' injections;
- to treat an acute episode of mental illness.

The midwife may visit clients who are in a mother and baby unit or work collaboratively with a local mental health team, supporting a woman and her family to stay at home during an acute psychotic phase (Oates, 1988).

Pregnancy and the puerperium are vulnerable periods for women with mental illness, due to both the physiological and psychosocial stresses associated. Women may be reassured to know that the risk of obstetric complications is not markedly increased in women with schizophrenia (Kendell et al, 2000). For women with enduring mental illness, it is possible that doses of medication will have been minimized during pregnancy, and this reduction of the 'pharmacological shield' will be insufficient to protect the mother in the puerperium.

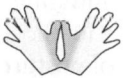 **Practice Point**

- Women with long term mental illness should be reviewed by their mental health practitioners soon after delivery, and regularly during the puerperium. Psychiatrists frequently need to adjust medication upwards during this period.

Some women may become non-compliant with prescribed anti-psychotic medication due to misplaced fears of damage to the fetus.

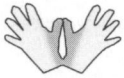 **Practice Points**

- For women with long term mental illness, non-compliance with prescribed anti-psychotic medication carries a high risk of relapse, which poses more danger to mother and baby than the adverse effects of the drugs (Pinkofsky, 1997).
- Women should be reassured that long term studies do not demonstrate that the traditional anti-psychotics have a significant teratogenic effect, and long term follow-up of infants has not demonstrated developmental delay (Loudon, 1995).
- An ultra-sound scan at 16–18 weeks will assist detection of congenital abnormalities.
- The effects of intra-muscular 'depot' injections persist for up to three months after the last dose. If injections are discontinued, symptoms may re-emerge around this time.

Actions and side effects of anti-psychotics

Many anti-psychotics are phenothiazines or related compounds. Therefore they have side effects similar to prochlorperazine (Stemetil ®) (see Chapter 5, anti-emetics). They act on many of the body's receptors to cause a range of side effects.

The hypotensive actions of these drugs may jeopardize the blood flow to the placenta (Pinkofsky, 1997).

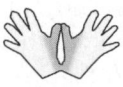 **Practice Point**

For many reasons, regular ante-natal checkups to monitor fetal growth are essential for women receiving anti-psychotic medication.

When phenothiazines or other anti-psychotics are used long term, for mental illness or hyperemsis, the **posture and movement side effects**, attributed to blockade of the dopamine (D_2) receptors, are extremely important. Women are particularly vulnerable to these side effects post-partum, due to the rapid decline in oestrogen levels at this time. Although the long acting intramuscular depot injections have the advantage of ensuring compliance in those with serious mental illness, they are associated with a high incidence of posture and movement side effects. These have also been reported in breastfed neonates (Loudon, 1995). There is a danger that some of these side effects, the tardive dyskinesias, associated with long term use, *may be irreversible.*

Table 16.2   Side effects of anti-psychotics

Dopamine (D2) antagonism	Posture and movement disorders Prolactin production Blunting of emotions Anti-emetic
Anti-muscarinic	Dry mouth, constipation, etc (Chapter 5, Table 5.2)
Anti-histaminic	Sedation
Antagonism of the alpha receptors	Hypotension Weight gain
Increased excitability	Risk of cardiac dysrhythmias or seizures (people with epilepsy)
Hypersensitivity responses	Agranulocytosis

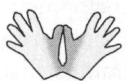 **Practice Point**

Women prescribed anti-psychotic medications for more than a few days should be regularly assessed for stiffness and abnormal movements which may herald the onset of pseudoparkinsonism and tardive dyskinesia. Scales, such as the AIMS (abnormal involuntary movement) scale have been devised to assist professionals in this (DoH & RCN, 1994; RCN, 1996).

With continuous use in the last three months of pregnancy, anti-psychotics can cause prolonged movement disorders in neonates, lasting for up to ten months (Cox & Nicholls, 1996). The neonate is less able to eliminate these drugs than adults, so is at risk of developing jaundice, gastro-intestinal obstruction, hyper-reflexia, restlessness, poor suckling, tremor and bradykinesia, even if the mother is free of side effects (Govoni & Hayes, 1990). Chlorpromazine may be associated with higher risks than other anti-psychotics.

The neuroleptic malignant syndrome is a rare complication of anti-psychotic therapy which can arise when medications are introduced or changed. It is characterized by fluctuating vital signs, autonomic instability, rigidity and muscle breakdown, leading to raised temperature and raised levels of creatine kinase (CPK) in the plasma. Early recognition of the syndrome and withdrawal of D_2 antagonists is life-saving (Sharma et al, 1995; *Drug & Therapeutics Bulletin*, 1995).

With long term use, anti-psychotics increase the production of **prolactin**. This may cause breast tenderness, galactorrhoea, hirsuitism and menstrual irregularities. Increased production of prolactin reduces, but does not abolish, fertility. Despite this, women with long term use of anti-psychotics should receive full contraceptive advice in the puerperium. Some breast tumours are prolactin dependent, contra-indicating the use of these drugs (Karch, 1992).

Effects on the fetus

Assessment of the effects of anti-psychotic drugs is complicated by the higher rates of fetal loss, perinatal complications and abnormalities in drug-naive women with serious mental illness (Austin & Mitchall, 1998). Exposure to phenothiazines in weeks four to ten may be linked with a small increase (0.4 per cent) in birth defects (Austin & Mitchell, 1998). US pregnancy category C.

Breastfeeding

When women are prescribed anti-psychotics, extreme caution should be exercised in breastfeeding as these drugs pass freely through breast milk and during this time high doses of drugs (>100 mgs chlorpromazine/day) are likely to be prescribed (Mortola, 1989). Animal studies have indicated that CNS development may be impaired (BNF, 2000). Dangers of developmental delay are increased if the mothers are prescribed more than one drug (Yoshida et al, 1999), if infants are small or premature, or intramuscular medication is prescribed (Campbell & Lees, 2000). Drowsiness, poor suckling and failure to feed and gain weight are the most common problems, particularly with chlorpromazine (Suri et al, 1998).

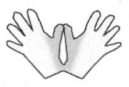 **Practice Point**

Where breastfeeding mothers are prescribed anti-psychotics or benzodiazepines, very careful records of weight gain and development must be kept. Review by paediatricians is advisable.

There is little information on the **newer**, **atypical anti-psychotic medications** (olanzapine, risperidone, quetiapine, zotepine), and therefore manufacturers advise against their use in pregnancy and lactation (BNF, 2000). Case study reviews found that five of 61 babies born to mothers taking clozapine had malformations, but many of the mothers were also taking other drugs. Only four breastfed babies were identified, of whom one developed agranulocytosis and another became excessively sleepy; on the basis of these alarming reports, authorities recommend bottle feeding with clozapine (Dev & Krupp, 1995).

Drug interactions with anti-psychotics

A comprehensive list of interactions is beyond the scope of this book (see Stockley, 1999), but the midwife should be aware that some of the drugs administered in labour can interact with anti-psychotics, particularly chlorpromazine. For example, opioids or prochlorperazine may induce problematic sedation, hypotension and respiratory depression. The reactive metabolite of pethidine may give rise to problems, including CNS toxicity, hypotension and profound respiratory depression in susceptible individuals (Baldessarini, 1996; Stockley, 1999). If local anaesthetics are used for pain relief, the risk of cardiac problems (heart block) is increased, necessitating careful monitoring.

Anxiolytics

Prescription of benzodiazepines is generally declining. In the management of anxiety, prescription is for a maximum of four weeks (BNF, 2000:164). The longer acting benzodiazepines, such as diazepam (Valium ®), are generally used to manage anxiety, and the shorter acting benzodiazepeines, such as temazepm, are generally used as hypnotics, but their actions are indistinguishable. Use during pregnancy is complicated by reports of microcephaly and cleft palate (Medawar, 1992). Diazepam reduces muscle tone, and, in the neonate, may cause the 'floppy baby syndrome', respiratory depression and hypothermia (Cox & Nicholls, 1996). Long term use of benzodiazepines in the mother may cause a withdrawal syndrome in the neonate (BNF, 2000). Neonates are less able to eliminate benzodiazepines than adults; use during lactation may unduly sedate a breastfed infant.

Lithium therapy

Lithium is a mood stabilizer or anti-manic agent. In young women, lithium is a drug of last resort, for manic depressive psychosis (Schou and Vestergaard, 1996). The action of lithium has been described as enhancing the uptake of norepinephrine/noradrenaline and serotonin. Lithium may help some clients, but it is only suitable for those who are able to comply closely with the prescribed regimen and attend for regular monitoring of venous blood samples. Withdrawal of lithium therapy, particularly if abrupt, is linked with a very high incidence of mania (Moncrieff, 1995; Silverstone & Romans, 1996).

The absorption of lithium is rapid and plasma concentrations peak two to four hours after ingestion. Lithium is distributed within the total body water, with slow passage across the blood/brain barrier. As lithium is primarily excreted by the kidney, adequate salt and fluid intake is essential in order to avoid accumulation and possible intoxication. The half-life of lithium in adults is 12–24 hours but may be much longer in neonates, due to immaturity of the kidneys.

Side effects of lithium

There have been consistent adverse effects reported, including:

- *gastrointestinal:* nausea, vomiting, diarrhoea, dry mouth, weight gain or loss;
- *neurological:* ataxia, tremor, weakness, muscle hyperirritability, facial muscle twitching, clonic movements, slurred speech, blurring of vision, headaches, seizures, psychomotor retardation, restlessness, stupor, coma, acute dystonia, EEG changes;
- *cardiovascular:* hypotension, dysrhythmias, oedema, electrolyte imbalance;
- *genitourinary:* glycosuria, polyuria, polydipsia, renal impairment;
- *dermatalogical:* dryness and thinning of hair, skin rash, leg ulcers;
- *haematological:* anaemia, leucocytosis;
- *endocrine:* thyroid imbalance.

Most drugs interact with lithium, including other drugs prescribed in mental illness.

The use of lithium in pregnancy, labour and the puerperium poses several problems:

- Lithium is teratogenic when administered during the first trimester. High resolution ultrasound scans and echocardiography (at 16–18 weeks) are needed to detect thyroid, renal and cardiac abnormalities, particularly defects in the tricuspid valve, which may be repaired *in utero* (Cox & Nicholls, 1996). US pregnancy category D.
- The haemodilution of pregnancy increases the risk of mania.
- The rapid decrease in circulatory volume following delivery may cause lithium toxicity, including damage to the kidneys and central nervous system.
- When lithium is discontinued during pregnancy, it is usually restarted within 24 hours of delivery, to protect the mother during this vulnerable period (Silverstone & Romans, 1996).
- The neonate is vulnerable to the side effects listed above. One infant exposed to lithium via breast milk was so hypoxic he became cyanosed (Suri et al, 1998). Should fluid and electrolyte imbalance occur, lithium causes potentially irreversible neurotoxicity in the neonate, and breastfeeding is usually not advised.

Ideally, women of child-bearing age should rarely be prescribed lithium, or be gradually withdrawn from lithium therapy prior to conception. In the second and third trimesters, lithium may be considered in preference to the alternative drug, carbamazepine, which also poses serious risks (see Chapter 19, anti-convulsants) (Austin & Mitchell, 1998).

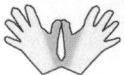 **Practice Points**

- Where there is no alternative drug, careful monitoring of mother, fetus and neonate is needed (Stewart et al, 1991).
- Monitoring should include serum lithium concentrations at least every month.

Implications for Practice: SSRIs in the puerperium

Potential Problem	Management
Agitation, anxiety, nervousness, insomnia, hypomania	Distinguish between side effects and 'normal' anxieties and sleep loss. Observe breastfed neonate for signs of irritability.
	Observe outstretched hands for a tremor before and during therapy.
	Advise regarding driving, in accordance with BNF guidelines.
Loss of libido	
Headache, migraine, tinnitus	Warn women to inform doctor if these side effects appear.
Gastro-intestinal disturbances	Warn women of potential nausea, gastro-intestinal upset, diarrhoea and constipation in themselves and breastfed babies.
Anorexia	Give firm advice regarding an adequate diet during pregnancy and lactation.
	Monitor weight of mother and neonates.
	Mouth care (risk of dry mouth).
	Inquire about taste disturbance.
Glucose disturbances (fluoxetine)	Monitor diabetics closely
Postural hypotension	Advise to stand slowly.
	Check sitting and standing BP.
Palpitations	Check heart rate.
Posture and movement disturbances (paroxetine)	Observe for motor signs of restlessness.
Menstrual irregularities	Advise that menstruation may be delayed.
Rash and pruritus; dyspnoea; bleeding and bruising	Warn women to inform doctor and discontinue SSRIs if any of these problems appear.
Convulsions	Vigilance in known epileptics.
	Concurrent ECT may be problematic.
Acne, herpes simplex, hair loss	Warn women to inform doctor if these side effects appear.
Rare side effects	Be prepared to take blood for liver function tests, amylase estimations and full blood counts if the patient develops abdominal pain and nausea or fever and sore throat.
Withdrawal reaction – headache, anxiety, sensory disturbance, fatigue	Discontinue medication gradually over several weeks, if possible.

Conclusion

The increasing importance of mental health in midwifery is illustrated by its inclusion in the *Report on Confidential Enquiries into Maternal Deaths* for the first time in 1998. During the last triennium, there were 29 maternal deaths recorded as attributable to psychiatric causes, exceeding the number due to hypertensive disorders (DoH, 1998). The management of women with enduring mental illness presents professionals with difficult choices: the prescriber is often aware that attempts to prescribe 'the lowest possible dose' may result in relapse of major psychotic illneess. Similarly, attempts to reduce doses two to three weeks before birth to minimize neonatal withdrawal symptoms may leave the woman vulnerable to recurrence of mental illness post-partum, unless very prompt action is taken to adjust medication on delivery.

Other issues are raised by women with less serious mental health problems, often in adverse social circumstances, where counselling, psychotherapy and social support may be more appropriate. Such women would benefit from a thorough post-partum examination, including thyroid function tests and a recognized screening instrument, such as the Edinburgh Post-natal Depression Scale (Cox et al, 1987). For a discussion see Chetley (1995), Medawar (1997).

Further research is needed to explore any connections between the medications administered in labour, such as ergometrine and corticosteroids, and post-partum illness.

Further Reading

Julien, R. (1998) *A Primer for Drug Action* 8th edition, New York. Freeman. (Discusses drugs relevant to mental health.)

Yoshida, K., Smith, B. & Kumar, R. (1999) Psychotropic drugs in mothers' milk: a comprehensive review of assay methods, pharmacokinetics and of safety of breast feeding, *Journal of Psychopharmacology* 13:1:64–80.

CHAPTER 17

Diabetes Mellitus and Pregnancy

SUE JORDAN

This chapter outlines the management of diabetes in pregnancy

---

Chapter Contents

- Diabetes
- Insulin needs in pregnancy
- Insulin
- Labour and diabetes
- Breastfeeding and diabetes
- Conclusion

Diabetes

Diabetes mellitus is a chronic metabolic disorder, arising from insulin deficiency or insulin resistance. Type I (juvenile onset) diabetes is characterized by an absolute deficiency of insulin, due to lack of beta cells in the islets of Langerhans; treatment is replacement therapy. Type II (maturity onset) diabetes is associated with varying degrees of insulin deficiency and insulin resistance; treatment may be by dietary control, oral hypoglycaemic drugs or insulin. To gain adequate control over blood sugar, all pregnant diabetic women receive insulin therapy.

Gestational diabetes arises when the woman's insulin reserves are insufficient to meet the extra demands of pregnancy. Fifty per cent of affected women develop type II diabetes in later life. Although the woman may be asymptomatic, it is important to detect gestational diabetes, otherwise fetal macrosomia and neonatal hypoglycaemia may not be recognized and managed appropriately. The risk of congenital anomalies is directly linked to the degree of hyperglycaemia at diagnosis (Schaefer-Graf et al, 2000). Undetected gestational diabetes is also associated with increased incidence of pre-eclampsia. Some authorities argue that all pregnant women should be screened for gestational diabetes by fasting plasma glucose estimations and/or glucose tolerance testing (Soares et al, 1997; Jarrett, 1997; Perucchini et al, 1999; Van Way, 1999; Dornhorst & Frost, 2000). However, the benefits of intensive investigation in women with borderline gestational diabetes (fasting plasma glucose 4.8–7.8 mmol/l) require further investigation (Bancroft et al, 2000).

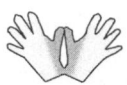 **Practice Points**

- Urine glucose measurements are not reliable, particularly in pregnancy.
- Diabetes mellitus is diagnosed by blood glucose estimations. If fasting plasma glucose is above 4.8 mmol/l (see above), the woman should be referred for further investigations, and/or repeat measurements (Griffith et al, 1996).
- A 'mini glucose tolerance test' may be arranged. This involves the woman drinking 50 g of glucose as Lucozade®, followed by a blood glucose measurement one hour later. If this value is >7.7 mmol/l, a full glucose tolerance test will be arranged (Campbell & Lees, 2000).
- Women with gestational diabetes should be retested for diabetes six weeks post-partum (Griffith et al, 1996).

Control of blood glucose

As the body alternates between the feeding and fasting states, insulin and glucagon are the main hormones keeping plasma glucose concentrations within normal limits. Insulin controls the storage and metabolism of ingested food and conserves the body's energy supplies. Without sufficient insulin, the metabolic pathways are unable to cope with glucose. Directly or indirectly, insulin affects the functioning of every tissue in the body. However, other hormones regulate plasma glucose concentrations, particularly during stress.

Stress causes an increase in blood glucose, due to the release of glucagon, cortisol, growth hormone and adrenaline (epinephrine). Therfore, stressors (such as infection, labour, illness, wounds, trauma or surgery) result in hyperglycaemia.

In hypoglycaemia, adrenaline (epinephrine) is rapidly released. This brings about the classic symptoms of hypoglycaemia: sweating, nausea and night-mares which, together, give 'hypoglycaemic awareness'. However, some diabetics lose hypoglycaemic awareness, and do not experience any symptoms when blood glucose falls. If these patients become hypoglycaemic, they develop, without warning, serious problems, including confusion, abnormal behaviour, convulsions and coma. Because of these dangers, once 'hypoglycaemic awareness' has been lost, the woman cannot receive intensive insulin therapy.

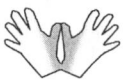 **Practice Points**

- Health care professionals should discuss loss of hypoglycaemic awareness with all diabetics and ensure that the family can manage hypoglycaemia (see pp. 372–3).
- Particular vigilance regarding the signs and symptoms of hypoglycaemia are needed at times when hypoglycaemia is very likely to occur: early pregnancy; changing from animal (porcine or bovine) to human insulin (BNF, 2000).

Insulin needs in pregnancy

The perinatal mortality rates and the incidence of major congenital malformations are 2–15 times greater than for non-diabetics, depending on whether care is received in a local hospital or a specialist setting (Vaughan, 1995; Casson et al, 1997). The higher the plasma glucose concentration at the first measurement in pregnancy, the worse the fetal outcome (Schaefer-Graf et al, 2000). In one series, 26 per cent of pregnancies had an adverse outcome (n = 113) (Hawthorne et al, 1997). These figures represent a considerable improvement in the management of diabetic pregnancy over the last 20 years. Much of the improvement is due to close glycaemic control *prior to conception* and throughout pregnancy.

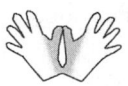 **Practice Points**

- Control is achieved by regular monitoring of blood glucose (four to eight times per day, before and after meals), strict attention to diet and dose titration. Computerized monitoring should also be considered (Parker, 1996).
- Early referral to diabetologist and obstetrician is essential.
- Ideally, the glycosated haemoglobin A_1 should be within the normal adult range prior to conception (Vaughan, 1995).

The complications of diabetes are listed in Box 17.1.

Box 17.1   Complications of diabetes

Hyperglycaemia

1. Hyperglycaemia is not easily recognized without regular measurements of blood glucose. Diabetics and their families should be alert for signs and symptoms, such as inability to 'cope', fatigue, failing memory, mood changes and blurred vision. Even moderate hyperglycaemia in pregnancy can jeopardize the outcome.

2. In hyperglycaemia, glucose adheres to various proteins, disrupting them to different degrees. Haemoglobin becomes glycosylated; this is measured as HbA_{1C}. This measure is a reflection of the glycaemic control over the preceding 8–12 weeks, and predicts the risk of fetal malformations, particularly cardiac malformations (Vaughan, 1995). Neural tube defects are more common, therefore folate supplements are prescribed pre-pregnancy and screening is undertaken.

3. Hyperglycaemia affects fetal growth, typically resulting in macrosomia. This, and the increased risk of shoulder dystocia, increases the rate of Caesarean section – to over 60 per cent in one series (Hawthorne et al, 1997). Fetal polycythaemia may cause neonatal jaundice when red cells are haemolysed at birth.

4. Hyperglycaemia damages tissues, for example lens of eye, nerves. Nerve damage may cause gastric paresis and hyperemesis.

5. Microvascular damage occurs, affecting the retina and the kidney. Damage to the kidney causes micro-albuminuria and hypertension, both of which should be monitored regularly. For women with elevated serum creatinine concentrations ($>180\,\mu mol/l$), the prognosis is poor, in terms of pregnancy outcome, renal function, life expectancy and eyesight. Retinopathy may arise or progress rapidly during pregnancy, therefore regular examinations must be undertaken (preferably by photograph) so that treatment can be initiated promptly. Sudden development or progression of retinopathy has been linked to rapidly improved glycaemic control (Pearson, 1993).

6. White blood cells become coated with glucose, making them less able to combat infection and promote healing. Infections, such as UTI, are a common complication of diabetes, which may explain the increased risk of miscarriage. Prophylactic antibiotics may be administered after Caesarean section (Gillmer, 1996).

Disordered fat metabolism

1. Atheroma is accelerated in diabetics, increasing the risks of cardiovascular, cerebrovascular and peripheral vascular disease at all ages. Lipid profile should be monitored.

Box 17.1 (*continued*)

2. Blood supply to the extremities is impaired by both atheroma and microvascular damage. Placental insufficiency, polyhydramnios and pre-eclampsia occur more frequently.

Ketoacidosis*

Ketoacidosis in pregnancy is an obstetric emergency, with fetal mortality around 50 per cent and maternal mortality around 5 per cent (Griffith et al, 1996). Pregnancy increases the risks of ketoacidosis. Vomiting may provoke ketosis. If vomiting cannot be prevented, admission to hospital and intensive care is urgently needed (Steel and Johnstone, 1996). The onset of impaired consciousness and confusion is usually gradual. Fetal death from acidosis may occur before the mother is seriously ill. Polyuria and vomiting lead to depletion of circulating fluids and electrolytes, and eventually circulatory collapse.

* *The first ketone produced in ketosis (beta-hydroxybutyric acid) is not detected by standard Ketostix. Therefore, ketosis can occur and not be detected.*

Risks of hypoglycaemia

The fetus is dependent upon glucose not only as an energy source but also for the synthesis of lipids. This extra demand increases the mother's dietary needs by around 2–300 kcals per day (more in thin women). The drain on plasma glucose may lead to hunger in non-diabetic women and to hypoglycaemia in diabetic women. During the first trimester, fasting plasma glucose concentrations fall by about 12 per cent, partly due to haemodilution; this sometimes reduces insulin requirements (Gillmer, 1996). Hypoglycaemia during the critical period of organ development (days 18–55) may give rise to malformations (Campbell & Lees, 2000).

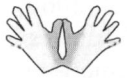 **Practice Point**

Pregnant diabetics should be advised against missing meals and being alone at night, when blood sugar is lowest (Steel & Johnstone, 1996).

Risks of hyperglycaemia

In pregnancy, the increased secretion of oestrogens, progesterone, prolactin and human placental lactogen shifts the metabolic pathways to promote the catabolism of fats, rather than glucose. The balance of the metabolic pathways is adjusted during normal pregnancy to promote the deposition of fat stores (3–4 kg) for lactation and to ensure that the fetus receives an adequate supply of glucose as demands rise during the third trimester. From about 24 weeks, maternal tissues develop a resistance to insulin, which inhibits the uptake of glucose from the plasma. As the concentration of glucose in the plasma rises, this helps the fetus absorb glucose. In those with a genetic predisposition to diabetes, the pancreas is unable to meet the increased demands imposed by a raised blood glucose, and gestational diabetes results.

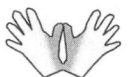 **Practice Point**

In diabetics, this demand for extra insulin must be met by increasing dosages, usually in increments of two units, eventually doubling or tripling the pre-pregnancy dose. Most of the extra insulin will be taken during the day (Steel & Johnstone, 1996). Obesity is likely to further increase insulin requirements.

Normal fetuses do not produce insulin. If maternal glucose concentrations rise, the excess glucose is transferred across the placenta to the fetus. Hyperglycaemia stimulates the fetal pancreas to produce insulin, causing:

- macrosomia, increased risk of shoulder dystocia and brachial plexus injury;
- congential malformations (cardiac and neural tube defects);
- delayed production of surfactant and increased risk of respiratory distress syndrome;
- neonatal hypoglycaemia;
- polycythaemia, leading to excess bilirubin in the neonate.

In all types of diabetes, maternal hyperglycaemia increases the incidence of congenital anomalies affecting all organ systems (Schaefer-Graf et al, 2000).

In contrast, women in whom the predominant complication of diabetes is microvascular disease (**retinal and renal disease**, see Box 17.1), demonstrate placental insufficiency and poor fetal growth rather than macrosomia. In these women, insulin needs in the third trimester are not markedly increased (Pearson, 1993).

Management of diabetes in pregnancy
(see Implications for Practice)

Ideally, this should start with preconception care. Good metabolic control maintaining normoglycaemia (4–6 mmol/l) over 24 hours is essential. In diabetics, poor glycaemic control has been associated with progression of maternal retinopathy (Lauszus et al, 2000). However if control is too strict, hypoglycaemia may prove harmful (Walkinshaw, 2000). Regular monitoring must be undertaken to adjust for the increased insulin requirements in pregnancy and after delievery. It is suggested that to achieve this level of control (4–6 mmol/l) without inducing hypoglycaemic attacks requires daily contact with health care professionals specializing in diabetes (Simmons, 1997). Others recommend that the woman should be seen at least every fortnight with additional telephone contacts, and weekly from 34 weeks (Vaughan, 1995).

Diet

All diabetics should obtain calories from high fibre carbohydrates such as rice and pasta, and restrict intake of refined sugars, including sweets, chocolates and soft drinks. At least 30–35 kcal/kg non-pregnant ideal body weight should be eaten to prevent ketosis. To keep glucose below 6 mmol/l, adherence to this diet should be very rigorous in pregnancy. Alcohol is contraindicated in all pregnancies but especially in diabetics.

It is advisable to ensure adequate intake of calcium and vitamin D, as the concentrations of these are lower in pregnant women with diabetes, and their infants (see p. 371) (Kuoppala, 1988).

Insulin

Insulin is only produced by the beta cells of the Islets of Langerhans of the pancreas. It is secreted into the hepatic portal vein, and therefore acts directly on the liver. This effect is not achieved when insulin is injected into peripheral sites. In health, about 50 per cent of the body's insulin is secreted at a basal rate, and the remainder in response to meals. It is not always possible to achieve this pattern by insulin injections.

A variety of insulin regimens are in current use. Doses are individually titrated to achieve normal blood glucose concentrations (normoglycaemia). Doses range from 0.2 units/kg per day in the very fit to 2.0 units/kg per day in the obese (Davis & Granner, 1996). Unfortunately, the therapeutic range for insulin is narrow: diabetics must steer between disabling hypoglycaemic episodes and hyperglycaemia causing long term complications. See Box 17.1.

Actions of insulin

Insulin acts on carbohydrates, fats and proteins to fundamentally alter the directions of the metabolic pathways so that sugars, fats and amino acids are stored and not burnt off. Without insulin, fats, sugars and amino acids cannot enter the cells, and therefore remain in the plasma. Consequently, the cells starve, and the plasma concentrations of glucose, cholesterol and fats rise. Some nutrients are subsequently lost via the urine. See Box 17.2.

Box 17.2   Actions of insulin

1. **Uptake of glucose by cells** – excluding brain, red blood cells, intestinal mucosa, renal tubules and placenta. Under the influence of insulin, the cells use glucose as a fuel, instead of fats or proteins. The main side effect of insulin is **hypoglycaemia**. During exercise, there is another mechanism whereby glucose is taken into exercising muscle, independent of insulin. Therefore, exercise is particularly important to diabetics, as it reduces insulin requirements.
2. **Increased synthesis** of glycogen from glucose in liver and muscle.
3. By removing glucose from the extra-cellular fluid, insulin reduces **infections**, such as thrush, and promotes wound healing. Gestational diabetes has been associated with an increased risk of wound infection following Caesarean section (Chaim et al, 2000).
4. It is said that diabetes is primarily a deficiency of **fat metabolism**. Insulin:
    ● promotes the formation of fatty acids in the liver and fat deposits in adipose tissue
    ● inhibits the breakdown of fat
    ● maintains low concentrations of free fatty acids, cholesterol and triglycerides in the plasma.
    Therefore, diabetics are at higher risk of thrombo-embolic events in childbirth and cardiovascular events after age 30.
5. Insulin is important in **preserving the protein** of the body. It has anabolic actions, essential for growth. Unlike the fetus of a non-diabetic woman, the fetus of a diabetic woman produces insulin, promoting growth. Pregnancy in diabetic women is associated with macrosomia, increasing the rate of Caesarean sections.
6. Insulin causes **potassium** ions to enter the cells. It is therefore important to monitor potassium ion concentration during insulin infusions. Glycosuria leads to loss of potassium and magnesium in the urine, possibly in association with diabetic nephropathy.

Calcium balance

In some diabetic women, mainly those who are poorly controlled, calcium metabolism becomes unstable. Together with low concentrations of magnesium, due to urine losses, this may suppress parathyroid function in neonates (Mehta et al, 1998). Parathyroid imbalance may be responsible for the low calcium and magnesium concentrations seen in neonates of diabetic mothers, 24–72 hours after delivery which can lead to tetany and convulsions (Tsang et al, 1975).

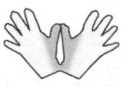 **Practice Points**

Neonates should be monitored for calcium and magnesium deficiencies, and excess bilirubin in addition to hypoglycaemia (Campbell & Lees, 2000).

Calcium gluconate

If necessary, calcium gluconate is administered *slowly*, to counter hypocalcaemia or magnesium toxicity. Reported hazards include: skin sloughing, bradycardia and even asystole (Mehta et al, 1998). Careful monitoring is essential.

Insulin regimens

Most pregnant diabetics receive human insulin. The three traditional types of insulin available are: short, intermediate and long acting (Table 17.3). The newly introduced insulin lispro and insulin aspart act more rapidly and transiently than short acting insulin. These preparations allow women to inject themselves shortly before eating, rather than 30 minutes prior to the meal (Rang et al, 1999). Most diabetics are prescribed a combination of insulins, in an attempt to replicate the physiological pattern of insulin secretion. Pen injectors allow soluble insulin to be administered 30 minutes before each of the three main meals plus a separate injection of intermediate insulin before bedtime; combined with frequent monitoring, this regimen is suitable in pregnancy (Nachum et al, 1999).

In pregnancy, the need for short acting insulin usually increases. The balance between short and intermediate acting insulins may need to be adjusted, making premixed formulations unsuitable.

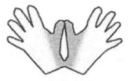 **Practice Points**

- An extra dose of short acting insulin may be introduced as a separate injection at lunch time, allowing the early morning intermediate insulin to be discontinued.
- After 36 weeks, blood glucose tends to fall, and the evening dose of intermediate insulin may be discontinued or reduced. A sudden fall in insulin requirements may indicate serious placental insufficiency.
- Some women with gestational diabetes may need only one injection of intermediate acting insulin per day, as they have sufficient endogenous hormone to maintain normoglycaemia overnight (Vaughan, 1995).

The 'dawn phenomenon' is morning hyperglycaemia; it occurs in most people, but may cause problems in diabetics. The timing of the evening insulin dose may need adjusting. The dawn phenomenon must be distinguished from the Somogyi effect, which is nocturnal hypoglycaemia, followed by rebound morning hyperglycaemia. This is treated by increasing the carbohydrate intake at supper time or reducing the insulin dose.

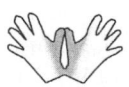 **Practice Point**

Pregnant diabetics should eat at least 25 g of carbohydrate at supper. Blood glucose measurements at 3 am are suggested to aid diagnosis of the cause of morning hypoglycaemia (Foster, 1991).

Side effects of insulin

Hypoglycaemia

The most important side effect of insulin is hypoglycaemia. Hypoglycaemic attacks are dangerous, and if repeated can lead to cerebral damage to the woman or neonate. The onset of hypoglycaemia may be abrupt. It is important that diabetics and their families recognize the prodromal signs and symptoms of hypoglycaemia (see Table 17.1). Hypoglycaemia causes a loss of consciousness, which may occur suddenly. It is therefore a particular hazard for drivers, who should check blood glucose concentrations before driving and every two hours, and have a supply of sugar available at all times (BNF, 2000).

Table 17.1 Signs and symptoms of hypoglycaemia

- *Accidents (cuts, falls or road traffic accidents)*
- Mood Changes
- Sleep Disturbances, Nightmares
- Night Sweats, Morning Headaches
- Nausea, Sweating
- Hunger *in the young*

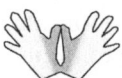 **Practice Points**

- If the patient is conscious, hypoglycaemia should be managed by oral administration of 10–20 g of glucose as 2–4 teaspoons of sugar, 2–400 ml of milk or 50–100 ml of Lucozade ®, repeated in ten minutes if necessary. An unconscious patient should receive either glucagon (see below) or intravenous glucose, for example 50 ml of 20 per cent glucose (BNF, 2000).
- Overstimulation of the fetal pancreas may cause persistent hypoglycaemia in the neonate, lasting 24–48 hours after delivery. Early instigation of glucose feeds and blood glucose monitoring (hourly for the first four hours) can control the situation. Breastfeeding is ideal.
- After delivery the infant is usually monitored in special care baby units for 24–48 hours (Campbell & Lees, 2000).
- In pregnancy, fluctuating glucose levels increase the risks of driving.
- The fetus is more tolerant of hypoglycaemia than hyperglycaemia.

Glucagon

This hormone is produced by the alpha cells of the Islets of Langerhans of the pancreas and by the gastro-intestinal tract. In health, glucagon is secreted between meals, as blood glucose concentrations begin to fall. Glucagon is rapidly released in response to hypoglycaemia; however, this mechanism fails in diabetes. Glucagon is sometimes administered to manage hypoglycaemia in diabetics. Glucagon (one unit) is given by injection (by any route) in hypo-glycaemic emergencies where intravenous glucose in impractical. However it will be ineffective in chronic hypoglycaemia or starvation. Glucagon may be prescribed on an 'as needed' basis.

Antibodies to insulin

The production of insulin antibodies is minimized (but not eliminated) by the use of human insulin. Antibodies delay and reduce the actions of insulin, necessitating higher doses. Some antibody formation occurs with porcine insulin, but changing to human insulin may cause problems with hypogly-caemic awareness (see above). Insulin antibodies may cross the placenta and damage the fetal pancreas; therefore human insulin is usually recommended in pregnancy.

Site reactions

Irritation at the injection site may be managed with anti-histamine creams. Both lipoatrophy and lipohypertrophy cause irregular absorption of insulin. Lipohypertrophy is fat deposition and storage due to overexposure to insulin. Lipoatrophy is rarer, and is an immune response.

Postural hypotension, which may result from diabetic autonomic neu-ropathy, is exacerbated by insulin.

Drug interactions with insulin

Drug interactions may raise or lower blood glucose. See Appendix 1.

- Diabetes complicates the management of **premature labour**. The admin-istration of β_2 agonists (such as ritodrine) is hazardous. The fetal lungs are particularly likely to be immature, but the administration of steroids dra-matically increases the woman's requirements for insulin. See Chapter 7.
- Nicotine reduces insulin absorption by causing vasoconstriction.
- Hypoglycaemic awareness is lost with beta blockers.

How the body handles insulin

Insulin has a short half-life of five minutes. It does not cross the placenta. Most diabetics administer their own insulin by subcutaneous injection. The amount of insulin absorbed depends upon the site and method of adminis-tration; (see Table 17.2) therefore a consistent pattern of rotation must be maintained.

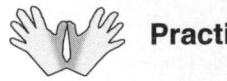 **Practice Point**

The abdomen is a good choice for the first injection of the day, because insulin is absorbed most rapidly from here unless the person exercises.

Table 17.2   Factors affecting insulin absorption
from subcutaneous injection

individual variation
amount of subcutaneous fat
site of administration (arm, abdomen, thigh)
blood supply which depends on:
   temperature of tissue
   massage
   exercise
depth of injection
tissue hypertrophy
volume of injection (slower from large volumes)
cloudy insulin ⎫
           ⎬ *avoid administering insulin in these conditions*
shaken insulin ⎭

Table 17.3   Types of insulins

Type of insulin	SOLUBLE	INTERMEDIATE	SLOW
Example	regular, soluble	isophane, lente insulin-zinc suspension	ultralente crystalline insulin-zinc suspension
ONSET of ACTION	30 mins	1–2 hrs	4–6 hrs
PEAK	2–4 hrs	6–12 hrs	16–18 hrs
DURATION	up to 8 hrs	18–24 hrs	20–36 hrs

The three traditional types of insulin are compared in Table 17.3.

Infusion pumps have been introduced into community care to improve glycaemic control in special situations, such as pregnancy. These have proved popular with some women, as they allow a more flexible lifestyle (Gabbe et al, 2000). Most devices deliver a continuous infusion of soluble insulin into the subcutaneous tissues of the abdomen, and bolus doses are administered at meal times which provides a more physiological replacement than repeated injections. The danger of nocturnal hypoglycaemia must be assessed, because a few deaths have occurred in the US (Foster, 1991). Technical problems can also occur, such as needle displacement, kinks in the tube, abscess formation and insulin reactions at the site. Pump failure can rapidly lead to ketoacidosis. To date, infusion pumps have not improved glycaemic control in pregnancy over regular pen injections (Steel & Johnstone, 1996).

Labour and diabetes

In the past, the problems posed by placental insufficiency, macrosomia, shoulder dystocia and pre-eclampsia have discouraged obstetricians from advising vaginal delivery. The woman should be in a position to make a fully informed decision on mode of delivery, as there is little evidence to support either elective delivery or expectant management at term (Boulvain et al, 2000).

Insulin needs fall rapidly with the onset of active labour and again on delivery of the placenta. Hence the demands for insulin and glucose change dramatically, necessitating two separate intravenous infusion lines. (Also, the infusions are incompatible.) Suggested regimens include a 10 per cent glucose infusion @ 1 litre every eight hours plus soluble insulin @ 1 unit per hour, adjusted in response to hourly bedside blood glucose measurements. This regimen may be started on the morning of a planned induction or section. Only short acting insulin is used in intravenous infusions.

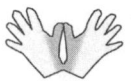 **Practice Points**

- The tendency for insulin to adhere to plastic tubing means that infusion is unpredictable and must be titrated against the patient's response.
- If oxytocin or opioids are used, there is a risk of fluid retention.

Effective analgesia is important, and epidural infusions are recommended (Steel & Johnstone, 1996). Continuous fetal heart rate monitoring is used routinely. Glucose infusion is continued until the next meal eaten without vomiting, as there is a danger of hypoglycaemia in the first 48–72 hours (Vaughan, 1995; Pangle, 2000).

Breastfeeding and diabetes

Breastfeeding reduces insulin requirements to below pre-pregnancy values and necessitates a high carbohydrate intake. Care should be taken to avoid hypoglycaemia when feeding at night. Although breastfeeding benefits the mother, careful glucose monitoring is required. The amount of insulin transferred to the neonate is considered too small to be harmful (BNF, 2000).

Implications for practice: diabetes in pregnancy

Potential Problem	Management
Congenital malformations and fetal loss	Maintain normoglycaemia 4–6 mmol/l from pre-conception. Pre-conception folate supplements. High resolution scans.

Implications for practice: (*continued*)

Potential Problem	Management
Hypoglycaemia	Rest and small meals. Minimize nausea.
	Do not miss meals. Avoid alcohol.
	Carry glucose and glucagon at all times. Instruct partner in administration.
	Measure 3.00 am blood glucose if nightmares or night sweats occur.
	Evaluate the risks of driving.
Vomiting	Reduce nausea. Replace carbohydrate. Immediate referral on vomiting.
Hyperglycaemia from 24 weeks	Monitor blood sugar. Be prepared to increase soluble insulin.
	Aim for weight gain as in normal pregnancy.
	Ensure client understands insulin regimen and injection administration techniques.
Vascular disease	Antenatal examination for cardiovascular disease, which could compromise labour. Risk of thromboembolism (Chapter 8).
Ketoacidosis and fetal loss	Regular monitoring, regular diet, avoid alcohol.
	Dosage adjustments. Consider introduction of pen injectors.
Diabetic retinopathy	Normoglycaemia, pre-conception and during pregnancy.
	Retinal examinations and treatment by specialists.
Diabetic nephropathy	Monitor urine for micoralbuminuria and albumin loss.
Increased risk of pre-eclampsia	Monitor BP very closely.
Placental failure	Deliver at or before 39 weeks. Fetal monitoring.
Potential Problem	**Management**
Macrosomia	Normoglycaemia during pregnancy. Establish definite date of conception.
Shoulder dystocia	Prepare for Caesarean section.
Fetal lung immaturity	Neonatal intensive care available.
Neonatal hypoglycaemia	Immediate feeds, preferably breastfeeding. Monitor blood glucose hourly for four hours, and four-hourly for 48 hours.
Neonatal hypocalcaemia or hypomagnesaemia	Monitor. Calcium and magnesium injections available.
Neonatal polycythaemia	Monitor. Exchange transfusion facilities available.
Infections	Urine testing, skin inspection, prophylactic antibiotics, good breastfeeding technique essential to prevent abscesses.

Conclusion

Although considerable progress has been made in specialist centres, women who are diabetic run a high risk of obstetric and medical complications. Successful outcome of pregnancy requires meticulous attention to diet, monitoring and insulin regimens, which in turn demand commitment from both multi-disciplinary teams and clients (see Implications for Practice).

Further Reading

Walkinshaw, S. (2000) Very tight versus tight control for diabetes in pregnancy. *Cochrane Database Systematic Review:* (issue 2) Oxford, Update Software. Accessed July 2000.

CHAPTER 18

Thyroid Disorders in Pregnancy

SUE JORDAN

This chapter discusses thyroid imbalance and its recognition in pregnancy. Other endocrine disorders are mentioned briefly.

Chapter Contents

- Thyroid hormones
- Thyroid function tests (TFTs) in pregnancy
- Hyperthyroidism
- Hypothyroidism
- Conclusion

After diabetes, thyroid disease is the commonest endocrine abnormality encountered in pregnancy. Like other endocrine disorders, thyroid imbalance may be a cause of infertility, but pregnancy can occur when thyroid imbalance has been corrected. Recognition of thyroid disorders in young women is not always easy, particularly when they arise *de novo* in pregnancy.

Thyroid hormones

The main function of the thyroid gland is to produce thyroid hormones (thyroxine (T_4) and tri-iodothyronine (T_3)). In the tissues, T_4 is converted to T_3. Most of the actions of the thyroid hormones are attributed to T_3. Thyroid disease disturbs the balance of thyroid hormone secretion, which upsets the regulation of:

- metabolic rate and heat production;
- the central and peripheral nervous systems;
- the sympathetic nervous system;

- heart rate and cardiac contractility;
- the absorption of glucose from the gastro-intestinal tract;
- reproduction and fertility;
- the development of the central nervous system;
- growth.

In health, the thyroid gland is controlled by thyroid stimulating hormone (TSH) from the anterior pituitary gland, which, in turn, is controlled by thyrotropin-releasing hormone (TRH) from the hypothalamus. The release of TSH and TRH is regulated in a negative feedback mechanism by circulating thyroid hormones (T_4 and T_3).

Fetal thyroid function is independent of the mother. However, iodine and anti-thyroid drugs cross the placenta. Therefore:

- maternal iodine deficiency causes neonatal cretinism;
- radioactive iodine (sometimes used to treat hyperthyroid conditions) destroys the fetal thyroid (Girling, 1996);
- large doses of iodine cause fetal goitre.

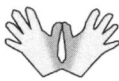 **Practice Point**

Handling or application of iodine-containing preparations such as povidone iodine while pregnant or breastfeeding may allow sufficient iodine to enter the circulation to cause fetal goitre.

Thyroid function tests (TFTs) in pregnancy

Thyroid function tests are undertaken when there is a family history of thyroid disorder or clinical suspicion of an abnormality. At present, it is not considered feasible to screen all pregnant women for thyroid disorders (Pop et al, 1999).

Thyroid hormones exist in two forms: free and bound to plasma proteins (mainly thyroid binding globulin). Only the free hormones are active (see Chapter 1). When interpreting thyroid function tests (TFTs) in pregnancy, it should be remembered that a goitre may be physiological and the concentrations of thyroid hormones are altered in normal pregnancy:

- the concentration of total thyroxine is raised;
- TSH is reduced;
- in the last trimester, the concentrations of the free hormones are reduced (Girling, 1996).

It is important that free thyroxine and tri-iodothyronine concentrations are measured. (Raised and lowered concentrations are indicative of hyper- and hypo-thyroidism respectively.) TFTs must be interpreted in relation to the normal values for pregnancy (see Box 18.1).

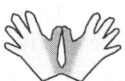 **Practice Points**

When blood is taken from a pregnant woman for TFTs:

- free hormone concentrations must be requested
- it must be clearly stated on the form that the patient is pregnant
- the dose and time of any thyroid related medications must be noted
- all medications taken must be noted, as several interfere with TFTs.

Box 18.1 Diagnostic tests for thyroid function

	Normal values*	
Test	**Nonpregnant**	**Pregnant**
Free serum thyroxine (T_4)	10–27 pmol/l	7–15 pmol/l (third trimester)
Total serum thyroxine (T_4)	64–142 nmol/l	64–256 nmol/l
Thyroid Stimulating Hormone (TSH)**	0.15–3.15 mU/l**	0.15–1.8 mU/l (first and second trimesters) 0.7–7.3 mU/l (third trimester)
Free serum tri-iodothyronine (T_3)	4–9 pmol/l.	3–5 pmol/l (third trimester)
Total serum tri-iodothyronine (T_3)	1.0–2.6 nmol/l	1.0–2.6 nmol/l
Thyroid antibody test	presence suggests Hashimoto's thyroiditis	

---

* exact values depend on the laboratory undertaking the tests
** in the first and second trimesters, the upper limit of the range for TSH is 1.8 mU/l, and in the third trimester the range is 0.7–7.3 mU/l

Hyperthyroidism

The commonest cause of hyperthyroidism is Graves' disease. Hyperthyroidism affects individuals in a variety of ways. The insidious onset of the disease may allow it to go unrecognized for years. The classic symptoms of heat intolerance, sweating, increased appetite, nervousness, insomnia, irritability and short temper can also be features of normal pregnancy: also the hands usually feel warm and the pulse is rapid and bounding. A tremor may be seen if the fingers are outstretched. Other common, and easily overlooked, features of hyperthyroidism include: fatigue, muscle weakness or cramps, over-active reflexes, increased frequency of bowel movements. Infrequent blinking and eyelid retraction give the classic 'staring' appearance of thyrotoxicosis.

The thyroid gland may be palpably enlarged but diagnosis of hyperthyroidism in pregnancy may be difficult, as a small goitre in pregnancy is normal, and is not usually a sign of Graves' disease.

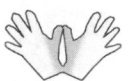 **Practice Point**

Hyperthyroidism should always be considered if hyperemesis occurs.

If the mother has Graves' disease, her autoantibodies cross the placenta. This may cause a goitre in the fetus and hyperthyroidism in the neonate. This is rare, but it is important that fetal growth and heart rate are monitored regularly by ultrasound. Fetal goitre may obstruct the airway or impede delivery. Untreated neonatal hyperthyroidism carries a poor prognosis. Therefore, the infants must be carefully monitored.

Management of hyperthyroidism in pregnancy

Like other autoimmune [glossary] diseases, hyperthyroidism may remit during pregnancy and rebound after delivery. Drug regimens must be monitored and adjusted accordingly. Hyperthyroidism in pregnancy is treated by antithyroid drugs alone, under specialist supervision. Antithyroid drugs cross the placenta, but thyroid hormones do not; therefore a blocking-replacement regimen would render the fetus hypothyroid. Propylthiouracil is sometimes preferred to carbimazole because placental transfer is less (Clark, 1995). The minimum effective dose is prescribed, often leaving a mild degree of maternal hyperthyroidism (Fitzgerald, 1995). Full TFTs must be taken at least monthly (Hague, 1995).

Antithyroid drugs may suppress fetal thyroid hormone production and stimulate TSH production, leading to fetal goitre and hypothyroidism. This is more likely with higher doses. In addition, carbimazole and methimazole are associated with aplasia cutis (BNF, 2000).

Although carbimazole is generally well tolerated by the mother, it has the potential to cause agranulocytosis [glossary], and patients are advised to inform their doctors should they develop any signs of infection, particularly a sore throat. If agranulocytosis is suspected, a venous blood sample should be taken for a white cell count (BNF, 2000). Carbimazole may also cause nausea, rashes and hair loss.

If hyperthyroidism cannot be controlled by drugs, surgery is carried out during the second trimester. However, ingestion of iodide in preparation for surgery may induce fetal goitre. Radioiodine is contra-indicated in pregnancy, breastfeeding and in children; four months should elapse between radioiodine treatment and pregnancy. Some endocrinologists prefer to avoid radioiodine in women under 40 (Conway & Betterbridge, 1996).

Uncontrolled or unrecognized hyperthyroidism may cause cardiac failure or even a thyroid storm.* This emergency carries a high mortality rate and is managed in intensive care units. High risk situations include stress, labour, infection, trauma or operative delivery.

* *Note:* A thyroid storm/crisis is a rare and dangerous medical emergency, where very high concentrations of circulating thyroid hormones cause hyper-pryrexia, delerium and extreme cardiovascular stress.

Breastfeeding

Both propylthiouracil and carbimazole appear in breast milk, and can cause thyroid enlargement and hypothyroidism in the infant. The transfer of pro-pylthiouracil to breast milk is considered to be too low to damage the infant. Breastfeeding may be permissible with low dose carbimazole. If possible, feeds should be given just before the mother takes the antithyroid drugs. The infant's development and thyroid function must be monitored (BNF, 2000), with the involvement of a paediatrician (Girling, 1996). Both iodine and tech-netium pass into breast milk and are concentrated in the thyroid gland of the infant. Therefore, women treated with radioactive isotopes of these elements are advised to discontinue breastfeeding.

Hypothyroidism

The symptoms of Hashimoto's thyroiditis often improve during pregnancy. However the increased TSH production can lead to enlargement of the pituitary gland. Pregnancies in women with untreated hypothyroidism are at increased risk of miscarriage and prematurity, but this may be due to the associated increased susceptibility to infection (Fitzgerald, 1995). Subnormal neonatal neurological development and low IQ in the infant are associated with untreated hypothyroidism in pregnancy (Hague, 1995). Pregnancy induced hypertension complicates 22–44 per cent of pregnancies in hypothyroid women (Montoro, 1997). Some features of hypothyroidism (weight gain, tiredness, lethargy, constipation, goitre, fluid retention, memory loss, joint pains) are easily confused with normal pregnancy; therefore TFTs are important in making a diagnosis. (In hypothyroidism, TSH is raised and free thyroid concentrations are reduced.)

Hypothyroidism is managed with thyroxine replacement therapy. If women are over-treated with thyroxine, the signs and symptoms of hyperthyroidism appear. Thyroxine does not cross the placenta. While some authors assert that most women who are euthyroid at conception do not require dose adjustment during pregnancy (Girling, 1996), others emphasize the importance of regular monitoring of thyroid function, and expect thyroxine requirements to rise during pregnancy (Monotoro, 1997). Neonatal encephalopathy, with permanent sequelae, may occur more frequently in hypothyroid women who do not receive regular monitoring during pergnancy (Badawi et al, 2000). A minimum of one full TFT each trimester is suggested (Hague, 1995).

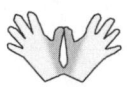 **Practice Point**

Women with hypothyroidism are unusually sensitive to opioids and may be rendered stuporous or even die if administered an average dose of opioids, for example 50 mg pethidine for pain relief in labour (Malseed et al, 1995).

Hypothyroidism is associated with post-partum depression, which may arise any time within the first year of birth (Campbell & Lees, 2000). Breastfeeding is not contra-indicated with replacement therapy.

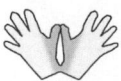 **Practice Points**

Thyroid function tests may be indicated in women with post-partum depression, as hypothyroidism is readily treatable.
Untreated hypothyroidism causes failure of lactation. If this is suspected, TFTs are essential.

Conclusion

If thyroid function is well controlled, the outcome of pregnancy is likely to be good. However poorly controlled thyroid disease may result in intrauterine growth retardation, premature labour, increased perinatal mortality or congenital abnormalities. It is important that health care professionals are aware of the Protean and often confusing manifestations of thyroid disorders, and instigate prompt measurement of thyroid function.

Post-partum thyroiditis

This occurs in up to 10 per cent of women, although the diagnosis is often unrecognized which causes much unnecessary distress. Post-partum thyroiditis is an autoimmune disorder, and many affected women develop thyroid disease later in life. The hyperthyroid phase of post-partum thyroiditis is usually self-limiting, but treatment of the hypothyroid phase (at four to eight months after delivery) may improve quality of life by relieving the symptoms of tiredness, lethargy and depression (Girling, 1996).

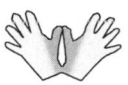 **Practice Point**

Hypothyroidism may cause psychosis and hallucinations, which can be mistaken for post-partum mental illness.

Other endocrine disorders

Pregnant women known to suffer from these relatively rare conditions, for example adrenal or parathyroid disorders, will be referred to tertiary centres. Diagnostic difficulties can arise if endocrine disorders present for the first time in pregnancy. For example, a raised blood pressure may be the only clue to an adrenal tumour. Disorders of the parathyroid glands and calcium metabolism are particularly threatening to the fetus. For further discussion, readers are referred to Hague (1995).

Further Reading

Jordan, S. & White, J. (1998) Systems and disease: hyperthyroidism. *Nursing Times*:94:24:48–51.

White, J. & Jordan, S. (1998) Systems and disease: hypothyroidism explained in words and pictures. *Nursing Times*:94:29:50–3.

CHAPTER 19

Epilepsy in Pregnancy

NICK CLERK AND SIMON EMERY

This chapter considers the difficult question of epilepsy in pregnancy. The reader will find that knowledge of the central nervous system and the normal physiological changes of pregnancy facilitates understanding of this chapter.

Chapter Contents

- Epilepsy
- Effect of pregnancy on epilepsy
- Effect of epilepsy on pregnancy
- Drugs used in epilepsy
- Management of epilepsy in pregnancy
- Conclusion

One in 200 women of childbearing age will suffer from epilepsy, making it one of the most common medical disorders encountered by maternity health workers (Donaldson, 1995). Pregnancy may influence the course of epilepsy by altering the seizure frequency. Epilepsy and its treatment with anti-epileptic drugs (anticonvulsants) can also affect the course and outcome of pregnancy.

Epilepsy

Epilepsy is a chronic disorder characterized by a recurrence of seizures that are often unprovoked and unpredictable (Pedley et al, 1995). An epileptic seizure* or fit is the result of a temporary physiologic dysfunction of the brain, caused by an abnormal electrical discharge of brain cells. There are different kinds of seizures. Each type is associated with a characteristic behavioural change and electrophysiological disturbance, usually detected by electroencephalography.

* *Note: A seizure is a transient event occurring in acute medical or neurologic illness. People who suffer a single unprovoked seizure will not usually receive extensive investigation and treatment.*

Epilepsy can be broadly be classified into three groups.

1 Partial (focal) seizures. These seizures originate from one part of the brain and may spread to become generalized seizures. These may or may not be associated with loss of consciousness.
2 Generalized seizures. These seizures involve the brain diffusely at onset. There is usually impaired consciousness and involuntary muscular activity.
3 Unclassified seizures. These do not fall into the two groups described above and include neonatal seizures and febrile convulsions (Commission, 1989).

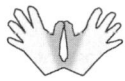 **Practice Point**

When an epileptic fit occurs for the first time in the latter half of pregnancy, eclampsia has to be excluded as a cause.

Effect of pregnancy on epilepsy

Epilepsy raises several clinical concerns in women. These include: menstrual cycle effects on seizure activity; antiepileptic-contraceptive interactions; antiepileptics' side effects, including teratogenesis; impact on breastfeeding and quality of life. In pregnancy, several factors may operate to increase seizure frequency either directly or by altering the serum antiepileptic concentrations. These include: altered hormone levels; physiological changes of pregnancy; sleep deprivation; women's reluctance to take drugs in pregnancy; nausea and vomiting in pregnancy (Swartjes et al, 1998; Malone and D'Alton, 1997).

In pregnancy, the rise in blood concentrations of oestrogens and progesterone can alter the brain threshold for seizures. Oestrogens are thought to decrease seizure threshold, whereas progesterone decreases neuronal excitability (Morrell, 1992). Changes in serum electrolyte levels can affect seizure frequency; the decreased sodium and magnesium concentrations found in pregnancy can predispose to seizures (Klingman, 1954).

Plasma concentrations of antiepileptics are reduced by:

- Expansion of the maternal extracellular fluid volume as well as the development of an 'extra' fetal compartment.
- Reduced intestinal absorption, due to:
  - reduced intestinal motility, which occurs in pregnancy (Chapter 13);
  - the chelating (binding) effects of substances commonly ingested in pregnancy such as iron and calcium supplements.
- Increased elimination of antiepileptics which can result from a combination of decreased plasma protein binding and increased renal excretion of antiepileptics. (The glomerular filtration rate is increased, see Chapter 1 and glossary.)
- Increased antiepileptic metabolism by maternal and fetal hepatic (liver) enzymes [glossary] and the placenta (Lander et al, 1977)

These effects combine to increase seizure frequency in pregnancy in some 25 per cent of women.

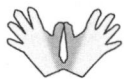 **Practice Points**

- Midwives should explain to women that they are likely to require an increased dose of antiepileptic drugs during pregnancy and for six to eight weeks afterwards.
- These changes in plasma concentrations can be monitored by venous blood samples (Schwartz, 1998).
- 'Midwives should check with relatives that they know what to do in the case of a fit and should provide instruction, particularly on the need to place the patient in the recovery position once the fit is over. Pregnant women who are at risk of fits should be advised not to bathe alone' (DoH, 1998: 116). Ignorance of such simple procedures may have contributed to two of the deaths reported in the latest *Confidential Enquiries*.

There is some evidence that the effect of pregnancy on seizure frequency can be predicted from the degree of pre-pregnancy control: women with long pre-pregnancy seizure-free periods are less likely to convulse in pregnancy. (Donaldson, 1995)

Effect of epilepsy on pregnancy

Although several obstetric complications have been reported to occur more frequently in women with epilepsy, there is little statistical evidence to support these observations. Reports suggest a two- to threefold increased incidence of vaginal haemorrhage, placental abruption, pre-eclampsia and breech presentation. Several authors have reported an increased rate of obstetric intervention during the delivery of women with epilepsy (Swartjes et al, 1998).

Generalized seizures are potentially dangerous for mother and fetus. Tonic-clonic seizures can cause fetal hypoxia and acidosis and cardiotocographic changes have been described (Paul et al, 1978). Seizures in early pregnancy may cause hypoxic damage to the embryo and result in malformations. Cognitive defects in infants may be linked to the number of seizures in pregnancy (Byrne et al, 2001).

Epilepsy and pregnancy outcome

Pregnancy outcome in women with epilepsy has been reported to be worse than in the general population. There is always the danger of trauma to mother and fetus with any seizures as well as an increased incidence of pre-term delivery, intrauterine growth restriction, asphyxia and perinatal mortality (Frederick, 1973). Status epilepticus [glossary] is one of the most serious complications of epilepsy in pregnancy.

Seizures, including status epilepticus, may result from abrupt discontinuation of antiepileptics. Incomplete compliance with antiepileptic drugs was reported in 62 per cent of pregnant women (Fairgrieve et al, 2000).

Case Report

Appropriate counselling can be life-saving:

> A woman whose epilepsy was controlled by sodium valproate had had a previous pregnancy terminated after a neural tube defect was diagnosed and attributed to the drug. It would appear that she abruptly discontinued therapy when she discovered that she was pregnant. This precipitated uncontrollable fits (DoH, 1998: 130).

This patient should have been clearly warned of the dangers of non-compliance and abrupt discontinuation of medication. It is always advisable to document such warnings in the patients' notes.

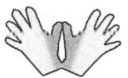 **Practice Point**

Women should be advised that seizures are far more likely to damage the fetus than are antiepileptics (in most cases).

Epilepsy and fetal malformations

Children of epileptic women are more frequently affected by congenital malformations. The incidence of fetal abnormalities in the general population is less than 3 per cent. There is a small (doubled) increased risk in offspring of epileptic mothers, only some of which is attributable to antiepileptics (Fairgrieve et al, 2000). The risk rises further with the number of antiepileptics taken (O'Brien and Gilmour-White, 1993). Several abnormalities have been described in relation to antiepileptic exposure, mainly cleft palate, glue ear, laryngeal problems, joint laxity, refractive error, squint, cardiac malformations and neural tube defects. *In utero* exposure to antiepileptic drugs can give rise to chararteristic facial features. Affected children are likely to experience developmental and speech delay and behavioural problems, including autism (Moore et al, 2000).

Causes of malformations

Although antiepileptics have been extensively studied, the mechanisms of teratogenesis are not clear (Lee and McManus, 1995). Genetic factors, both fetal and parental, probably play a part, as evidenced by the high rate of recurrence of malformations in sibships (Moore et al, 2000).

One proposed mechanism of teratogenesis is folic acid deficiency. Folic acid is a cofactor in the synthesis of DNA and cell division. Antiepileptics decrease serum folate levels by decreasing absorption and accelerating hepatic metabolism. Low serum folate levels have been correlated with increased malformation rates, most specifically neural tube defects. Up to 90 per cent of women receiving phenytoin, carbamazepine or barbiturates have reduced serum folate concentrations. Folate supplementation in these women can reduce the incidence of neural tube defects by up to 60 per cent (Mulinare, 1988), but as few as 11 per cent are taking folate supplementation appropriately (Fairgrieve et al, 2000).

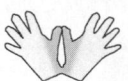 **Practice Points**

- Women prescribed the established antiepileptics should consult specialists, as they may require folate supplementation at the higher dose, 5 mg (the usual dose is 400 micrograms) preferably pre-conception (BNF, 2000).
- It is important that this is commenced under medical supervision, because folic acid can induce convulsions.

However, some authors question the role of folic acid deficiency in neural tube defects associated with antiepileptics (see Byrne, 2001). Another possible mechanism involves the formation of unstable oxides, with known mutagenic properties, during the metabolism of antiepileptics. There may be a limitation in the ability of some fetuses to detoxify these oxides, resulting in abnormalities. Tests on fetal cells obtained by amniocentesis may determine the susceptibility of the fetus to toxic metabolites (Byrne, 2001).

The formation of free radicals [glossary] during the metabolism of antiepileptics has also been proposed as a cause of malformations. These free radicals can be teratogenic and a genetic defect in the pathways responsible for their metabolism can contribute to fetal malformations. It would therefore seem advisable to increase the dietary intake of vitamin C as fresh fruit and vegetables. There is some evidence to suggest low socioeconomic class in epileptic mothers increases the risk of teratogenesis, possibly via malnutrition (Malone and D'Alton, 1997, Blume, 1997).

Management of epilepsy

Therapy of epilepsy generally has three goals (Pedley et al, 1995):

1 To eliminate seizures or reduce their frequency to the maximum extent possible;
2 To avoid the side effects associated with long term therapy;
3 To assist the woman achieve normal psychosocial and vocational adjustment.

In women of reproductive age, therapy should aim to reduce the risk to the developing fetus by appropriate dosage and nutritional supplements. Antiepileptics should be prescribed when the benefits of treatment outweigh the risks of uncontrolled seizures. The ideal antiepileptic would suppress seizures without causing any untoward effects. Drugs in current use cure or reduce seizures in about 75 per cent of women but frequently cause side effects. The degree of success depends on several factors such as seizure type, family history, neurological abnormalities, patient compliance and drug pharmacokinetic [glossary] properties, which are notably altered in pregnancy (McNamara, 1996)

Drugs used in epilepsy

Almost all epileptic women seen in midwifery will be prescribed antiepileptics. In general, therapy with a single drug (monotherapy) carries less risk than multiple drug therapy (polytherapy), as all antiepileptics are potentially teratogenic.

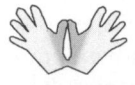 **Practice Point**

To reduce the risk of teratogenicity further in monotherapy, where possible, antiepileptics must be given in slow release preparations or divided doses to avoid drug concentration peaks in maternal plasma.

Two broad groups of antiepileptic drugs will be described: the older, well tried 'first generation' drugs and the newer but less tried 'second generation' drugs.

Mode of action of antiepileptic drugs

There are three main mechanisms by which antiepileptics exert their effects.

- One is to limit the sustained repetitive firing of neurones, an effect mediated by altering the axon membrane channels for the transport of ions such as sodium (carbamazepine, phenytoin, valproate and lamotrigine).
- The second mechanism appears to involve enhancing gamma-aminobutyric acid (GABA) mediated synaptic inhibition [glossary]. This may be achieved by modifying chloride ion transport channels at synaptic junctions [glossary] raising the seizure threshold (benzodiazepines, barbiturates and valproate). Newer antiepileptics appear to act directly at presynaptic junctions to increase GABA released at nerve endings (gabapentin). Other drugs effectively increase the amount of GABA at synapses by inhibiting the enzyme responsible for the breakdown of GABA (vigabatrin).
- Antiabsence antiepileptics appear to utilize a different mechanism (ethosuximide and valproate). They act on calcium ion channels to inhibit neuronal transmission in the thalamus*, which plays an important role in the generation of electrical waves characteristic of absence seizures (McNamara, 1996)

* *Note: The thalamus is the region of the brain just above the mid-brain.*

First generation antiepileptic drugs

With the exception of phenobarbitone, plasma concentrations are useful in monitoring therapy. Patients on phenobarbitone develop tolerance. All these antiepileptics are metabolized in the liver and the kidneys excrete the more soluble conjugated forms [glossary].

Summary of antiepileptics

A detailed consideration of each of the commonly prescribed antiepileptics is outside the scope of this book, but relevant information, not all of which is readily available elsewhere, is summarized below.

Carbamazepine (Tegretol®)

This is the drug of choice for partial seizures, secondary generalized seizures and trigeminal neuralgia. It is used in the treatment of bipolar affective disorders as an alternative to lithium.

Side effects Some of the unpleasant side effects of carbamazepine may subside within the first few weeks of use. Other side effects, such as acne and hirsuitism, may affect the woman's body image, a problem which may be intensified in pregnancy and the puerperium. The most severe reaction is bone marrow damage, which can lead to fatal agranulocytosis or aplastic anaemia.

- *central nervous system*: dizziness, double vision, headaches, confusion and agitation.
- *gastro-intestinal tract*: dry mouth, decreased appetite, diarrhoea or constipation, cholestatic jaundice.
- *skin*: pruritus, acne, hair loss or hirsuitism, hypersensitivity reactions.
- *blood*: thrombocytopenia (reduced platelet count), erythrocytopenia (reduced red cell count) and leucocytopenia (reduced white cell counts) and thromboembolism. Rarely, aplastic anaemia can occur.
- *cardiovascular system*: oedema. Hypotension. Thrombophlebitis.
- *metabolic*: hypocalcaemia with rickets and osteomalacia. Vitamin K deficiency. Folate deficiency.

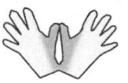 **Practice Points**

- Any signs of sore throat, fever, abnormal bruising or bleeding should be reported to the prescriber immediately. A full blood count should be arranged as an urgency.
- Weight gain in pregnancy must be monitored carefully if appetite is impaired.
- Oedema should be reported to prescribers: it should not be dismissed as a physiological response to pregnancy.
- Supplements of folic acid, calcium, vitamin D and vitamin K are important for the health of the woman and neonate. Folic acid can cause convulsions (see p. 278).

In overdose, carbamazepine causes tremors, excitation, convulsions, blood pressure changes and cardiac dysrhythmias.

Effects on the fetus can be severe, including a 1 per cent risk of neural tube defects; craniofacial defects; digital defects; cardiac malformations; and developmental delay. US pregnancy category C.

Many drugs interact with carbamazepine, due to induction of liver enzymes. Carbamazepine reduces the effectiveness of oral contraceptives [Chapter 1 p. 19]. Side effects are enhanced by alcohol, erythromycin, grapefruit juice and cimetidine.

There is no consensus on breastfeeding. Although some authorities say it is contra-indicated (Muir, 1998), the BNF (2000) states it is probably not harmful, while reporting one case of a severe skin reaction. Cases of liver damage (two) and poor feeding (four) in breastfed infants have been documented (Chaudron & Jefferson, 2000).

Sodium valproate (Epilim, Convulex®)

Valproate is widely prescribed for generalized seizures and partial seizures. Due to its effects on the fetus, valproate is usually a second line drug in pregnancy.

Side effects   Valproate is generally well tolerated; however, serious liver disorders or bleeding problems can arise.

- *central nervous system*: ataxia, tremors, sedation, hyperactivity and hallucinations.
- *gastro-intestinal tract*: increased appetite and weight gain, gastric irritation, liver dysfunction and pancreatitis.
- *skin*: rash and transient hair loss.
- *blood*: thrombocytopenia and inhibition of platelet aggregation. Leucopenia and erythrocytopenia.
- *cardiovascular system*: oedema

A neonatal withdrawal syndrome with severe hypoglycaemia has been reported.

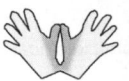 **Practice Points**

- Weight should be continuously monitored to pre-empt excessive weight gain.
- Any bruising and bleeding should be reported to the prescriber. A full blood count should be arranged as an urgency.

- Liver function tests are advisable, as pregnancy may compound any hepatic abnormalities.
- Oedema should be reported to prescribers: it should not be dismissed as a physiological response to pregnancy.
- Severe vomiting and abdominal pain should be reported to prescriber, as it could represent pancreatitis. A venous blood sample for serum amylase and glucose estimations should be arranged as an urgency.
- Delivery should take place where paediatricians are available. Neonatal blood glucose should be estimated (Ebbesen et al, 2000).

In overdose, valproate causes sedation, loss of consciousness and respiratory depression which may be fatal.

Effects on the fetus can be severe, and a 'fetal valproate syndrome' has been described, including: facial dysmorphic features; impaired psychomotor development; neural tube defects (up to 10 per cent in some reports); digital defects; phocomelia; urogenital malformations (Pangle, 2000). US pregnancy category D.

Drugs interacting with sodium valproate include: anticoagulant drugs, erythromycin; anti-psychotics (including prochlorperazine); anti-depressants.

The literature offers no consensus on breastfeeding. While some authorities consider the amount of drug passed into breast milk too small to be harmful (BNF, 2000), others advise caution (Muir, 1998). The half-life of valproate is prolonged in breastfed infants, particularly in the first ten days of life; therefore the drug may accumulate. A case is reported of a breastfed infant developing a low platelet count and anaemia which resolved on discontinuation of breast feeding (Chaudron & Jefferson, 2000).

Phenytoin (Epanutin®)

Phenytoin is indicated for partial and generalized seizures, except absence seizures. It is occasionally used in the management of status epilepticus and cardiac dysrhythmias. Phenytoin is becoming less popular, due to its narrow therapeutic range, complicated pharmacokinetics [glossary], serious side effects and numerous drug interactions.

Side effects

- *central nervous system*: nystagmus, slurred speech, ataxia, confusion, twitching, nervousness, insomnia and dystonic reactions.
- *gastro-intestinal tract*: nausea, vomiting and constipation.

- *skin*: morbilliform rash with fever, bullous dermatitis, hirsuitism, toxic epidermal necrolysis.
- *face*: gingival (gum) and lip hyperplasia and coarsening of facial features
- *blood*: megaloblastic anaemia responsive to folic acid, aplastic anaemia, lymphadenopathy thrombocytopenia, leucocytopenia, erythrocytopenia.
- *metabolic*: hypocalcaemia with rickets and osteomalacia. Vitamin K deficiency. Folate deficiency.
- *other*: systemic lupus erythromatosus. Dupuytren's contracture.

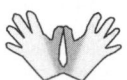 **Practice Points**

- The physiological changes of pregnancy and the puerperium alter the plasma concentration of phenytoin. The woman should be carefully checked for signs of central nervous system toxicity such as balance problems and confusion.
- Scrupulous attention to dental hygiene is required to minimize the risk of unsightly gum hyperplasia. (This problem occasionally arises with carbamazepine.)
- Supplements of folic acid, calcium, vitamin D and vitamin K are important for the health of the woman and neonate. Folic acid can cause convulsions (see p. 278).

In overdose, phenytoin causes hyperglycaemia, nystagmus, ataxia, dysarthria, coma, cardiac dysrhythmias, hypotension and respiratory depression. The lethal dose is 2–5 g, which is four to ten times the maximum recommended daily dose.

Effects on the fetus give rise to concern. There is evidence of 'fetal hydantoin syndrome' in 10–30 per cent of neonates. This comprises craniofacial and limb or digital abnormalities, hernias, learning disability and intrauterine growth restriction. There is also a reported risk of malignant tumours in children with a history of intrauterine exposure. US pregnancy category D.

Most drugs interact with phenytoin, including oral contraceptives, alcohol, antacids and other antiepileptrics.

The literature offers no consensus on breastfeeding. While some authorities consider the amount of drug passed into breast milk too small to be harmful, the manufacturers advise against breastfeeding (BNF, 2000).

Table 19.1 Diazepam

Indication	Main obstetric indication is the treatment of acute epileptic fit. It is not currently favoured for seizure prophylaxis.
Preparations	*Per rectum* 0.5 mg/kg body weight, intravenous, 10–20 mg slowly.
Contraindications	Previous drug sensitivity. Respiratory depression, severe hepatic impairment.
Side Effects	Hypotension, apnoea and respiratory depression. Thrombophlebitis if administered into a vein (see Chapter 2).
Overdose	CNS and severe respiratory depression, coma.
Fetal Effects	CNS and respiratory depression. Neonatal withdrawal symptoms. Hypotonia and hypothermia.
Breastfeeding	Avoid if possible, too sedating (BNF, 2000).

Diazepam (Diazemuls®, Valium®)

Diazepam is the main benzodiazepine commonly used in the emergency treatment of epileptic seizures. Diazemuls® is diazepam formulated to reduce the risk of thrombophlebitis, associated with the intravenous administration of benzodiazepines. Benzodiazepines are also prescribed for short term treatment of acute anxiety.

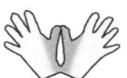 **Practice Points**

- Diazemuls® or an alternative benzodiazepine should be available and protocols should be in place in the event of a seizure during or following labour.
- Facilities for resuscitation of mother and neonate must be in place.

Barbiturates

Barbitures, including primidone, are prescribed as drugs of 'last resort'. All barbiturates are so sedating that they interfere with learning. They also interact with several nutrients, resulting in deficiency of vitamins D and K. Supplementation is necessary for both mother and neonate. Some authorities consider that barbiturates are less teratogenic than other antiepileptic drugs. However, the neonate may experience a severe withdrawal reaction. Breastfeeding is contra-indicated.

Ethosuximide

Ethosuximide is prescribed for absence seizures. Since these often resolve in adulthood, most prescribers review the need for medication as the woman approaches reproductive age. Ethosuximide is associated with fetal malformations. Breastfeeding is contra-indicated.

Second generation antiepileptic drugs

The new or second generation drugs include felbamate, gabapentin, lamotrigine, oxcarbazepine, tiagabine, topiramate, and vigabatrin. There have been no trials involving pregnant women to establish their safety in pregnancy. Data on their pharmacokinetics suggest a better safety profile compared to the well-tried first generation antiepileptics (Morrell, 1996). Outcomes of 53 pregnancies in women prescribed lamotrigine were reassuring (Pangle, 2000). However, animal studies indicate that vigabatrin and topiramate are teratogenic (Byrne, 2001).

Lamotrigine passes into breast milk, and concerns have been expressed regarding the possibility of rashes developing in infants (Chaudron & Jefferson, 2000).

With the exception of tiagabine, the rest have little or low protein binding and produce few, if any, oxide intermediates known to contribute to teratogenesis. Their use, at present, in pregnancy cannot be endorsed as evidencebased. To date only gabapentin, lamotrigine, oxcarbazepine, tiagabine, topiramate, and vigabatrin are listed in the British National Formulary (BNF, 2000).

Management of epilepsy in pregnancy

Up to 90 per cent of babies born to epileptic mothers will be normal with appropriate management. Antiepileptics are perhaps the best studied teratogens. As a result there are several recommendations to reduce their undesired effects. The main aim of management involves reducing the risks of teratogenicity from antiepileptics while maintaining seizure control despite the physiological changes of pregnancy. (See Implications for Practice.) All women should have the option of receiving combined care from an obstetrician and a neurologist. The neonates of women taking antiepileptics frequently experience drug withdrawal reactions, which make breastfeeding difficult to establish (Schwartz, 1998).

Preconceptional

- defer pregnancy until seizure control is optimal;
- re-evaluate the need for antiepileptic;
- antiepileptic monotherapy if possible;
- folic acid supplementation (5 mg daily), under supervision;

- lowest possible antiepileptic in divided doses if possible (Nulman et al, 1999);
- genetic counseling may be offered;
- discuss the risks associated with medication and the methods of anomaly detection.

Pregnancy

- care by obstetrician and neurologist/epileptologist;
- ultrasound screening for congenital abnormalities;
- continue folic acid supplement;
- consider vitamin D and calcium supplements;
- offer serum screening for congenital anomalies;
- antiepileptic blood levels to allow appropriate dosage adjustment;
- close obstetric monitoring looking out for known complications, for example fetal growth restriction;
- appropriate treatment of seizures;
- offer oral vitamin K supplement in the last trimester of pregnancy.

Labour and delivery

- deliver in hospital with anaesthetists and obstetrician and neonatal intensive care facilities;
- treatment of seizures;
- parenteral administration of antiepileptic if necessary;
- active management of third stage;
- avoid fetal scalp blood sampling if possible where vitamin K has not been given.

Post-partum

- offer intramuscular vitamin K to the neonate. See Chapter 8, anticoagulants;
- examine the neonate for congenital abnormalities and assess for signs of CNS depression;
- observation of the neonate for antiepileptic withdrawal symptoms;
- breastfeeding – particular caution with phenobarbitone and ethosuximide;
- offer extended hospital puerperium or discharge home to adequate domestic support;
- offer practical advice on care to avoid trauma to mother and neonate, for example avoid bathing infants alone;
- antiepileptic concentrations and dosage adjustment may be required;

- discuss contraceptive options. Antiepileptics reduce the efficiency of all oral contraceptives;
- regular consultant follow-up for three to six months to monitor blood concentrations and supervise dose titration towards pre-pregnancy requirements.

(See Swartjes et al, 1998; Malone et al, 1997.)

Case Report

Accurate appreciation of changing dose requirements facilitates care:

Following seizures at 27 weeks' gestation, a woman's dose of carbamazepine was increased from 600 to 800 mg/day. This was decreased immediately after delivery. Death occurred 17 days later. Carbamazepine was below the therapeutic range at post-mortem.

This patient had followed advice, but the advice had been dangerously inaccurate. Dosage reductions to pre-pregnancy levels should take place six to eight weeks after delivery. There was no evidence of therapeutic drug monitoring in this case (DoH, 1998: 130).

Implications for Practice: epilepsy in pregnancy

Due to the complexities of medication management, midwives should advise women to receive care from medical specialists, both an obstetrician and a neurologist or an epileptologist.

Potential Problem	Management
Increased risks of seizures	Ensure that a record of all seizures is maintained.
	Encourage medication compliance. Discourage abrupt discontinuation of antiepileptics.
	Ensure the woman's family are able to manage seizures.
	Minimize stress, allow plenty of rest and undisturbed sleep.
Need to adjust medication	Advise women that antiepileptic requirements are likely to increase during pregnancy, and fall during the puerperium.
	Liaise with physicians so that appropriate venous blood samples are taken and collected.
	Arrange help, if needed, for women to attend all appointments.
	Advise regarding the hazards of driving during periods of dose adjustment.

Implications for Practice (*continued*)

Potential Problem	Management
Appearance of side effects when doses are changed	Observe for side effects, particularly drowsiness/tiredness, constipation or nausea which may be mistaken for signs and symptoms of pregnancy. Women prescribed carbamazepine or phenytoin should be checked for nystagmus [glossary].
Loss of oral medication during vomiting	If vomiting occurs, ask the woman to note the time in relation to medication administration. Report problems to medical personnel.
Drug-induced nausea	Advise taking new tablets or increased doses with food to reduce the risk of nausea. Valproate should not be taken with milk.
Appetite changes	Monitor weight gain. Valproate may cause excessive weight gain, whereas carbamazepine may suppress appetite.
Dietary deficiencies	An optimal diet, rich in vitamins B, C, D and K, calcium and folates is important. Referral to a dietitian may be appropriate.
Emergency admission	Ensure patients wear identification with details of their medication.
Teratogenesis	Offer reassurance. Encourage screening – ultrasound and alpha-fetoprotein. Encourage compliance with folate and vitamin K supplements.
Contraception in the puerperium	Several anti-convulsants (phenytoin, carbamazepine, phenobarbitone) interact with oral contraceptives. High doses of oral contraceptives are normally required, but this may be ill-advised during breastfeeding or prior to the establishment of regular menstrual cycles.

Conclusion

If possible, antiepileptics should be reviewed prior to conception, with a view to gradual withdrawal and discontinuation if no fits have occurred for five years (Malseed et al, 1995) or four years (Dichter, 1991) or even less (Bloomfield, 1996). This may take several months. All patients should be on the minimum effective doses. If medication is needed, monotherapy is associated with much lower risks for the fetus.

Women should realize that the risks associated with seizures are greater than those of the drugs. Sudden withdrawal of anticonvulsants may precipitate fits. Also, if untreated, epilepsy tends to worsen. The risk of fetal abnormality is above that of the general population in people with untreated epilepsy. This may not be greatly increased by the use of monotherapy, in association with careful adherence to practice guidelines, such as outlined above (Implications for Practice).

Further Reading

Byrne, B. (2001) Management of Epilepsy in Pregnancy. In Bonnar, J. (ed.) *Recent Advances in Obstetrics and Gynaecology 21*. Edinburgh, Churchill Livingstone.

Nulman, I., Laslo, D. & Koren, G. (1999) Treatment of epilepsy in pregnancy. *Drugs*: 57:535–44.

PART VI

NON-PRESCRIPTION MEDICATIONS

A wide range of drugs can be purchased without prescription from chemists' shops. In the UK, prior to the advent of the NHS, this was the usual means of obtaining medicines. Old traditions die hard. Pregnancy and childbirth can be a time of discomfort and 'minor' ailments, when women resort to such medicines as are easily available. Unfortunately, they do not always seek the advice of pharmacists. This last part of the book addresses this by setting out the pharmacists' perspective on the use of non-prescription medicines in pregnant and lactating women.

CHAPTER 20

Over-the-Counter Medicines

CHERYL DAVIES, SCOTT PEGLER AND SUE JORDAN

This chapter offers a brief account of some of the medications available without prescription.

Chapter Contents

▦ Use of OTCs in pregnancy

▦ Drug use in breastfeeding

▦ Coughs and colds

▦ Pain

▦ Haemorrhoids

▦ Skin conditions and topical corticosteroids

▦ Allergic rhinitis and hayfever

▦ Threadworms

▦ Scabies and lice

▦ Conclusion

Remedies for nausea, constipation and indigestion are considered in chapters 5, 13 and 12.

Use of OTCs in pregnancy

It is estimated that over one-third of women take self-administered over-the counter (OTC) drugs during pregnancy. Many products readily available from pharmacies, supermarkets and garages are neither suitable nor safe for use in pregnancy. There is often no clear evidence as to the safety or otherwise of OTC products in pregnancy: randomized controlled trials would be considered unethical and case control studies are confounded by recall bias. As the thalidomide disaster indicated, safety in animal studies is no guarantee of safety in human pregnancy. Although total abstinence from self-medication would be ideal, the pragmatic solution is to advise and guide the choice of medication so as to minimize any potential risks.

In pregnancy, drug choice may be based on an assessment of drug safety to the fetus, rather than efficacy in managing a particular condition. Therefore, the drugs chosen to treat a pregnant woman may differ from those that would empirically be the drugs of first choice in a non-pregnant person. Treatment tends to be based on long established products which have come to be generally regarded as safe, although research-based evidence is often unobtainable.

Principles of drug use in pregnancy

- Wherever possible, non-drug treatments should be tried first.
- In general, older established drugs with a proven safety record are generally preferred to drugs marketed more recently.
- Compound preparations should be avoided if possible, preferring remedies based on single ingredients.
- Avoid OTC therapy in the first trimester unless there are compelling reasons.
- Use the lowest dose of drug for the shortest duration possible.

Drug use in breastfeeding

Although only a few drugs are thought to be hazardous to the suckling infant, it is prudent to minimize drug exposure. If medication is clinically essential, it should be taken immediately after feeding. If a drug is taken orally, the peak concentration appears in the milk one to three hours later. If possible, feeding should be reduced during these times (Pangle, 2000).

- Drug administration to the lactating mother should be restricted to essential medication after a careful risk: benefit assessment has been made.
- Select drug and dosage regimen that will minimize the infant's exposure.
- Infants are most vulnerable in the first few weeks of life, until the liver and kidneys have reached a level of maturity. Specialist advice should be sought if premature infants are involved.
- The infant should be carefully monitored for predictable potential side effects, for example drowsiness with antihistamines.
- If medication is considered essential and is passed into breast milk in sufficient quantities to be hazardous to the infant, it may be necessary to suspend breastfeeding, if a suitable alternative therapy is not available.

Coughs and colds

Cough and cold remedies are among the most commonly used drugs in pregnancy. Most cold remedies contain a sympathomimetic agent [glossary] (see ephedrine, Chapter 4) such as pseudoephedrine or phenylpropanolamine, or an antihistamine, such as diphenhydramine (Chapter 5). Sympathomimetics help to relieve congestion by constricting the blood vessels of the nasal mucosa. Cough and cold remedies also commonly contain an analgesic and/or expectorant. Although there is no evidence of problems when these drugs are used in pregnancy, equally there is little proof of safety, and in view of their questionable efficacy, their use is best avoided (Folb & Dukes, 1990; BNF, 2000).

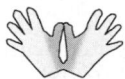 **Practice Points**

- Rebound congestion and 'runny nose' frequently follow use of sympathomimetics.
- Nasal decongestants may cause dryness and stinging of the mucosa.
- Large doses can cause side effects, such as headache, insomnia, nervousness, hypertension and tachycardia. Therefore, use is ill-advised.

Similarly, many of the commonly used cough medicines have questionable efficacy and in general, there is a lack of evidence of safety. For these reasons, they are best avoided in pregnant women. Cough suppressants containing opioids, such as codeine, are unsuitable as OTC preparations in pregnancy and breastfeeding due to potential problems of neonatal withdrawal. However, in certain circumstances, codeine may be prescribed as an analgesic. (see Chapter 13)

Demulcent or soothing preparations, such as simple linctus or cough sweets, are unlikely to have any adverse effects on the fetus and can be used if required. Women should bear in mind the increased risk of dental caries in pregnancy before they self-medicate with preparations containing sugar.

Pain

Pain can often be managed using non-pharmacological measures, such as immobilization, warmth and, if appropriate, reassurance. However, some conditions, including headache or dental pain, may require medical treatment.

Paracetamol is the analgesic of first choice during pregnancy and lactation (Byron, 1995; Folb & Dukes, 1990), as this has been used for many years without evidence of teratogenicity. Side effects from paracetamol are unusual but include rashes, blood disorders (BNF, 2000) and, rarely, deterioration of asthma (Po & Po, 1992).

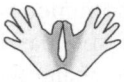 **Practice Points**

- The maximum paracetamol dose of 4 g (eight tablets) per day should never be exceeded, as pregnancy renders the liver vulnerable to injury. It is advisable to use the lowest possible use for the shortest possible time.
- Many OTC analgesics contain multiple ingredients, such as caffeine or phenylephrine, and these are best avoided.

A daily intake of 600 mg caffeine, from all sources, has been associated with low birthweight and fetal malformations (see McKenry & Salerno, 1998).

Non-steroidal anti-inflammatory drugs (NSAIDs) such as aspirin, ibuprofen (Nurofen®, Cuprofen®) should be used under medical supervision during pregnancy and should be avoided altogether in the third trimester, due to risks of bleeding complications and premature closure of the ductus arteriosis which can lead to pulmonary hypertension and lung damage (Lee & Schofield, 1994). Aspirin in the third trimester is also associated with reduction in fetal urine output and olighydramnios. Low dose aspirin is sometimes prescribed for pre-eclampsia prophylaxis, where the benefits are thought to outweigh the risks (see Chapter 9, Box 9.3).

NSAIDs (such as Ibugel® (ibuprofen) Gel) or counter-irritants applied topically to the skin, retain the potential for systemic adverse effects (BNF, 2000) and the same cautions apply as for the oral preparations.

Migraine

Since migraine symptoms remit in a significant number of pregnant women, prophylaxis may not be necessary during pregnancy. Paracetamol is recommended for migraine in pregnancy (Campbell & Lees, 2000). Soluble or liquid preparations may be preferred for a more rapid action (see Chapter 1, p. 7).

Haemorrhoids

Women may experience haemorrhoids for the first time during pregnancy. Any woman with rectal bleeding should be referred to her doctor for a definite diagnosis. Haemorrhoids are exacerbated by constipation. Advice on fluid intake and diet may help (see Chapter 13).

Ice-packs may provide some temporary relief. Bland soothing creams containing a mild astringent without a local anaesthetic, for example Anusol Cream® (bismuth oxide, zinc oxide and Peru Balsam) and Anusol Ointment® (ABPI, 2000) may be useful; the dose of bismuth is considered too low to be harmful in normal application. If a local anaesthetic is applied to the haemorrhoids, it may be absorbed in sufficient quantities to cause fetal side effects, including bradycardia (see Chapter 15).

Skin conditions and topical corticosteroids

Hydrocortisone 0.1 per cent and 1 per cent is used for a variety of skin complaints such as pruritus, nappy rash and eczema. It is available OTC, but use without prescription is not recommended in children under ten or pregnant women. Use should be restricted to five to seven days, avoiding the face or broken skin. A variety of additives are present in different preparations, any of which may cause allergy: for example Hydrocortisyl® contains wool fat. The more potent topical steroids are more likely to cause side systemic effects (for example Betamethasone 0.1 per cent, Clobetasol 0.05 per cent); these are only available on prescription. Absorption is greatest through thin or occluded skin, particularly in infants.

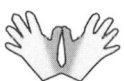 **Practice Point**

If an occlusive dressing is applied over corticosteroid prepations, more of the steroid will be absorbed, and side effects are more likely.

If corticosteroids are applied to the skin, women should be alerted to potential problems:

- local spread of infection;
- dermal atrophy and thinning;
- hirsuitism;
- striae;
- perioral dermatitis if the steroid is applied near the mouth;
- acne;
- depigmentation of the area.

It is important that such problems are detected before permanent scarring occurs.

Allergic rhinitis and hayfever

Allergic rhinitis and hayfever occur commonly in pregnancy. Trigger factors should be identified and avoided if possible (see Chapter 15, Table 15.1). Glasses and topical chromoglycate eye drops are useful for allergic conjunctivitis.

Topical treatments should be recommended before systemic therapy is given. Topical corticosteroid preparations may alleviate the symptoms of allergic rhinitis. There is a risk of nose bleeds with these preparations.

Chlorpheniramine (Piriton®) and promethazine (Phenergan®) remain the anti-histamines of choice during pregnancy and may be needed if topical treatment proves ineffective. See anti-histamines, Chapter 5.

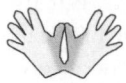 **Practice Points**

- These 'first generation' anti-histamines are very sedating, and may impair ability to drive.
- These drugs interact with all other sedatives, including alcohol and opioids.

There is insufficient evidence of safety to recommend the OTC use of newer, non-sedating anti-histamines.

Threadworms

Threadworm infection during pregnancy is surprisingly common, possibly because pregnant women are often in close contact with young children. The life cycle of the parasite can last up to six weeks. Spread of threadworm infection involves anal to oral transmission of the eggs. Thus, with strict adherence to good hygiene, the life cycle of the parasite can be broken, and this represents the safest method of management, particularly in the first trimester of pregnancy.

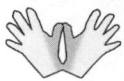 **Practice Points**

- Women should be advised to wash their hands and scrub their nails thoroughly before each meal and after using the lavatory.
- Infection can be spread via clothing. Bed linen should be washed daily.
- A morning shower will remove any eggs laid overnight.

In some women however, symptoms are intolerable and drug therapy may be necessary. In these circumstances, therapy should be delayed if possible until the end of the first trimester. Piperazine (Pripsen®) has been used over many years without any evidence of hazard (Welsh Drug Information Centre, 1996). In pregnancy, piperazine must be administered under medical supervision: the packs on sale to the public carry a warning against self-medicating in pregnancy.

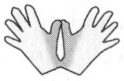 **Practice Points**

- Piperazine may stimulate (sometimes violent) contraction of the gastrointestinal tract, causing vomiting and diarrhoea.
- It is absorbed from the gut and passes into the central nervous system. If the therapeutic dose is exceeded, piperazine can cause incoordination, memory defects and convulsions.
- Hypersensitivity responses have occurred (see Chapter 1).
- Piperazine is contra-indicated in people with epilepsy, renal or liver impariment (Malseed et al, 1995).

Scabies and lice

Aqueous malathion preparations are the preferred products for managing both scabies and head lice during pregnancy. Malathion (an organophosphate) has been available in the UK for longer than other insecticides, for example pyrethroids, and hence experience of its use in pregnancy is greater. Some authorities consider exposure in pregnancy to be safe (Thomas et al, 1992). Aqueous preparations, such as Derbac M® and Quellada M®, are preferred to alcoholic preparations as exposure to noxious fumes is avoided, and systemic absorption may be less. Each product should be used strictly in accordance with the instructions provided by the manufacturer.

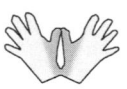 **Practice Points**

- Malathion should not be applied to broken, infected or hot skin.
- Co-administration with oils or creams will increase absorption and should be avoided.
- Gloves should be warn by pregnant women applying these preparations to others.
- Malathion can cause a contact dermatitis.
- Ingestion or absorption of malathion can cause central nervous system disturbance and convulsions.
- Applications should be no more frequent than once a week or for more than three weeks (BNF, 2000).
- Malathion should be left to dry: hairdryers should not be used.

The itching of scabies may persist for some time after eradication and calamine lotion and a sedative antihistamine, for example chlorpheniramine or promethazine, may be helpful.

Conclusion

The use of all medication requires a careful risk: benefit assessment. Very few products available OTC are licensed for use during pregnancy or lactation. In most circumstances, drug therapy, including 'alternative medicines', during pregnancy and lactation should be undertaken under medical supervision.

Reference to the Data Sheet or Summary of Product Characteristics will provide some indication of the likely risks of drug use, while also giving the medico-legal standpoint. The appendices to the BNF provide brief guidance. In the UK, independent information may be sought by contacting the local Medicines' Information Centre, based in Pharmacy Departments of many large hospitals.

Further Reading

Pfaffenrath, V. & Rehm, M. (1998) Migraine in pregnancy: what are the safest treatment options? *Drug Safety*: 19:383–8.

Quick Reference for Major Drugs

The most important drugs in midwifery are summarized under the headings: uses, side effects; cautions and contra-indications; interactions. The drugs are listed alphabetically.

Contents:

- Beta$_2$ adrenorceptor agonists
- Corticosteroids
- D$_2$ antagonist anti-emetics
- Ergometrine
- Heparin
- Histamine$_1$ receptor antagonists (anti-emetics)
- Insulin
- Iron (oral preparations)
- Laxatives
- Local anaesthetics
- Magnesium
- Methyldopa
- Nifedipine
- Nitrous oxide
- Opioids
- Oxytocin
- Prostaglandins
- SSRIs (selective serotonin reuptake inhibitors)
- Vitamin K
- Warfarin

BETA₂ ADRENORECEPTOR AGONISTS

USES:
Rescue medication for asthma   Premature labour

SIDE EFFECTS:
Cardiovascular system
Bleeding tendency   Postural hypotension
Cardiac dysrhythmias   Pulmonary oedema
Chest pain   Raised systolic BP
Lowered diastolic BP   Sweating, erythema
Over-active thyroid worsened   Tachycardia
Peripheral vasodilation   Transient fall in pO_2

Central nervous system
Anxiety   Insomnia
Behaviour disturbances   Irritability
Dizziness   Paranoia
Hallucinations   Tension
Headache   Tremor

Smooth muscle inhibition
Constipation   Nausea
Heartburn   Urine retention/dysuria
Ileus   Vomiting

Metabolic
Drying of mucous secretions   Increased lactate and free
Hyperglycaemia – rarely ketoacidosis   fatty acids
Hypokalaemia – cramps, weakness,   Neonatal hypoglycaemia
    cardiac dysrhythmias

Hypersensitivity Responses
Anaphylaxis   LFT changes
Bronchospasm   Rash

CAUTIONS AND CONTRA-INDICATIONS:
Acute angle glaucoma   Hyperthyroidism
Cardiac disease, high risk of myocardial   Hypokalaemia
    infarction   Intrauterine infection
Cardiac Dysrhythmias   Phaeochromocytoma
Diabetes   Pregnancy and lactation
Haemorrhage   Severe asthma
Hypertension of any cause

(continued)

(BETA$_2$ ADRENORECEPTOR AGONISTS continued)

INTERACTIONS:

Amphetamines
Atropine
Beta blockers
Cocaine
'Cold cures'
Digoxin
Diuretics
Glycopyrronium

MAOIs
Oxytocin
Salbutamol
Steroids
TCAs
Terbutaline
Theophylline

CORTICOSTEROIDS

USES:

Arthritis
Asthma
Dermatology
Emesis
Immunosuppression

Inflammatory bowel disease
Neoplastic disease
Prematurity
Replacement therapy

SIDE EFFECTS:

Anti-inflammatory

Acne
Impaired healing

Infections

Metabolic

Avascular necrosis
Bruising
Fluid retention
Hypertension
Hypocalcaemia
Hypokalaemia
Hyperglycaemia
Muscle wasting
Oesophageal ulceration
Osteoporosis

Pancreatitis
Peptic ulceration
Raised intracranial pressure
Striae
Telangiectasia
Tendon rupture
Thin skin
Thromboembolism
Weight gain

Endocrine

Adrenal suppression
Hirsuitism

Oligomenorrhoea

Eyes

Cataracts
Glaucoma

Papilloedema

(continued)

(CORTICOSTEROIDS continued)

Central nervous system

Hiccups	Nausea
Insomnia	Psychoses
Malaise	Seizures

CAUTIONS AND CONTRA-INDICATIONS:

Diabetes	Liver failure
Epilepsy	Mental illness
Glaucoma	Migraine
Heart failure	Myasthenia gravis
Hypertension	Osteoporosis
Hypothyroidism	Peptic ulceration
Infections	Renal insufficiency
Live vaccines	TB

INTERACTIONS:

Alcohol	Erythromycin
Antacids	Hypoglycaemia agents
Anticoagulants	NSAIDs
Anticonvulsants	Oestrogens
Anti-hypertensives	Salt (in food or ivi)
Beta$_2$ adrenoreceptor agonists	Sympathomimetics
Cyclosporin	Vaccines

D$_2$ ANTAGONIST ANTI-EMETICS (E.G. PROCHLORPERAZINE, BUT SEE ALSO HISTAMINE ANTAGONISTS)

USES:

Anaesthetics	Hyperemesis gravidarum
Emesis due to labour	Migraine
Ergotamine	Opioids

SIDE EFFECTS:

Alterations in BP	Hypokalaemia
Anxiety	Impaired fertility
Breast tenderness	Insomnia
Cardiac dysrhythmias	Neuroleptic malignant
Diarrhoea	syndrome

(continued)

(D$_2$ ANTAGONIST ANTI-EMETICS continued)

Fluid retention   Restlessness
Hypersensitivity responses   SIADH

Depression of
  Alertness   Respiration
  Cough   Thermoregulation
  Mood

Posture and movement disorders
  Abnormal movements   Parkinsonism
  Acute Dystonia   Tremors

CAUTIONS AND CONTRA-INDICATIONS:

Blood dyscrasias   Hepatic impairment
Breast cancer   Masking serious pathology
Breastfeeding   Phaeochromocytoma
Cardiovascular disease   Porphyria
Diabetes   Pregnancy
Epilepsy   Renal impairment
For three to four days after   Respiratory disorders
  gastro-intestinal surgery   Young people

INTERACTIONS:

All CNS depressants   Corticosteroids
Anti-coagulants   Desferoxamine
Anti-convulsants   Diuretics
Anti-histamines   Drugs for Parkinsonism
Anti-hypertensives   Insulin
Anti-psychotics   Lithium
Beta$_2$ agonists   Ritodrine

HEPARIN

USES:

Prevention and mangement of thromboembolic disorders
Reducing plasmia hyperlipidaemia

(continued)

(HEPARIN continued)

SIDE EFFECTS:
Bleeding

Thrombocytopenia
Delayed – severe   Increased diuresis @ 36–48 hrs
Early – mild   Vasospastic reaction (rare)

Hypersensitivity responses
Anaphylaxis   Nasal congestion
Bronchospasm   Pruritus
Chills   Pyrexia
Diarrhoea   Rash
Lacrimation   Urticaria

Long term use only
Decreased renal function   Hyperkalaemia
Hair loss   Osteoporosis
Heparin resistance   Raised liver enzymes

CAUTIONS AND CONTRA-INDICATIONS:
Aortic aneurysm   Liver disease/alcoholism
Bleeding tendencies   Pericarditis
Cerebral aneurysm   Prematurity
Cerebrovascular haemorrhage   Renal impairment
Deficiency of vitamin K or C   Severe diabetes
Drainage tubes *in situ*   Threatened abortion
Epidural or spinal puncture   Thrombocytopenia
Haemophilias   Thrombophilias
Hypertension   Trauma/surgery
Lesions in GI, GU or respiratory tracts   Tuberculosis

INTERACTIONS:
Acid-citrate-dextrose   Oral anticoagulants
Alcohol   Oral hypoglycaemics
Blood   Penicillins
Cephalosporins   Quinine
Dextrans   Salicylates
Ketorolac   Thrombolytic therapy
Nitrates   Tobacco
NSAIDs   Valproic acid

HISTAMINE$_1$ RECEPTOR ANTAGONISTS (ANTI-EMETICS)

USES:
Allergic disorders   Sedation
Anti-emetics

SIDE EFFECTS:
Central nervous system
   Confusion   Sedation
   Inco-ordination   Seizures
   Insomnia   Tinnitus
   Irritability

Drying of secretions
   Blurred vision   Risk of chest infection
   Dry eyes   Sore mouth
   Dry skin   Xerostomia (dry mouth)
   Inability to sweat

Cardiovascular system
   Hypotension   Tachycardia

Gastro-intestinal system
   Anorexia   Gastric upset
   Constipation   Ileus

Renal system
   Dysuria   Urine retention

Hypersensitivity responses (rare)
   Blood dyscrasia   Rash
   Photosensitivity

CAUTIONS:
Asthma   Hypertension
Breastfeeding   Hyperthyroidism
Cardiovascular disease   Liver impairment
Diabetes   Peptic ulcer
GI or bladder obstruction   Pregnancy
Glaucoma   Renal impairment
History of seizures

(continued)

(HISTAMINE₁ RECEPTOR ANTAGONISTS continued)

INTERACTIONS:

Anaesthetics   Opioids
Anti-psychotics   Ototoxic drugs
Epinephrine (adrenaline)   Sedatives, for example alcohol
MAOIs   Tricyclic anti-depressants

INSULIN

USES:
Ketoacidosis
Maintenance of normoglycaemia in diabetics

SIDE EFFECTS:
Antibody formation   Loss of hypoglycaemic
Hypoglycaemia   awareness
Hypokalaemia (infusions only)   Postural hypotension
Insulin resistance

Injection site problems
   Lipoatrophy   Lipohypertrophy

CAUTIONS AND CONTRA-INDICATIONS:
Hypersensitivity   Hypoglycaemia

INTERACTIONS:
Drugs causing hyperglycaemia
   Caffeine (large doses)   Phenytoin
   Calcium antagonists   Steroids (oestrogens,
   Diuretics   progesterone,
   Lithium   glucocorticoids)
   Marijuana   Sympathomimetics
   Nicotine   Thyroxine

Drugs causing hypoglycaemia
   ACEIs   Salicylates
   Alcohol   Some NSAIDs
   Anabolic steroids   Tetracyclines
   MAOIs

Loss of hypoglycaemic awareness
   Beta Blockers

IRON (ORAL PREPARATIONS)

USES:
Iron deficiency anaemia

SIDE EFFECTS:
Gastro-intestinal system

Anorexia	Painful swallowing
Constipation	Stomach cramps
Diarrhoea	Stool and urine discolouration
Indigestion	Teeth staining
Nausea	Vomiting

Impaired absorption

Phosphate deficiency (rare)	Zinc deficiency

Haematological

Folic acid deficiency	Iron overload
Headache	

CAUTIONS AND CONTRA-INDICATIONS:

Haemolytic anaemia	Peptic ulcer
Haemosiderosis	Sensitivity to iron
Liver disease	Ulcerative colitis

INTERACTIONS:

Alcohol	Methyldopa
Antacids	Milk, eggs
Calcium supplements	Ranitidine
Cereals (phytates)	Tea (tannins)
Chloramphenicol	Tetracyclines (including
Cholestyramine	doxycycline)
Cimetidine	Vitamin C
Ciprofloxacin	Vitamin E
Coffee	

LAXATIVES

USES:

Bowel disease and investigations	Failure to pass faeces within three days of delivery

(continued)

(LAXATIVES continued)

SIDE EFFECTS:

Abdominal cramps	Flatulence
Dehydration	Hypokalaemia
Diarrhoea	Intestinal obstruction

Prolonged use

Absorption of the laxative	Loss of protein, calcium and
Colonic atony	other minerals
Dependence	

CAUTIONS AND CONTRA-INDICATIONS:

Debility	Intestinal obstruction
Dehydration	Lactation
Hypersensitivity	Pregnancy

INTERACTIONS:

Administer at least two hours apart from other drugs and food	Loss of other drugs due to diarrhoea

---

LOCAL ANAESTHETICS

USES:

Dental procedures	Subcutaneous
Epidural	Suturing and minor
Intravenous regional anaesthesia	procedures
Nerve block	Topical
Spinal (intrathecal) analgesia	

SIDE EFFECTS: MATERNAL

Cardiovascular

Cardiovascular collapse	Hypotension

Central nervous system

Confusion	Restlessness
Convulsions	Shivering
Nausea	Thermoregulation failure
Paraesthesia/paralysis	Tremor

(continued)

(LOCAL ANAESTHETICS continued)

Smooth muscle relaxation
Incontinence of urine or faeces   Retention of urine
Prolongation of labour

Hypersensitivity reactions

Problems associated with dural puncture such as headache or backache

SIDE EFFECTS: FETAL/NEONATAL
Depression of CNS   Neonatal hypothermia
Fetal bradycardia   Respiratory depression

CAUTIONS:
Bradycardia, heart block   Malignant hyperthermia
Epilepsy   Previous hypersensitivity
Hypovolaemia
Liver, kidney or thyroid
  disease

INTERACTIONS:
Anti-arrhythmics   Cimetidine, possibly ranitidine
Anti-rheumatics alcohol   Diuretics
Benzodiazeipines   Muscle relaxants
Beta antagonists (blockers)   Sedatives (alcohol,
Calcium antagonists   prochlorperazine)

MAGNESIUM

USES:
Anticonvulsant prophylaxis in eclampsia   Hypomagnesemia
Cardiac dysrhythmias   Tocolysis

SIDE EFFECTS: MATERNAL
Nervous system
Dizziness   Respiratory paralysis
Drowsiness/sedation   Reduced muscle tone
Flaccid paralysis   Tetany
Headache   Weakness, lethargy, depression
Loss of deep tendon reflexes

(continued)

(MAGNESIUM continued)

Cardiovascular system

Asystole
Chest pain
Complete heart block
Flushing
Hypotension
Hypothermia

Hypoxia
Impaired coagulation
Palpitations
Pulmonary oedema
Sweating

Smooth muscle relaxation

Abdominal cramps
Ileus
Nausea

Tocolysis
Vomiting

Renal system

Dry mouth
Osmotic diuresis

Protein loss

Other

Decreased bone density with long
  term use

Urticaria with iv use

SIDE EFFECTS: NEONATAL/FETAL

Blunting of reflexes
Congenital rickets with long term use
Convulsions
Decreased HR variability
Drowsiness
Hypothermia

Neonatal convulsions
Meconium ileus
Poor muscle tone
Respiratory depression/
  apnoea

CAUTIONS AND CONTRA-INDICATIONS:

Cardiac disease
Heart block
Hepatic impairment

Myasthenia gravis
Renal impairment
Respiratory impairment

INTERACTIONS:

Aminoglycosides
Benzodiazepines
β_2 adrenoreceptor agonists (salbutamol)
Calcium antagonists
General anaesthetics

Local anaesthetics
Muscle relaxants
Opioids
Phenothiazines

METHYLDOPA

USES:
Hypertension

SIDE EFFECTS:
Central nervous system

Depression
Galactorrhoea
Headache
Loss of libido
Loss of memory
Nightmares

Paraesthesia
Posture and movement
 disorders
Sedation
Tremors in the neonate
Weakness

Gastro-intestinal system

Abdominal distention
Constipation
Dry mouth
Fever

Liver impairment
Nausea
Tongue discolouration
Weight gain

Cardiovascular system

Angina
Bradycardia
Hypertension, if intravenous
Nasal stuffiness

Nocturia
Oedema
Orthostatic hypotension

Haematological disturbances

Haemolytic anaemia
Leukopenia

Thrombocytopenia

Hypersensitivity responses

Arthralgia
Myocarditis

Rash
Retrolental fibroplasia

CAUTIONS AND CONTRA-INDICATIONS:

Anaemia
Angina
Blood dyscrasias
Breastfeeding
Endocrine disorders
History of depression

Liver disease
Parkinson's disease
Phaeochromocytoma
Porphyria
Renal impairment

(continued)

(METHYLDOPA continued)

INTERACTIONS:

Amphetamines	Lithium
Anaesthetics	NSAIDs
Antidepressants	OTC cold cures
Antihypertensives	Sedatives, for example
Antipsychotics	alcohol, opioids
Benzodiazepines	Steroids
Digoxin	Tolbutamide
Iron salts	

NIFEDIPINE

USES:

Angina	Raynaud's phenomenon
Hypertension	Tocolysis

SIDE EFFECTS: MATERNAL

Blurred vision	Oedema
Dizziness	Pulmonary oedema
Eye pain	Tachycardia
Flushing	Tinnitus
Headache	Vasodilation
Hypotension	

Gastro-intestinal

Constipation	Nausea
Heartburn	

Other

Cramps/stiffness	Insomnia
Fatigue	Nervousness
Frequency of micturition	Prolongation of labour

Hypersensitivity

Hepatotoxicity	Urticaria
Rashes	

SIDE EFFECTS: NEONATAL/FETAL

Possibly IUGR	Possibly prematurity

(continued)

(NIFEDIPINE continued)
CAUTIONS AND CONTRA-INDICATIONS:
Abrupt withdrawal
Breastfeeding
Diabetes
Heart failure

Ischaemic heart disease
Liver impairment
Porphyria

INTERACTIONS:
Alcohol
All anti-hypertensives
Anitconvulsants
Cimetidine, ranitidine
Cyclosporin
Digoxin
Grapefruit juice
Ionic X-ray contrast media
Magnesium sulphate

Muscle relaxants (non-
  depolarizing)
Rifampicin
Some antiemetics
  (prochlorperazine)
Sympathomimetics (including
  OTC cold cures)
Theophylline
Vancomycin

NITROUS OXIDE

USES:
Anaesthesia when combined with
  other agents
Dressing changes

Inhalation analgesia
Trauma

SIDE EFFECTS: MATERNAL
Alkalosis
Dizziness
Hallucinations
Hypoxia

Light-headedness
Nausea
Sedation
Vomiting

SIDE EFFECTS: NEONATAL
Hypoxia

Sedation

SIDE EFFECTS: HEALTH CARE WORKERS
Impaired fertility
Leucopenia
Peripheral neuropathy

Subacute combined
  degeneration of the spinal
  cord

Vitamin B$_{12}$ deficiency
  Megaloblastic anaemia

(continued)

(NITROUS OXIDE continued)

CAUTIONS:

Air embolism	Intoxication
Bowel distension	Occluded middle ear
Family history of malignant hyperthermia	Pneumothorax
	Respiratory impairment
First 16 weeks of pregnancy	Storage precautions

INTERACTIONS:

Methotrexate	Other sedatives
Opioids	Vitamin B_{12}
Other anaesthetics (such as halothane)	

OPIOIDS

USES:

Acute pulmonary oedema	Cough
Analgesia	Diarrhoea
Anxioloysis	Sedation

SIDE EFFECTS:

Depression of

Confusion and hallucinations	Pruritus
Miosis (except meperidine/pethidine)	Retention of urine
Nausea	SIADH [glossary]
Prolonged labour	

Depression of

Blood pressure	Respiration
Central nervous system	Thermoregulation
Heart rate	
GI tract motility – delayed gastric emptying, ileus, constipation	

CAUTIONS AND CONTRA-INDICATIONS:

Addison's disease	Hypotension
Convulsions (particularly meperidine (pethidine))	Hypothyroidism
	Kidney failure
Decreased respiratory reserve/ asthma attack	Known allergy to opioids
	Liver failure
Head injury	Paralytic ileus

(continued)

(OPIOIDS continued)
INTERACTIONS:

Aciclovir	MAOIs
All central nervous system depressants	Metoclopramide
Anti-arrhythmics	Midazolam (with fentanyl)
Antidepressants	Nitrous oxide
Antiepileptics	Non-sedating anti-histamines
Anti-malarials	Phenothiazines
Benzodiazeipines	Promethazine
Cimetidine	Rifampicin
Cyclizine	Ritonavir
Erythromycin	Selegiline
Including alcohol	SSRIs
Ketoconazole	Tobacco

OXYTOCIN

USES:
Augmentation of labour   Post-partum haemorrhage
Induction of labour
Missed or incomplete abortion

SIDE EFFECTS: MATERNAL
Overstimulation of the uterus

Abruptio placenta	Post-partum haemorrhage
Amniotic fluid embolus	Trauma
Pelvic haematoma	Uterine rupture

Cardiovascular system

Cardiovascular collapse	Hypotension
Cerebrovascular accident	Nausea and vomiting
Fluid retention	Water intoxication
Hypertension	

SIDE EFFECTS: FETAL/NEONATAL

Acidosis	Cardiac dysrhythmias
Asphyxia	Hypoxia
Birth trauma	Neonatal jaundice

(continued)

(OXYTOCIN continued)

CAUTIONS AND CONTRA-INDICATIONS:
Cephalopelvic disproportion
Difficult delivery (prolapsed cord,
  placenta praevia)
Eclampsia/pre-eclampsia
Fetal distress
Fetal malposition
Grande multiparae
History of uterine sepsis
Hypersensitivity

Hypertonic uterus
Obstetric emergencies
Over-distension of uterus
Placental abruption
Premature labour
Undilated cervix
Uterine inertia
Uterine or cervical surgery

INTERACTIONS:
Adrenaline
Anaesthetics
Carbamazepine
Cyclophosphamide

Ephedrine
Opioids
Prostaglandins

PROSTAGLANDINS

USES IN CHILDBIRTH:
Evacuation of the uterus
Induction of labour

Post-partum haemorrhage

SIDE EFFECTS:
Gastro-intestinal
  Abdominal pain
  Diarrhoea

  Hiccups
  Nausea, vomiting

Uterine hyperstimulation
  Fetal compromise
  Pain

  Rupture of uterus

Cardiovascular
  Cardiac dysrhythmias
  Diuresis
  Flushing
  Hypertension
  Hypotension

  Hypoxia
  Pulmonary oedema
  Pyrexia/chills
  Sweating
  Tachycardia

Respiratory system
  Bronchospasm
  Choking

  Wheezing

(continued)

(PROSTAGLANDINS continued)

Nervous system

Back pain	Tremor
Increase in intra-ocular pressure	Seizures

CAUTIONS AND CONTRA-INDICATIONS:

Asthma	High risk of uterine rupture
BP abnormalities	Hypersensitivity
Cardiac disease	Kidney disease
Epilepsy	Liver disease
Fetal compromise	Pulmonary disease
Glaucoma/raised intra-ocular pressure	Ruptured membranes

INTERACTIONS:

Alcohol	Oxytocin
Aspirin/NSAIDs	

SSRIS (SELECTIVE SEROTONIN REUPTAKE INHIBITORS FOR EXAMPLE FLUOXETINE/PROZAC®)

USES:

Bulimia nervosa	Panic disorder
Depression	Social phobia
Obsessive/compulsive disorders	

SIDE EFFECTS:

Central nervous system

Aggression	Indigestion
Agitation	Insomnia
Amnesia	Loss of libido
Anorexia	Migraine
Anxiety	Neuroleptic malignant
Constipation	syndrome
Convulsions	Palpitations
Diarrhoea	Parkinsonian movements
Frequent micturition	Restlessness
Glucose changes	Taste disturbance
Hallucinations	Tinnitus
Headache	Tremor
Hypomania	Weight changes

(continued)

(SSRIs continued)

Cardiovscular system
Hypersalivation   SIADH
Nasal congestion   Sweating
Postural hypotension

Hypersensitivitiy responses:
Angioedema   Lung damage
Arthralgia   Myalgia
Bleeding   Pancreatitis
Bone marrow damage   Pins and needles
Bruising   Pruritus
Hair loss   Rash
Liver damage   Vasculitis

CAUTIONS AND CONTRA-INDICATIONS:
Abrupt withdrawal   Hepatic impairment
Agitation   History of mania
Bleeding   Pregnancy
Breastfeeding   Renal impairment
Cardiac disease   Risk of convulsions
ECT

INTERACTIONS:
Alcohol   LSD
Anti-convulsants   Other anti-depressants
Anti-histamines   Pentazocine
Anti-psychotics   Prochlorperazine
Benzodiazepines   Sumatriptan
Calcium blockers   Theophylline
Cannabis   Tramadol
Lithium   Warfarin

VITAMIN K

USES:
In pregnancy for women receiving   Prophylaxis against
   anti-convulsant therapy   haemorrhagic disease of the
Malabsorptive states (menadiol)   newborn
Overdose of warfarin (not heparin)

(continued)

(VITAMIN K continued)

SIDE EFFECTS:
Oral administration

Depression of liver function

Haemolysis in G6PD or vitamin E
deficiency (menadiol)

Headache, flushing

Nausea

Thrombo-embolism

Intramuscular administration

Alterations in blood viscosity

Dyspnoea

Hypersensitivity reactions

Hypertension

Hypothermia

Pain and swelling at injection
site

RBC aggregation

Sweating

Tachycardia

Intravenous administration

Anaphylaxis

Cardiovascular collapse (rare)

Chest pain

Cyanosis

Flushing

Rashes

Vasodilation

In neonates

Hacmolysis

Hyperbilirubinaemia and jaundice

CAUTIONS AND CONTRA-INDICATIONS:
G6PD deficiency

Intravenous administration

Vitamin E deficiency

INTERACTIONS:
Antibiotics

Anticonvulsants

Cefamandole

Cholestyramine

Laxatives

Mineral oils

Oral anti-coagulants

Salicylates

WARFARIN

USES:
Management of thromboembolic disorders,
atrial fibrillation

Prophylaxis in patients with artificial heart
valves (even if pregnant)

(continued)

(WARFARIN continued)

SIDE EFFECTS:

Bleeding	Gut disturbances
Coumarin induced skin necrosis of fat tissue	Hepatic or renal damage
	Mouth ulcers
Discolouration of feet	

Hypersensitivity

Agranulocytosis	Hair loss
Fever	Rash

CAUTIONS AND CONTRA-INDICATIONS:

Atopy [glossary]	Malnutrition
Bacterial endocarditis	Pancreatic disorders
Bleeding tendencies	Radiation exposure
GI tract abnormalities	Risk of CVA eg. hypertension
Heart failure	TB
Hypothyroidism	Thrombocytopenia
Liver disease	Vitamin. C or K deficiency
Malabsorption	

INTERACTIONS (NOT A COMPLETE LIST):

Increased risk of bleeding

Alcohol acute ingestion	Liquid paraffin
Anabolic steroids	NSAIDS, prolonged
Antibiotics	paracetamol
Anti-histamines	Oral hypoglycaemics
Cimetidine	Thyroid hormones
Influenza vaccine	Vitamin E
Lipid-lowering drugs	

Increased risk of clotting

Alcohol, chronic ingestion	Oestrogens
Cabbage and similar vegetables	Potassium
Caffeine	Quinine
Corticosteroids	Vitamins C & K
Nicotine	

Others

Antacids	Anticonvulsants
Antibiotics	

US Classification of Drug Safety in Pregnancy

The FDA (Food and Drug Administration) has established a 'risk scale' for drugs in pregnancy, although this is due to be revised shortly. Not all drugs are included in this scale, as the information is not always available: for example aspirin, paracetamol (acetaminophen). However for established drugs the ratings are a useful guide, more detailed than the information in the BNF.

Category A
No risk indicated from existing studies.

Category B
No information for humans. No problems observed in animal fetuses.

Category C
No information for humans. Adverse effects observed in animal fetuses.
Examples: corticosteroids, baclofen, vitamin D, vitamin B_{12}.

Category D
Possible risk to fetus in humans. However, use is justified where potential benefits outweigh risks.

Examples: warfarin, phenytoin, sodium valproate, diazepam, most drugs prescribed for cancer.

Category X
Drugs to be avoided in pregnant women. Fetal abnormalities reported. Risk identified from animal and/or human studies.

Examples: alcohol, isotretinoin (for acne), oestrogens, androgens, live vaccines such as smallpox, measles, mumps, rubella).

Sources: Mackenry & Salerno, 1995; Malseed et al, 1995.

Glossary

achlorhydria Deficiency in hydrochloric acid production by the stomach.

acidosis A pathological condition resulting from accumulation of acid or loss of base, and characterized by increase in hydrogen ion concentration (and decrease in pH).

adsorption The formation of a layer of a substance on the surface of a solid by chemical attraction.

agonist A substance having a specific cellular affinity that produces a predictable response; also, a chemical capable of stimulating a cell receptor.

agranulocytosis A marked reduction in the number of circulating granular leukocytes, particularly neutrophils. This renders the patient very liable to serious infections. Unrecognized and untreated, these overwhelming infections can be fatal.

AIDS Acquired Immune Deficiency Syndrome, a disease associated with the HIV virus.

alkalosis A pathological condition resulting from accumulation of base or loss of acid, and characterized by decrease in hydrogen ion concentration (and increase in pH).

alpha (α) agonist A drug which stimulates the alpha receptors. These receptors normally respond to norepinephrine/noradrenaline and epinephrine/adrenaline. One of their important functions is the control of blood pressure.

anaesthetic An agent causing reversible loss of sensation.

anaphylaxis A severe hypersensitivity response (allergic reaction) to a chemical introduced into the body. The response is characterized by histamine release in the tissues, causing bronchospasm, swelling and severe hypotension. Immediate treatment is needed to avert fatality.

antagonist A chemical that can occupy a cell receptor without stimulating it and thereby block the action of agonists for that receptor.

antibacterial A substance that inhibits the growth of, or kills, a bacterium.

antibiotic A natural substance that inhibits the growth of, or kills, a bacterium. Sometimes widened to substances that inhibit all micro-organisms.

antifungal A substance that inhibits the growth of, or kills, a fungus.

antimicrobial A substance that inhibits the growth of, or kills, a micro-organism.

antimuscarinic A substance that blocks the actions of the parasympathetic nervous system by acting on the postganglionic muscarinic receptors.

antiviral A substance that inhibits the replication of, or destroys, a virus.

apgar score This system was named after Virginia Apgar, an anaesthetist. It was introduced to standardize the observation of all neonates. It combines measures of heart rate and respiratory effort with observations of muscle tone, skin colour and reflex irritability. A score of 9 or 10 indicates a healthy baby. A score of 4–6 indicates mild or moderate neonatal depression. A non-responsive baby will score 4 or less. Assessments are made one, five and ten minutes after delivery.

aPTT Activated partial thromboplastin time. A coagulation test of the entire coagulation mechanism which detects deficiencies in the formation of thromboplastin (factor Xa). Normal range 30–40 seconds.

atelectasis In adults, collapse of the lungs, usually the lower lobes. At birth, incomplete expansion of the lungs.

atopy/atopic A condition characterized by hypersensitivity responses, including asthma, eczema, hay fever.

autoimmune diseases Disorders of the body's defence system in which components of the immune system attack the body's own tissues. Rheumatoid arthritis and systemic lupus erythematosis are examples.

bacteraemia The presence of bacteria in the blood.

beta (β) lactamase A penicillin-degrading enzyme produced by some bacteria.

beta (β) agonist A drug which stimulates the beta receptors. These receptors normally respond to epinephrine/adrenaline and norepinephrine/noradrenaline. Their important functions include the control of the heart, bronchioles and blood vessels. There are several sub-types of beta receptors. The best studied are the β_1 (mainly in the heart) and β_2 receptors, which are associated with the fright and flight response.

bioequivalence Two forms of a drug are said to be bioequivalent if their rates and extent of absorption of their active ingredients are the same under test conditions.

blood/brain barrier The structure separating the blood from the brain tissue and the cerebro-spinal fluid. It is composed of the capillary endothelium and the astrocyte end-feet. In adults, it protects the brain tissue from fluctuations in the plasma. It is not fully developed in neonates.

broad-spectrum antibiotic An antibiotic that is active against many types of gram-positive and gram-negative bacteria.

capsule A gelatine case surrounding an oral preparation.

cardiac dysrhythmias Disordered rhythms of the heart, usually due to disturbance of the conducting system. They range in severity from benign to lethal. They may be symptomless, or give rise to vague symptoms such as breathlessness or palpitations.

cardiac output Cardiac output is the volume of blood pumped into the dorsal aorta each minute by the left ventricle of the heart. This is the quantity of blood flowing through the circulation each minute, transporting substances (including oxygen and carbon dioxide) to and from the tissues.

chemotherapeutic agent An antimicrobial that is used to treat infections inside the human body.

Common Law This refers to legal principles derived from cases decided in the higher courts, which are then binding on lower courts through a system of precedence. This allows for a degree of certainty in the law to be maintained.

confidence limits/intervals The range of values around the mean, within which the true mean is located.

conjugation The joining of two compounds to produce another compound. The compound produced is usually less toxic than the original. This occurs in the liver, where glucuronic acid is added to drug molecules to make them water soluble, so that they can be eliminated by the kidneys.

contra-indicated Not recommended for clinical use.

cytokines Any soluble factor secreted by cells of the lymphoid system that act as signals to other lymphoid cells.

dystocia Abnormal labour or childbirth.

dystocia, shoulder Due to failure of rotation, after delivery of the baby's head, the shoulders impact on the pelvic brim, with the anterior shoulder trapped under the pubis. Without very prompt action to deliver the baby, intra-partum death will occur.

endothelial cells/endothelium The layer of epithelial cells lining the heart, blood vessels, lymph vessels and serous cavities of the body.

enteric coating A layer of material on the outer surface of a tablet or capsule which prevents dissolution in the stomach, and thereby both delays absorption and protects the lining of the stomach.

entero-hepatic recycling Several substances, including steroids and bile salts, are excreted in the bile and reabsorbed into the liver lower down the intestine via the hepatic protal vein. This recycling and reusing reduces the loss in the faecaes.

enzymes Enzymes are proteins which act as catalysts in biochemical reactions. Each enzyme is specific to one reaction or a group of similar reactions. Catalysts are substances which increase the rate of chemical reactions without undergoing any permanent change.

free radical A free radical is an atom or a group of atoms with an unpaired valence electron. Because of the unpaired electron, free radicals are extremely reactive, and can easily damage cell membranes.

general anaesthetic An anaesthetic causing loss of consciousness in addition to loss of sensation.

glomerular filtration rate (GFR) The quantity of fluid passing into the Bowman's capsules each minute in all nephrons in both kidneys is the glomerular filtration rate. The normal value is about 125 ml/minute or 180 litres/day. Normally, 99 per cent of this is reabsorbed by the renal tubules. GFR is measured by inulin or creatinine clearance. Serum creatinine values give an approximation of GFR.

gram-negative A major class of bacteria that have a thin cell wall and an outer membrane on their surface.

gram-positive A major class of bacteria that have a thick cell wall and no outer membrane on their surface.

ground substance The intercellular matrix of connective tissue in which cells and fibres are embedded. It is composed of mucopolysaccharides/proteoglycans, such as chondroitin-4-sulphate, chondroitin-6-sulphate and hyaluronic acid.

haemolysis Destruction of the red blood cells, liberating haemoglobin into the surrounding fluid.

half-life The time it takes for one-half of an observed change to occur. In pharmacology, the half-life usually referred to is the 'elimination half-life'. Elimination half-life is the time taken for the concentration of the drug in blood or plasma to fall to half its maximum value. For some drugs, elimination half-life has three distinct phases (is triphasic). 1. Distribution phase, where the drug enters the tissues. 2. A phase where the drug is moving from the tissues into the circulation and simultaneously being excreted. 3. Excretion phase, where the drug is removed from the body.

heterozygous Describing an organism with two different alleles (genes) at a given locus on a pair of homologous chromosomes.

homozygous Describing an organism with two identical alleles (genes) at a given locus on a pair of homologous chromosomes.

hypersensitivity A response quantitatively greater than is usual for a given dose.

hypertonic A hypertonic solution has a higher osmotic pressure than normal plasma.

hyponatraemia Serum sodium ion concentration below normal values. In the third trimester these are 133–143 mmol/litre. Serious symptoms develop if serum sodium concentration falls below 120 mmol/l.

hypotonic A hypotonic solution has a lower osmotic pressure than normal plasma.

international normalized ratio (INR) The ratio of the prothrombin time of the patient's blood sample to the prothrombin time of a standard blood sample. The prothrombin time is a measure of the time taken for clot formation when a tissue thromboplastin reagent is added. It effectively measures the activity of prothrombin, fibrinogen and factors V, VII & X.

intrathecal administration The introduction of a drug or other substance into the cerebro-spinal fluid.

ionized Containing ions. An ion is an atom or group of atoms that carries either a positive or a negative charge as a result of either losing or gaining an electron.

isotonic An isotonic solution has the same osmotic pressure as normal plasma.

kernicterus High plasma concentrations of bilirubin in the neonate, leading to neurological damage.

leucocytosis An increased concentration of white blood cells in the circulation. Normal value 4000–11 000 cells/microlitre.

ligand Any substance that binds to a particular type of receptor.

lipophilic Having an affinity for lipids (fats). A lipid is a substance insoluble in water, but soluble in ether; examples include fats, fatty acids, steroids, phospholipids, oils.

macrocytosis Circulating red blood cells are larger than normal. Normal red cell volume is 78–95 femto-litres. The commonest causes of macrocytosis are folate or vitamin B_{12} deficiency.

methaemoglobinaemia Methaemoglobin is formed, in genetically susceptible individuals, when the iron atoms in haemoglobin are oxidized, usually as a result of ingesting oxidizing drugs. Methaemoglobin cannot transport oxygen around the body. Therefore, if it builds up in the circulation (methaemoglobinaemia), the patient will develop a life-threatening cyanotic condition.

Microflora The community of micro-organisms in a micro-environment such as the gut.

Micro-organism An organism that can only be seen with the aid of a microscope.

mOsm/kg (milli-osmoles / kilogram) Unit of measurement for osmotic pressure. In health, human plasma has an osmotic pressure 280–296 mOsm/kg.

MRSA Methicillin-resistant staphylococcus aureus.

narrow-spectrum antibiotic An antibiotic that is active against a narrow range of bacteria.

nocebo Harmful effects brought on by administration of a placebo treatment (see below). Usually common ailments such as headache, nausea.

nystagmus Involuntary rapid movements of the eyeballs. Movements may be horizontal, vertical or rotatory.

obtunding Rendering dull or reducing sensitivity, for example to pain.

opportunistic pathogen A normally harmless micro-organism that can cause disease when the body is weakened.

osmosis The movement of water across a differentially permeable membrane separating two solutions of unequal concentration of solutes or osmotic pressure.

osmotic pressure or osmolality of a solution The force or pressure required to prevent the movement of pure water into that solution. This depends on the number of osmotically active particles in the solution, or its effective concentration.

over-the-counter drug (OTC) A medicine sold directly to the public, without a prescription.

oxytocic An agent which hastens the evacuation of the uterus by increasing contraction of the myometrium.

partial pressure of a gas This refers to mixtures of gases. It is the pressure that gas would exert, if it were present alone, occupying the same volume. The 'partial pressure' is effectively the concentration of the gas.

pathogen A micro-organism that causes disease.

peptidoglycan The polymer which makes up most bacterial cell walls.

pH The pH scale is a logarithmic scale of hydrogen ion concentration expressing the acidity or alkalinity of a solution. A neutral solution at 25°C has a pH of 7. An acid solution has a pH below 7. An alkaline solution has a pH above 7. The pH of normal adult arterial blood is 7.35–7.45. Venous blood has a lower pH.

pharmacodynamics The science and study of the actions and effects of chemicals on living material.

pharmacokinetics The science and study of the factors that determine the amount of a drug present at biologically effective sites at various times after its introduction to a biological system.

placebo An inactive preparation administered in the guise of a therapeutic agent, originally as a placating measure.

polymer A substance made up of large molecules, which consist of repeating units of identical chemical composition (the monomers). Examples include polysaccharides and plastics.

receptor A specialized configuration of molecules on the cell membrane or within the cell which responds to neurotransmitters, hormones, paracrines or drugs with similar structures.

renin-angiotensin-aldosterone axis Renin is secreted by the juxtaglomerular apparatus of the kidneys, in response to changes in blood pressure, salt and water balance and the sympathetic nervous system. Renin triggers the release of several other hormones which regulate blood pressure and salt and water balance. See Chapter 7, beta$_2$ adrenoreceptor agonists.

serum Plasma with the clotting factors removed.

shock Inadequate delivery of oxygen to the tissues, due to acute failure of the peripheral circulation. Causes include: excessive fluid loss such as haemorrhage; acute cardiac failure; sepsis; and adrenal failure.

SIADH Syndrome Inappropriate ADH (anti-diuretic hormone). Production of ADH in excess of the body's requirements, leading to water retention and eventually water intoxication.

side effect   A physiological effect other than that for which a given drug is administered.

status epilepticus   A state of repeated epileptic fits with no period of consciousness between them. About 30 per cent of survivors have permanent brain damage.

sympathomimetic   A sympathomimetic is a drug whose actions resemble those of the stimulant neurotransmitters of the sympathetic nervous system.

synapse / synaptic junction   The contact between two neurones, where action potentials are transmitted from one neurone to the next.

synaptic inhibition   Inhibiting the transmission of excitatory signals between neurones at the synapse.

tablet   A preparation of powdered drug compressed or moulded into discs. In addition to the active drug, a tablet usually contains excipients, such as binders or lubricants.

teratogen   A chemical that causes malformation of a fetus.

teratogenesis   Teratogenesis is the impaired development of fetal organs, leading to structural or functional abnormalities

thrombocytopenia   A concentration of platelets in the circulation below the normal limits (150 000–400 000/micro-litre). If the concentration falls below 50 000/micro-litre, severe bleeding disorders will ensue.

thrombosis   Blood vessel occlusion by a platelet aggregate and/or a fibrin clot.

thromboxanes   Derivatives of the phospholipids of plasma membranes, which promote platelet aggregation and vasoconstriction.

tocolytic   An agent which delays evacuation of the uterus by inhibiting contraction of the uterine muscle.

tolerance   Decreased responsiveness acquired after exposure to a drug.

tort   A civil wrong for which one may seek compensation in a court of law.

underpowered   This is a term used in statistics. It refers to studies with too few subjects to be able to determine whether there or not there are statistically significant differences between the study groups in the variable under consideration. Studies examining the occurrence of rare events, such as eclamptic fits or certain congenital malformations, must recruit large numbers of women to avoid being underpowered.

vaccine   A suspension of inactivated or dead micro-organisms that stimulates the body to develop immunity to a disease.

venous return   This is the quantity of blood flowing into the right atrium each minute. Generally, this is equal to the cardiac output.

ventilation   The ventilation rate is the volume of air breathed in per minute, that is, the volume of air inspired times the number of breaths per minute.

References

ABPI (2000) *Compendium of Data Sheets and Summaries of Product Characteristics 1999–2000.* London, Datapharm Publications Ltd.

Abramsky, L., Botting, B., Chapple, J. & Stone, D. (1999) Has advice on periconceptual folate supplementation reduced neural tube defect? *The Lancet* (research letter):354:998.

Adair, C., Weeks, J., Barrilleaux, S., Edwards, M., Burlison, K. & Lewis, D. (1998) Oral or vaginal misoprostol administration for induction of labor. *Obstetrics and Gynecology*:92:5:810–3.

Alberta Medical Association (1993) Clinical practice guidelines: guidelines for the use of commercially prepared PgE2 gel as a cervical ripening agent. Committee on Reproductive Care of the Alberta Medical Association: Alberta http://www.amda.ab.ca/cpgs/pge2gel.htm

Aldrich, C.J., D'Antona, D., Spencer, J., Wyatt, J.S., Peebles, D.M., Delpy, D.T. & Reynolds, E.O.R. (1995) The effect of maternal posture on fetal cerebral oxygenation during labour. *British Journal of Obstetrics and Gynaecology*:102:14–19.

Alef, K. (1999) Clostridium difficile-associated disease. *Journal of Nurse Midwifery*:44:19–29.

Alfirevic, Z., Howarth, G. & Gaussmann, A. (2000) Oral misoprostol for induction of labour with a viable fetus. Oxford, *The Cochrane Pregnancy and Childbirth Database*, Issue 2 Update software. Accessed Nov 2000.

Allman, A.C., Genevier, E.S., Johnson, M.R. & Steer, P.J. (1996) Head-to-cervix force: an important physiological variable in labour. *British Journal of Obstetrics and Gynaecology*:103:763–8.

Al-Mufti, R., Morey, R., Shennan, A. & Morgan, B. (1997) Blood pressure and fetal heart rate changes with patient-controlled combined spinal epidural analgesia while ambulating in labour. *British Journal of Obstetrics and Gynaecology*:104:554–8.

Amant, F., Spitz, B., Timmerman, D., Corremans, A. & Assche, F. (1999) Misoprostol compared with methylergometrine for the prevention of postpartum haemorrhage. *British Journal of Obstetrics and Gynaecology*:106:1066–70.

Amedee-Manesme, O., Lambert, W.E., Alagille, D. & De Leenheer, A.P. (1992) Pharmacokinetics and safety of a new solution of vitamin K1(20) in children with cholestasis. *Journal of Paediatric Gastroenterology and Nutrition*:14:160–5.

American Journal of Hospital Pharmacy (1994) ASHP therapeutic position statement on the institutional use of 0.9% sodium chloride injection to maintain patency of peripheral indwelling intermittent infusion devices. *American Journal of Hospital Pharmacy*:51:1572–4.

Andrew, M., Blanchette, U.S., Adams, M., Ali, K., Barnard, D., Chan, K.W., De Veber, L.B., Esseltine, D., Israels, S., Korbinsky, N., Luke, B., Milner, R.A., Woloski, M.R. & Vegh, P. (1992) A multicenter study of the treatment of childhood chronic idiopathic thrombocytopenia purpura with Anti-D. *Journal of Paediatrics*:120:522.

Ansell, P., Bull, D. & Roman, E. (1996) Childhood leukaemia and intramuscular vitamin K: findings from a case control study. *BMJ*:313:204–5.

Anthony, D. (1999) *Understanding Advanced Statistics.* Edinburgh, Churchill Livingstone.

Arfeen, Z., Armstron, P.J. & Whitfield, A. (1994) The effects of Entonox and epidural analgesia on arterial oxygen saturation of women in labour. *Anaesthesia*:49:1:32–4.

Arkoosh, V. (1991) Guidelines for regional anesthesia in obstetrics: viewpoint of an anesthesiologist in a tertiary care center. Cleveland Clinic Foundation, sector for anaesthesia for obstetrics, http://www.anes.ccf.org:8080/soap/guideline.htm

Armand, S., Jasson, J., Talafre, M. & Tison, C. (1993) The effects of regional analgesia on the newborn. In: Reynolds, F. (ed.) *Effects on the Baby of Maternal Analgesia and Anaesthesia.* Saunders, London.

Arner, S. & Meyerson, B. (1988) Lack of analgesic effect of opioids on neuropathic and idiopathic forms of pain. *Pain*:33:11–23.

Assaley, J., Baron, J. & Cibils, L. (1998) Effects of magnesium sulphate infusion upon clotting parameters in patients with pre-eclampsia. *Journal of Perinatal Medicine*:26:2:115–19.

Austin, M. & Mitchell, P. (1998) Psychotropic medications in pregnant women: treatment dilemmas. *Medical Journal of Australia*:169:8:428–31.

Babe, K. & Serafin, W. (1996) Histamine, bradykinin and their antagonists. In: Hardman, J., Limbard, L., Molinoff, P., Ruddon, R. & Goodman Gilman, A. (eds) *Goodman & Gilman's: The Pharmacological Basis of Therapeutics*, 9th edition. New York, McGraw-Hill.

Badawi, N., Kurinczuk, J., Mackenzie, C., Keogh, J., Burton, P., Pemberton, P. & Stanley, F. (2000) Maternal thyroid disease: a risk factor for newborn encephalopathy in term infants. *British Journal of Obstetrics and Gynaecology*:107:798–801.

Badr, K. & Brenner, B. (1991) Vascular injury to the kidney. In: Wilson, J., Braunwald, E., Isselbacher, K., Petersdorf, R., Martin, J., Fauci, A. & Root, R. (eds) *Harrison's Principles of Internal Medicine*, 12th edition. New York, McGraw-Hill.

Baldessarini, R. (1996) Drugs and the treatment of psychiatric disorders: psychosis and anxiety. In: Hardman, J., Limbard, L., Molinoff, P., Ruddon, R. & Goodman Gilman, A. (eds) *Goodman & Gilman's: The Pharmacological Basis of Therapeutics*, 9th edition. New York, McGraw-Hill.

Bancroft, K., Tuffnell, D., Mason, G., Rogerson, L. & Mansfield, M. (2000) A randomised controlled pilot study of the management of gestational impaired glucose tolerance. *British Journal of Obstetrics and Gynaecology*:107:959–63.

Barbour, L., Kick, S., Steiner, J., LoVerde, M., Heddleston, L., Lear, J., Baron, A. & Barton, P. (1994) A prospective study of heparin-induced osteoporosis in pregnancy using bone densitometry. *American Journal of Obstetrics and Gynaecology*:170:862–9.

Barker, D., Bull, A., Osmond, C. & Simmonds, S. (1990) Fetal and placental size and risk of hypertension in adult life, *BMJ*:301:259–62.

Barrett, J., Whittaker, P., Williams, J. & Lind, T. (1994) Absorption of non-haem iron from food during normal pregnancy. *BMJ*:309:79–82.

Barzo, B., Moretti, M., Mareels, G., van Tittelboom, T. & Koren, G. (1999) Reporting bias in retrospective ascertainment of drug-induced embryopathy. *Lancet*:354:1700–1.

Baxi, L.V., Petrie, R.H. & James, L.H. (1988) Human fetal oxygenation, heart rate variability and uterine activity following maternal administration of meperidine. *Journal of Perinatal Medicine*:16:23–30.

Bayer plc (1995) Adalat. In: *ABPI Data Sheet Compendium*. London, Datapharm Publications.

Beecher, H. & Boston, M. (1955) The powerful placebo. *JAMA*:159:1602–6.

Begley, C. (1990a) A comparison of 'active' and 'physiolgocial' management of the third stage of labour. *Midwifery*:6:3–17.

Begley, C. (1990b) The effect of Ergometrine on breast feeding. *Midwifery*:6:60–72.

Begley, C. (1990c) The effect of Ergometrine on breast feeding. (reply to letter) *Midwifery*:6:232–3.

Beischer, N., Mackay, E. & Colditz, P. (1997) *Obstetrics and the Newborn*, 3rd edition. London, Saunders.

Bell, G. (1996) Psychological medicine. In: Axford, J. (ed.) *Medicine*. Oxford, Blackwell, 15.1–25.

Bem, M., Roddam, P. & Wheatley, R. (1996) Patient controlled analgesia in critically ill patients. *Care of the Critically Ill*:12:1:10–14.

Ben-Arush, M. & Berant, M. (1996) Retention of drugs in venous access port chamber: a note of caution. *BMJ*:312:496–7.

Bennett, V.R. & Brown, L.K. (1993) *Myles Textbook for Midwives*. Edinburgh, Churchill Livingstone.

Bhatia, S.C. & Bhatia, S.K. (1999) Depression in women: diagnostic and treatment considerations. *American Family Physician*:60:239–40.

Blair, D.T. & Dauner, A. (1992) Extrapyramidal symptoms are serious side-effects of antipsychotics and other drugs. *Nurse Practitioner*:17:11:56–67.

Blair, F., Tassone, S., Pearman, C., St Cyr, M. & Rayburn, W. (1998) Inducing labor with a sustained-release PGE2 vaginal insert. *Journal of Reproductive Medicine*:43:5:408–12.

Blanch, G., Lavender, T., Walkinshaw, S. & Alfirevic, Z. (1998) Dysfunctional labour: a randomised trial. *British Journal of Obstetrics and Gynaecology*:105:117–20.

Bloomfield, T. (1996) Principles of prescribing in pregnancy. *Prescriber*:7:1:66–70.

Blume, W.T. (1997) Epilepsy: advances in management. *European Neurology*:38:198–208.

BOC (1995) *Entonox Data Sheet*. Guildford, BOC Gases Medical.

BOC (1996) *Entonox: Suggested Protocol Document*. Guildford, BOC Gases Medical.

Bootman, L. & Milne, R. (1996) Costs, innovation and efficiency in anti-infective therapy. *Pharmacoeconomics*:9:suppl 1:31–9.

Boseley, S. (1999) Prozac: can it make you kill? *The Guardian Weekend*:30 October:13–16.

Boulvain, M., Stan, C. & Irion, O. (2000) Elective delivery in diabetic pregnant women. *Cochrane Database Systematic Review*: (issue 2) Update Software, Oxford, accessed July 2000.

Bowdle, T. (1998) Adverse effects of opioid agonists and agonist-antagonists in anaesthesia. *Drug Safety*:19:3:173–89.

Bowman, J.M. & Pollock, J.M. (1987) Failures of intravenous Rh immune globulin prophylaxis: an analysis of the reasons for such failures. *Transfusion Medicine Reviews*:1:101–12.

Bramadat, I.J. (1994) Induction of labor: an integrated review. *Health Care for Women International*:15:2:135–48.

Brancazio, L., Laifer, S. & Schwartz, T. (1997) Peak expiratory flow in normal pregnancy. *Obstetrics and Gynecology*:89:383–6.

Breathnach, S. (1993) Management of drug eruptions. *Update*:19:10:553–61.

Brennan, A. (1991) The enigma of puerperal psychosis. *Nursing Standard*:6:1:33–6.

British National Formulary (BNF) (2000) *British National Formulary no. 40*. London, British Medical Association and the Royal Pharmaceutical Society of Great Britain.

Brocklehurst, P., Gates, S., McHarg, K.M., Alfirevic, Z. & Chamberlain, G. (1999) Are we prescribing multiple courses of antenatal corticosteroids? A survey of practice in the UK. *British Journal of Obstetrics and Gynaecology*:106:977–9.

Broussard, C. & Richter, J. (1998) Treating gastro-oesophageal reflux diseaase during pregnancy and lactation: what are the safest therapy options? *Drug Safety*:19:4:325–37.

Brown, M. (1997) Pre-eclampsia: a case of nerves? *The Lancet*:349:297–8.

Brown, M. & Buddle, M. (1996) Hypertension in pregnancy. *Med. J. Australia*:165:7:360–5.

Brownridge, P. (1991) Treatment options for the relief of pain during childbirth. *Drugs*: 41:1:69–80.

Brucker, M. & Faucher, M. (1997) Pharmacologic management of common gastrointestinal health problems in women. *Journal of Nurse Midwifery*:42:3:145–62.

Brunton, L. (1996) Agents affecting gastrointestinal water flux and motility: emesis and antiemetics: bile acids and pancreatic enzymes. In: Hardman, J., Limbard, L., Molinoff, P., Ruddon, R. & Goodman Gilman, A. (eds) *Goodman & Gilman's: The Pharmacological Basis of Therapeutics*, 9th edition. New York, McGraw-Hill, 917–36.

Buchan, P.C. (1979) Pathogenesis of neonatal hyperbilirubinaemia after induction of labour with oxytocin. *BMJ*:2:1255–7.

Buckley, K. (1990) Abnormalities of the postpartum period. In: Buckley, K. & Kulb, N. (eds) *High Risk Maternity Nursing Manual*. Baltimore, Williams and Wilkins.

Bunn, H. (1991) Disorders of haemoglobin. In: Wilson, J., Braunwald, E., Isselbacher, K. et al *Harrison's Principles of Internal Medicine*, 12th edition. New York, McGraw Hill, 1543–52.

Bushnell, T. & Justins, D. (1993) Choosing the right analgesic. *Drugs*:46:394–408.

Busowski, J.D. & Parsons, M.T. (1995) Amniotomy to induce labor. *Clinical Obstetrics and Gynecology*:38:2:232–45.

Byrne, B. (2001) Management of epilepsy in pregnancy. In: Bonnar, J. (ed.) *Recent Advances in Obstetrics and Gynaecology 21*. Edinburgh, Churchill Livingstone. 21–34.

Byrne, C., Saxton, D., Pelikan, P. & Nugent, P. (1986) *Laboratory Tests: Implications for Nursing Care*. Menlo Park, Addison-Wesley.

Byron, M. (1995) Treatment of rheumatic diseases. In: Rubin, P. (ed.) *Prescribing in Pregnancy*. London, BMJ Group. 59–71.

Cammu, H. & Eeckhout, E.V. (1996) A randomised controlled trial of early versus delayed use of amniotomy and oxytocin infusion in nulliparous labour. *British Journal of Obstetrics and Gynaecology*:103:313–18.

Campbell, D., Zwack, R., Crone, L. & Yip, R. (2000) Ambulatory labor epidural analgesia: bupivacaine versus ropivacaine. *Anesthetic Analgesia*:90:6:1384–9.

Campbell, S. & Lees, C. (eds) (2000) *Obstetrics by Ten Teachers*, 17th edition. London, Arnold.

Campbell, W. & Halushka, P. (1996) Lipid-derived autacoids. In: Hardman, J., Limbard, L., Molinoff, P., Ruddon, R. & Goodman Gilman, A. (eds) *Goodman & Gilman's: The Pharmacological Basis of Therapeutics*, 9th edition. New York, McGraw-Hill.

Canales, E., Garrido, J., Zarate, A., Mason, M. & Soria, J. (1976) Effect of ergonovine on prolactin secretion and milk letdown. *Obstetrics and Gynecology*:48:228–9.

Cao, Z., Bideau, R., Valdes, R. & Elin, R. (1999) Acute hypermagnesemia and respiratory arriest following infusion of MgSO4 for tocolysis. *Clinica Chimica Acta*:285:191–3.

Capogna, G. & Celleno, D. (1993) The effects of anaesthetic agents on the newborn. In: Reynolds, F. *Effects on the Baby of Maternal Analgesia and Anaesthesia*. London, Saunders, 221–37.

Capogna, G., Celleno, D., Fusco, P., Lyons, G. & Columb, M. (1999) Relative potencies of bupivacaine and ropivacaine for analgesia in labour. *British Journal of Anaesthesia*:82:3:371–3.

Capogna, G., Celleno, D., Lyons, G., Columb, M. & Fusco, P. (1998) Minimum local analgesic concentration of extradural bupivacaine increase with progression in labour. *British Journal of Anaesthesia*:80:1:11–13.

Cappell, M. & Garcia, A. (1998) Gastric and duodenal ulcers during pregnancy. *Gastroenterological Clinics of North America*:27:1:169–95.

Carli, F., Creagh-Barry, P., Gordan, H., Logue, M.M. & Dore, C.J. (1993) Does epidural analgesia influence the mode of delivery in primiparae managed actively? *International. Journal of Obstetric Anesthesia*:2:15–20.

Carlson, J. & Byington, K. (1998) Fundamental principles of pharmacology. In: Williams, B. & Baer, C. (eds) *Essentials of Clinical Pharmacology in Nursing*, 3rd edition. Springhouse, Pennsylvania, Springhouse Corporation, 11–30.

Carr, D. & Goudas, L. (1999) Acute Pain. *Lancet*:353:2151–8.

Carson, R. (1996) The administration of analgesics. *Modern Midwife*:Nov.:12–16.

Carstoniu, J., Levytam, S. & Norman, P. (1994) Nitrous oxide in early labour. Safety and analgesic efficacy assessed by a double-blind, placebo-controlled study. *Anesthesiology*:80:1:30–35.

Casson, I., Clarke, C., Howard, C., McKendrick, O., Pennycook, S., Pharoah, P., Platt, M., Stanisstreet, M., van Velszen, D. & Walkinshaw, S. (1997) Outcomes of pregnancy in insulin dependent diabetic women: results of a five year population cohort study. *BMJ*:315:275–8.

Catterall, W. & Mackie, K. (1996) Local anaesthetics. In: Hardman, J., Limbard, L., Molinoff, P., Ruddon, R. & Goodman Gilman, A. (eds) *Goodman & Gilman's: The Pharmacological Basis of Therapeutics*, 9th edition. New York, McGraw-Hill, 349–60.

Cederholm, I. (1997) Preliminary risk-benefit analysis of ropivacaine in labour and following surgery. *Drug Safety*:16:6:391–402.

Chaim, W., Bashiri, A., Bar-David, J., Shoham-Vardi, I. & Mazor, M. (2000) Prevalence and clinical significance of postpartum endometritis and wound infection. *Infectious Disease in Obstetrics and Gynecology*:8:2:77–82.

Chamberlain, G. (1975) *Lecture Notes on Obstetrics*, 3rd edition. Oxford, Blackwell Scientific.

Chamberlain, G., Gibbings, C.R. & Dewhurst, J. (1989) *Illustrated Textbook of Obstetrics*. New York, Gower Medical Publishing.

Chamberlain, G. & Zander, L. (1999) Induction. *BMJ*:318:995–8.

Chambers, C., Anderson, P., Thomas, R., Dick, L., Felix, R., Johnson, K. & Jones, K.L. (1999) Weight gain in infants breastfed by mothers who take fluoxetine. *Pediatrics*:104:5:1010–15.

Chambers, C., Johnson, K., Dick, L., Felix, R. & Jones, K.L. (1996) Birth outcomes in pregnancy women taking fluoxetine. *New England Journal of Medicine*:335:1010–15.

Chambers, H. & Sande, M. (1996) Antimicrobial agents – general considerations. In: Hardman, J., Limbard, L., Molinoff, P., Ruddon, R. & Goodman Gilman, A. (eds) *Goodman & Gilman's the Pharmacological Basis of Therapeutics*, 9th edition. New York, McGraw-Hill, 1029–56.

Chappell, L., Poulton, L., Halligan, A. & Shennan, A. (1999) Lack of consistency in research papers over the definition of pre-eclampsia. *British Journal of Obstetrics and Gynaecology*:106:983–5.

Chaudron, L. & Jefferson, J. (2000) Mood stabilisers during breastfeeding. *Journal of Clinical Psychiatry*:61:79–90.

Chen, F.P., Chang, S.D. & Chuu, K.K. (1995) Expectant management in severe pre-eclampsia: does magnesium sulfate prevent the development of eclampsia? *Acta Obstetricia et Gynecologica Scandinavia*:74:181–5.

Cherny, N. (1996) Opioid analgesics. *Drugs*:51:713–37.

Chetley, A. (1995) *Problem Drugs*. London, Zed Books.

Chien, P., Khan, K. & Arnott, N. (1996) Magnesium sulphate in the treatment of eclampsia and pre-eclampsia: an overview of the evidence from randomised trials. *British Journal of Obstetrics and Gynaecology*:103:1085–91.

Choy, J. (2000) Mortality from peripartum meningitis. *Anaesthesia and Intensive Care*:28: 328–30.

Chrubasik, J., Chrubasik, S. & Martin, E. (1992) Patient-controlled spinal opiate analgesia in terminal cancer. *Drugs*:43:799–804.

Clark, A.J. (1933) *The Mode of Action of Drugs on Cells*. London, Edward Arnold.

Clark, D. & Lipworth, B. (1997) Dose-response of inhaled drugs in asthma. *Clinical Pharmacokinetics*:32:1:58–74.

Clark, J. (1995) Current management of thyroid disease. *Prescriber*:6:5:31–42.

Clarke, C.A. & Sheppard, P.M. (1965) Prevention of rhesus haemolytic disease. *Lancet:* 1965;ii:343.

CLASP Collaborative Group (1994) A randomised trial of low-dose aspirin for the prevention and treatment of pre-eclampsia among 9364 pregnant women. *Lancet*:343:619–29.

Clayton, B. & Stock, Y. (1993) *Basic Pharmacology for Nurses*. 10th edition, London, Mosby.

Clayworth, S. (2000) The nurse's role during oxytocin administration. *MCN: American Journal of Maternal and Child Nursing*:25:2:80–5.

Clyburn, P. & Rosen, M. (1993) The effects of opioid and inhalational analgesia on the newborn. In: Reynolds, F. *Effects on the Baby of Maternal Analgesia and Anaesthesia*. London, Saunders, 169–90.

Cochrane, G. & Rees, P. (1989) *A Colour Atlas of Asthma*. London, Wolfe Medical.

Coetzee, E., Dommisse, J. & Anthony, J. (1998) A randomised controlled trial of intravenous magnesium sulphate versus placebo in the management of women with severe pre-eclampsia. *British Journal of Obstetrics and Gynaecology*:105:300–3.

Cole, P.V. (1975) Entonox at St Bartholomew's Hospital. In: Proceedings of Symposium on Entonox held at St Bartholomew's Hospital, 1975, London. In: *Entonox Digest*. London, Medishield.

Collins v Hertfordshire County Council (1947) 1 All ER 633.

Commission on Classification and Terminology of the International League against Epilepsy (1989) *Epilepsia*:25:582–93.

Congenital Disabilities (Civil Liability) Act 1976.

Contreras, M. (1998) The prevention of Rh haemolytic disease of the fetus and newborn. *British Journal of Obstetrics and Gynaecology*:105:Supplement 18:7–10.

Conway, G. & Betteridge, D. (1996) Endocrine disease. In: Axfor, J. (ed.) *1996 Medicine*. Oxford, Blackwell Science: 12.1–12.50.

Cook, C., Spurrett, B. & Murray, H. (1999) A randomized clinical trial comparing oral misoprostol with synthetic oxytocin or syntometrine in the third stage of labour. *Australian and New Zealand Journal of Obstetrics and Gynecology*:39:4:414–19.

Cornelissen, M., von Kries, R., Loughnan, P. & Schubiger, G. (1997) Prevention of vitamin K deficiency bleeding: efficacy of different multiple oral dose schedules of vitamin K. *European Journal of Paediatrics*:156:2:414–19.

Cousins, D.H. (1994) Stop these parenteral blunders. *Hospital Pharmacy Practice*: 4:10:387–9.

Cousins, D.H. (1995) A patient dies after receiving vancomycin. *Hospital Pharmacy Practice*:5:5:227–8.

Cousins, D.H. (1996) Medication errors. epidural analgesia needs you. *Pharmacy in Practice*: 6:2:53.

Coutts, A. (2000) Nutrition and the life cycle: maternal nutrition and pregnancy. *British Journal of Nursing*:9:1133–8.

Coverdale, J.H., Chervenak, F., McCullough, L. & Bayer, T. (1996) Ethically justified clinically comprehensive guidelines for the management of depressed pregnant patients. *American Journal of Obstetrics & Gynaecology*:174:169–73.

Cox, J., Holden, J. & Sagovsky, R. (1987) Detection of postnatal depression. Development of the 10-item Edinburgh Postnatal Depression Scale. *British Journal of Psychiatry*:150: 782–6.

Cox, J. & Nicholls, K. (1996) Prescribing psychotropic drugs for pregnant patients. *Prescribers' Journal*:36:4:192–7.

Crowell, M.K., Hill, P. & Humenick, S. (1994) Relationship between obstetric analgesia and time of effective breast feeding. *Journal of Nurse-Midwifery*:39:3:150–6.

Crowley, P. (1999) Corticosteroids prior to preterm delivery. In: *The Cochrane Database of Systematic Reviews*. Issue 3. P.14 Update software, Oxford. Accessed July 2000.

Crowther, C. (1990) Magnesium sulphate versus diazepam in the management of eclampsia: a randomised controlled trial. *British Journal of Obstetrics and Gynaecology*:97:110–17.

Crowther, C.A. & Keirse, M. (2000) Anti-D administration for preventing rhesus alloimmunisation (Cochrane Review). In: *The Cochrane Library*:1, 2000. Oxford:Update Software. http://www.update-software.com.cochrane.htm

CSM (Committee on Safety of Medicines) (1998) Focus on corticosteroids. *Current Problems in Pharmacovigilance*:24:5–10.

Cuervo, L., Rodreguez, M. & Delgado, M. (2000) Enemas during labor. *Cochrane Database Systematic Review*: (issue 2) Software Update, Oxford. accessed July 2000.

Cuskelly, G., McNulty, H. & Scott, J. (1996) Effect of increasing dietary folate on red-cell folate: implications for prevention of neural tube defects. *The Lancet*:347:657–9.

Czarnocka, J. & Slade, P. (2000) Prevalence and predictors of post-traumatic stress symptoms following childbirth. *British Journal of Clinical Psychology*:39:35–51.

Czeizel, A. & Dudas, I. (1992) Prevention of the first occurrence of neural-tube defects by periconceptual vitamin supplementation. *New England Journal of Medicine*:327:1832–5.

Dahlman, T.C. (1993) Osteoporotic fractures and the recurrence of thromboembolism during pregnancy and the puerperium in 184 women undergoing thromboprophylaxis with heparin. *American Journal of Obstetrics and Gynecology*:168:1265–70.

Dahlman, T.C., Sjoberg, H. & Ringertz, H. (1994) Bone mineral density during long-term prophylaxis with heparin in pregnancy. *American Journal of Obstetrics and Gynecology*: 170:1315–20.

Dailland, P. (1993) Analgesia and anaesthesia and breast feeding. In: Reynolds, F. (ed.) *Effects on the Baby of Maternal Analgesia and Anaesthesia*. London, Saunders.

Daly v Wolverhampton Health Authority (1986) CLY 1050.

Daly, S., Mills, J., Molloy, A., Conley, M., Lee, Y., Kirke, P., Weir, D. & Scott, J. (1997) Minimum effective dose of folic acid for food fortification to prevent neural tube defects. *The Lancet*:350:1666–9.

Dargaville, P. & Campbell, N. (1998) Overdose of ergometrine in the newborn infant. *Journal of Paediatric Child Health*:34:1:83–9.

Darroca, R., Buttino, L., Miller, J. & Khamis, H. (1996) Prostaglandin E2 gel for cervical ripening in patients with an indication for delivery. *Obstetrics and Gynecology*:87:228–30.

Davis, N.M. (1992) Local and topical anaesthetic agents. In: Baer, C. & Williams, B. (eds) *Clinical Pharmacology and Nursing*, 2nd edition. Springhouse, Pennsylvania, Springhouse Corporation.

Davis, S. & Granner, D. (1996) Insulin and the pharmacology of the endocrine pancreas. In: Hardman, J., Limbard, L., Molinoff, P., Ruddon, R., Goodman Gilman, A. (eds) *Goodman & Gilman's: The Pharmacological Basis of Therapeutics*, 9th edition. New York, McGraw-Hill, 1487–517.

Davis, W., Wells, S., Kuller, J. & Thorp, J. (1997) Analysis of the risks associated with calcium channel blockade: implications for the obstetrician-gynecologist. *Obstetric and Gynecological Survey*:52:198–201.

Dawood, M.Y. (1995) Pharmacologic stimulation of uterine contraction. *Seminars in Perinatology*:19:1:73–83.

Dean, B. (1996) Are incompatibilities a problem? *Pharmacy in Practice*:November:371–2.

De Arcos, F., Gratacos, E., Palacio, M. & Cararach, V. (1996) Toxic hepatitis: a rare complication associated with the use of ritodrine during pregnancy. *Acta Obstetricia et Gynecologica Scandinavica*:75:4:340–2.

De Groot, A., van Dongen, P., Vree, T., Hekster, Y. & van Roosmalen, J. (1998) Ergot alkaloids. *Drugs*:56:523–35.

de Jong, P., Johanson, R., Baxen, P., Adrians, V., Westhuisen, S. & Jones, P.W. (1997) Randomised trial comparing the upright and supine positions for the second stage of labour. *British Journal of Obstetrics and Gynaecology*.104:567–71.

Dennesen, P., Bonten, M. & Weinstein, R. (1998) Multiresistant bacteria as a hospital epidemic problem. *Annals of Medicine*:30:2:176–85.

De Swiet, M. (1995a) Anticoagulants. In: Rubin, P. (ed.) *Prescribing in Pregnancy*, 2nd edition. London, BMJ Group.

De Swiet, M. (1995b) *Medical Disorders in Obstetric Practice*, 3rd edition. Oxford, Blackwell Science.

De Swiet, M. (2000) Maternal blood pressure and birthweight. *Lancet*:355:81–2.

Dev, V. & Krupp, P. (1995) Adverse event profile and safety of clozapine. *Review of Contemporary Pharmacotherapeutics*:6:197–208.

Dever, L., China, C., Eng, R., O'Donovan, C. & Johanson, W. (1998) Vancomycin-resistant *Enterococcus faecium* in a Veterans' Affairs Medical Center: association with antibiotic usage. *American Journal of Infection Control*:26:1:40–6.

Dewan, D. & Cohen, S. (1994) Epidural analgesia and the incidence of Caesarean section. *Anesthesiology*:80:6:1189–92.

Dharmasena, R., Salvage, C. & Godman, B. (1995) Developing a 'standard' for midwives for medically induced labour with prostaglandin E2 gel. *British Journal of Midwifery*:3:2:92–8.

DHSS (1986) *Neighbourhood Nursing – a Focus for Care*. Committee headed by Cumberlege, J., London, HMSO.

Dichter, M. (1991) The epilepsies and convulsive disorders. In: Wilson, J. et al (eds) *Harrison's Principles and Practice of Medicine*. New York, McGraw Hill.

Dickersin, K. (1989) Pharmacological control of pain during labour. In: Chalmers, I., Enkin, M. & Kierse, M.J.N.C. (eds) *Effective Care in Pregnancy and Childbirth*. Oxford, Oxford Medical, 913–50.

DoH (1991) *Report on Confidential Enquiries into Maternal Deaths in the United Kingdom 1985–7*. London, HMSO.

DoH (1994) *Report on Confidential Enquiries into Maternal Deaths in the United Kingdom 1988–90*. London, HMSO.

DoH (1996) *Report on Confidential Enquiries into Maternal Deaths in the United Kingdom 1991–3*. London, HMSO.

DoH (1998) *Why Mothers Die. Report on Confidential Enquiries into Maternal Deaths in the United Kingdom 1994–6*. London, HMSO.

(DoH) Department of Health (1999) *Review of Prescribing, Supply & Administration of Medicines: Final Report* (Chair: Dr June Crown). London, DOH.

DoH & National Assembly of Wales (2000) *Sale, Supply and Administration of Medicines by Health Professionals Under Patient Group Directions – Consultation on Draft Guidance* (CNO (00) 04).

DoH & RCN (1994) *Good Practice in the Administration of Depot Neuroleptics: A Guidance Document for Mental Health and Practice Nurses*. London, HMSO.

Donaldson, J.O. (1995) Neurologic disorders. In: de Swiet, M. (ed.) *Medical Disorders in Obstetric Practice*, 3rd Edition. Oxford, Blackwell Science, 535–9.

Donders, G. (2000) Treatment of sexually transmitted bacterial diseases in pregnant women. *Drugs*:59:477–85.

Dornhorst, A. & Frost, G. (2000) Jelly-beans, only a colourful distraction from gestational glucose-challenge tests. *Lancet*:355:674.

Dounas, M., O'Kelly, B., Jamali, S., Mercier, F. & Benhamou, D. (1996) Maternal and fetal effects of adrenaline with bupivacaine (0.25%) for epidural analgesia during labour. *European Journal of Anaesthesiology*:13:6:594–8.

Downing, J. & Ramasubramanian, R. (1993) Effects of analgesia and anaesthesia on fetal acid-base balance and respiratory gas exchange. In: Reynolds, F. (ed.) *Effects on the Baby of Maternal Analgesia and Anaesthesia*. London, Saunders, 125–47.

Dresser, G., Spence, J. & Bailey, D. (2000) Pharmacokinetic-pharmacodynamic consequences and clinical relevance of cytochrome P450 3A4 inhibition. *Clinical Pharmacokinetics*: 38:41–57.

Drife, J.O. (1996) Choice and instrumental delivery. *British Journal of Obstetrics and Gynaecology*:103:7:608–11.

Drug and Therapeutics Bulletin (1995) The drug treatment of patients with schizophrenia. *Drug and Therapeutics Bulletin*:33:11:81–6.

Drug and Therapeutics Bulletin (1998) Which vitamin K preparation for the newborn? *Drug and Therapeutics Bulletin*:36:3:17–19.

Drugs and Therapy Perspectives (1993a) Antiemetic selection depends on cause of emesis. *Drugs and Therapy Perspectives*:1:8:9–11.

Drugs and Therapy Perspectives (1993b) Opioid analgesics interact with a variety of drugs. *Drugs and Therapy Perspectives*:2:2:12–14.

Drugs and Therapy Perspectives (1996) Plenty of scope for individualised pain control during labour and delivery. *Drugs and Therapy Perspectives*:7:4:7–10.

Drugs and Therapy Perspectives (1997) Asthma in pregnancy. *Drugs and Therapy Perspectives*:9:3:5–7.

Duley, L. (1996) Magnesium sulphate regimens for women with eclampsia: messages from the Collaborative Eclampsia Trial. *British Journal of Obstetrics and Gynaecology*:103:103–5.

Duley, L. (1999) Aspirin for preventing and treating pre-eclampsia. *BMJ*:318:751–2.

Duley, L., Gulmezoglu, A. & Henderson-Smart, D. (2000) Anticonvulsants for women with pre-eclampsia. *The Cochrane Pregnancy and Childbirth Database* (issue 2). Oxford, Update Software.

Duley, L. & Neilson, J. (1999) Magnesium sulphate and pre-eclampsia. *BMJ*:319:3–4.

Dwyer v Rodrick and Others (1983) 127 Sol Jo 805.

Eastwood, M. (1992) *Human Nutrition – A Continuing Debate*. London: Chapman and Hall.

Ebbesen, F., Joergensen, A., Hoseth, E., Kaad, P., Moeller, M., Holsteen, V. & Rix, M. (2000) Neonatal hypoglycaemia and withdrawal symptoms after exposure in utero to valproate. *Archives of Disease in Childhood. Fetal & Neonatal Edition*:83:2:F124–9.

Ebden, P. & Evans, E. (1996) Management of asthmatic conditions in pregnancy. *Prescriber*: 7:3:21–5.

Eberle, R. & Norris, M. (1996) Labour analgesia. A risk-benefit analysis. *Drug Safety*: 14:4:239–51.

Eclampsia Trial Collaborative Group (1995) Which anticonvulsant for women with Eclampsia? Evidence from the Collaborative Eclampsia Trial. *Lancet*:345:1455–63.

Edwards, G. & Anderson, I. (1999) Systematic review and guide to selection of selective serotonin reuptake inhibitors. *Drugs*:57:507–33.

Egerman, R., Mercer, B., Doss, J. & Sibai, B. (1998) A randomized controlled trial of oral and intramuscular dexamethasone in the prevention of neonatal respiratory distress syndrome. *American Journal of Obstetrics & Gynecology*:179:1120–3.

Einarson, A., Ho, E. & Koren, G. (2000) Can we use metronidazole during pregnancy and breastfeeding? *Canadian Family Physician*:46:1053–4.

Elbourne, D. & Wiseman, R. (2000) Types of intra-muscular opioids for maternal pain relief. *Cochrane Database Systematic Review*: (issue 2) Oxford, Update Software, accessed July 2000.

Elliot, S., Gerrard, J. & Holden, J. (1994) *The Management of Postnatal Depression in Primary Care*. London, Sainsbury Centre for Mental Health.

Ellis, M., Manandhar, N., Manandhar, D. & Costello, A. (2000) Risk factors for neonatal encephalopathy in Kathmandu, Nepal, a developing country. *BMJ*:320:1229–36.

Ellison, J., Walker, I. & Greer, I. (2000) Antenatal use of enoxaparin for prevention and treatment of thromboembolism in pregnancy. *British Journal of Obstetrics and Gynaecology*: 107:1116–21.

El-Refaey, H., Nooh, R., O'Brien, P., Abdalla, M., Geary, M., Walder, J. & Rodeck, C. (2000) The misoprostol third stage of labour: a randomised controlled comparison between orally administered misoprostol and standard management. *British Journal of Obstetrics and Gynaecology*:107:1104–10.

Engstrom, J. & Sittler, C. (1994) Nurse-midwifery management of iron-deficiency anaemia during pregnancy. *Journal of Nurse Midwifery*:39:2 (supplement):20S–43S.

Evidence-Based Medicine (EBM) Working Group (1992) Evidence-based medicine: a new approach to teaching the practice of medicine. *JAMA*:268:2420–5.

Fairgrieve, S., Jackson, M., Jonas, P., Walshaw, D., White, K., Montgomery, T., Burn, J. & Lynch,

S. (2000) Population based, prospective study of the care of women with epilepsy in pregnancy. *BMJ*:321:674–5.

Fairlie, F., Walker, J., Marchall, L. & Elbourne, D. (1999) Intramuscular opioids for maternal pain relief in labour: a randomised controlled trial comparing pethidine with diamorphine. *British Journal of Obstetrics and Gynaecology*:106:1181–7.

Fernandez, S. (2000) *Hamochromatosis Mutations*. Unpublished research project, Cardiff, University of Wales.

Findley, I. & Chamberlain, G. (1999) Relief of pain. *BMJ*:318:927–30.

Finn, R., Clarke, C.A., Donohoe, W.T.A., McConnel, R.B., Sheppard, P.M., Lehane, D. & Kulke, W. (1961) Experimental studies on the prevention of Rh haemolytic disease. *BMJ*:1486–90.

Fischer, C., Blanie, P., Jaouen, E., Vayssiere, C., Kaloul, I. & Coltat, J. (2000) Ropivacaine, 0.1%, plus sufentanil. *Anesthesiology*:92:6:1588–93.

Fitzgerald, P. (1995) Endocrine disorders. In: Tierney, L., McPhee, S. & Papadakis, M. (eds) *Current Medical Diagnosis and Treatment*. Norwalk: Appleton and Lange, 943–81.

Folb, P. & Graham Dukes, M.N. (1990) *Drug Safety in Pregnancy*. Amsterdam, Elsevier.

Forster, M., Nimmo, G. & Brown, A. (1996) Prolapsed intervertebral disc after epidural analgesia in labour. *Anaesthesia*:51:8:773–5.

Foster, D. (1991) Diabetes Mellitus. In: Wilson, J., Braunwald, E., Isselbacher, K., Petersdorf, R., Martin, J., Fauci, A. & Root, R. (eds) *Harrison's Principles of Internal Medicine*, 12th edition. New York: McGraw Hill, 1739–59.

Foster, P.R., McIntosh, R.V. & Welch, A.G. (1995) Hepatitis C infection from anti-D immunoglobulin. *Lancet*:345:372.

Fowler, L. (1998) Corticosteroids. In: Williams, B. & Baer, C. (eds) *Essentials of Clinical Pharmacology in Nursing*, 3rd edition. Springhouse, Philadelphia, Springhouse 488–501.

Fox, R. & Draycott, T. (1996) Diazepam is more useful than magnesium for immediate control of eclampsia. (letter) *BMJ*:312:1668–9.

Fraser, C. & Arieff, A. (1990) Water metabolism and its disorders. In: Cohen, R., Lewis, B., Alberti, K. & Denman, A. (eds) *The Metabolic and Molecular Basis of Acquired Disease*. London, Bailliere Tindall.

Fraser, W., Vendittelli, F., Krauss, I. & Breasrt, G. (1998) Effects of early augmentation of labour with amniotomy and oxytocin in nulliparous women: a meta-analysis. *British Journal of Obstetrics and Gynaecology*:105:189–94.

Frederick, J. (1973) Epilepsy and pregnancy: a report from the Oxford record-linkage study. *British Medical Journal* 1973;2:442–8.

French, N.P., Hagan, R., Evans, S., Godfrey, M. & Newnham, J. (1999) Repeated antenatal corticosteroids: size at birth and subsequent development. *American Journal of Obstetrics and Gynecology*:180:114–21.

Friedman, L. & Isselbacher, K. (1991) Anorexia, nausea, vomiting and indigestion. In: Wilson, J., Braunwald, E., Isselbacher, K., Petersdorf, R., Martin, J., Fauci, A., Root, R. (eds) *Harrison's Principles of Internal Medicine*, 12th edition. New York, McGraw-Hill.

Friedman, L. et al (1978) Factors influencing the incidence of neonatal jaundice. *BMJ*:1978;1:1235–7.

Frigoletto, F., Lieberman, E., Lang, J., Cohen, A., Barss, V., Ringer, S. & Datta, S. (1995) A clinical trial of active management of labor. *New England Journal of Medicine*:333:745–50.

Fujii, Y., Tanaka, H. & Toyooka, H. (1998) Prevention of nausea and vomiting with granisetron, droperidol and metoclopramide during and after spinal anaesthesia for caesarean section. *Acta Anaesthesiologica Scandinavia*:42:8:921–5.

Fung, B. (2000) Continuous epidural analgesia for painless labor does not increase the incidence of cesarean delivery. *Acta Anaesthesiologia Sinica*:38:79–84.

Gabbe, S., Holing, E., Temple, P. & Brown, Z. (2000) Benefits, risks, costs, and patient satisfaction associated with insulin pump therapy for the pregnancy complicated by type 1 diabetes mellitus. *American Journal of Obstetrics and Gynecology*:182:1283–91.

Gahart, B. (1992) *Intravenous Medications*, 8th edition. London, Mosby.

Gaiser, R., Cheek, T. & Gutsche, B. (1998) Comparison of three different doses of intrathecal fentanyl and sufentanil for labor analgesia. *Journal of Clinical Anesthesetics*:10:488–93.

Galbraith, A., Bullock, S., Manias, E., Hunt, B. & Richards, A. (1999) *Fundamentals of Pharmacology*. Harlow, Essex, Addison Wesley Longman.

Gallery, E. (1995) Hypertension in Pregnancy. *Drugs*:49:555–62.

Ganong, W.F. (1999) *Review of Medical Physiology*, 19th edition. East Norwalk, Connecticut, Appleton Lange.

Garland, H.O. (1985) Maternal adjustments to pregnancy. In: Case, R.M. (ed.) *Variations in Human Physiology*. Manchester, Manchester University Press.

Gautier, P., Derby, F., Fanard, L., van Steenberge, A. & Hody, J. (1997) Ambulatory CSE analgesia for labor. *Regional Anesthesia*:22:143–9.

Geerts, W., Jay, R., Code, K., Chen, E., Szalai, J., Saibil, E. & Hamilton, P. (1996) A comparison of low-dose heparin with low-molecular weight heparin as prophylaxis against venous thromboembolism after major trauma. *New England J. of Medicine*:335:701–7.

Gerber v Pines (1934) 79 Sol Jo 13.

Gibb, D. & Arulkumaran, S. (1997) *Fetal Monitoring in Practice*, 2nd edition. Oxford, Butterworth-Heinemann.

Gillmer, M. (1996) Management of pre-existing disorders in pregnancy: diabetes mellitus. *Prescribers' Journal*:36:159–64.

Ginsberg, J. (1996) Management of Venous Thromboembolism. *New England Journal of Medicine*:335:1816–28.

Girling, J. (1996) Thyroid disease in pregnancy. *British Journal of Hospital Medicine*:56:316–20.

Girling, J. & De Swiet, M. (1996) Pre-eclampsia. *Update*:16:10:338–42.

Golding, J. (1998) A randomised trial of low dose aspirin for primiparae in pregnancy. *British Journal of Obstetrics and Gynaecology*:105:293–9.

Golding, J., Greenwood, R., Birmingham, K. & Mott, M. (1992) Childhood cancer, intramuscular vitamin K, and pethidine given during labour. *BMJ*:305:341–6.

Golding, J., Paterson, M. & Kinlen, L.J. (1990) Factors associated with childhood cancer in a national cohort study. *British Journal of Cancer*:62:304–8.

Gonser, M. (1995) Labor induction and augmentation with oxytocin: pharmacokinetic considerations. *Archives of Gynecology and Obstetrics*:256:63–6.

Goorkani v Tayside Health Board (1991) 3 Med LR 33.

Govoni, L. & Hayes, J. (1990) *Drugs and Nursing Implications*. New York, Prentice Hall.

Govoni, L. & Hayes, J. (1998) *Drugs and Nursing Implications*. London, Prentice Hall.

Graham, K. (1998) Magnesium sulphate in eclampsia. *Lancet*:351:1061.

Graves, C. (1996) Agents that cause contraction or relaxation of the uterus. In: Hardman, J., Limbard, L., Molinoff, P., Ruddon, R. & Goodman Gilman, A. (eds) *Goodman & Gilman's: The Pharmacological Basis of Therapeutics*, 9th edition. New York, McGraw-Hill, 939–54.

Greaves, M. (1999) Antiphospholipid antibodies and thrombosis. *Lancet*:353:1348–53.

Greer, F., Marchall, S., Severson, R., Smith, D.A., Shearer, M., Pace, D. & Joubert, P. (1998) A new mixed micellar preparation for oral vitamin K prophylaxis. *Archives of Disease in Childhood*:79:4:300–5.

Greer, I. (1999) Thrombosis in pregnancy: maternal and fetal issues. *Lancet*:353:1258–65.

Griffith, D., Betteridge, D. & Axford, J. (1996) Diabetes mellitus, lipoprotein disorders and other metabolic diseases. In: Axford, J. (ed.) *Medicine*. Oxford, Blackwell, 13.1–56.

Groer, M. & Shekleton, M. (1989) *Basic Pathophysiology*. St. Louis, Mosby.

Grohmann, R., Ruther, E., Engel, R. & Hippius, R. (1999) Assessment of adverse drug reactions in psychiatric inpatients. *Pharmacopsychiatry*:32:1:21–8.

Grossman, E., Messerli, F., Grodzicki, T. & Kowey, P. (1996) Should a moratorium be placed on sublingual nifedipine capsules given for hypertensive emergencies and pseudoemergencies? *JAMA*:276:1328–31.

Guidolin, L., Vignoli, A. & Canger, R. (1998) Worsening in seizure frequency and severity in relation to folic acid administration. *European Journal of Neurology*:5:301–3.

Gulmezoglu, A. (2000) Prostaglandins for prevention of postpartum harmorrhage. *Cochrane Database Systematic Review*: (issue 2) Oxford, Update Software. Accessed July 2000.

Gupta, S. (1998) Selective serotonin reuptake inhibitors in pregnancy and lactation. *Obstetric & Gynaecology Review*: December:53:733–6.

Guyton, A. (1996) *Textbook of Medical Physiology*, 9th edition. Philadelphia, Saunders. *Gynaecology*:103:4:313–18.

Gyetvai, K., Hannah, M., Hodnett, E. & Ohlsson, A. (1999) Tocolytics for preterm labor: a systematic review. *Obstetrics and Gynecology*:94:869–77.

Haberg, M. & Matheson, I. (1997) Antidepressive agents and breastfeeding, *Tidsskr Nor Laegeforen*:117:27:3952–5.

Hague, W. (1995) Treatment of endocrine diseases, 2nd edition. In: Rubin, P. *Prescribing in Pregnancy*. London, BMJ Group, 85–96.

Hall, D., Odendaal, H. & Smith, M. (2000) Is the prophylactic administration of magnesium sulphate in women with pre-eclampsia indicated prior to labour? *British Journal of Obstetrics and Gynaecology*:107:903–8.

Hall, J., Pauli, R. & Wilson, K.M. (1980) Maternal and fetal sequelae of anti-coagulation during pregnancy. *American Journal of Medicine*:68:122–40.

Hall, R. (1996) Intrathecal opioids for labor analgesia in a community hospital. Cleveland Clinic Foundation, sector for anaesthesia for obstetrics. *http://www.anes.ccf.org:8080/soap/itnarc.htm*

Halligan, A., Bell, S. & Taylor, D. (1999) Dipstick proteinuris: caveat emptor. *British Journal of Obstetrics and Gynaecology*:106:1113–15.

Halpern, S., Leighton, B., Ohlsson, A., Barrett, J. & Rice, A. (1998) Effect of epidural vs. parenteral opioid analgesia on the progress of labour: a meta-analysis. *JAMA*:280:24:2105–10.

Halpern, S., Levine, T., Wilson, D., MacDonell, J., Katsiris, S. & Leighton, B. (1999) Effect of labor analgesia on breastfeeding success. *Birth*:26:2:83–8.

Hannah, M., Ohlsson, A., Farine, D., Hewson, S., Hodnett, E., Myhr, T., Wang, E., Weston, J. & Willan, A. (1996) Induction of labor compared with expectant management for prelabor rupture of the membranes at term. *New England Journal of Medicine*:334:1005–10.

Hansen, D., Lou, H. & Olsen, J. (2000) Serious life events and congential malformations: a national study with complete follow-up. *Lancet*:356:875–80.

Haram, K., Hervig, T., Thordarson, H. & Aksnes, L. (1993) Osteopenia caused by heparin treatment in pregnancy. *Acta Obstetrica et Gynecologica Scandanavia*:72:8:674–5.

Harms, C., Sigemund, M., Marsch, S., Surbek, D., Hosli, I. & Schneider, M. (1999) Initiating extradural analgesia during labour: comparison of three different bupivacaine concentrations used as the loading dose. *Fetal Diagnostics and Therapeutics*:14:368–74.

Harris, B. (1996) Psychiatric disorders of the puerperium, *Primary Care Psychiatry*:2:25–36.

Harsten, A., Gillberg, L., Hakansson, L. & Olsson, M. (1997) Intrathecal sufentanil compared with epidural bupivacaine analgesia in labour. *European Journal of Anaesthesiology*:14:642–5.

Haste, F., Brooke, O., Anderson, H. & Bland, J. (1991) The effect of nutritional intake on outcome of pregnancy in smokers and non-smokers. *British Journal of Nutrition*:65:3:347–54.

Hauth, J., Golenberg, R., Andrews, W., Dubard, M. & Copper, R. (1995) Reduced incidence of preterm delivery with metronidazole and erythromycin. *New England Journal of Medicine*:333:1732–6.

Hawthorne, G., Robson, S., Ryall, E., Sen, D., Roberts, S. & Platt, M.P.W. (1997) Prospective population based survey of outcome of pregnancy in diabetic women: results of the Northern Diabetic Pregnancy Audit (1994) *BMJ*:315:279–81.

Hayashi, R. (1990) The role of prostaglandins in the treatment of postpartum haemorrhage. *Journal of Obstetrics and Gynaecology*:10:S2:S21–4.

Heaton, D. & Pearce, M. (1995) Low molecular weight versus unfractionated heparin. *Pharmacoeconomics*:8:2:91–9.

Helewa, M., Burrows, R., Smith, J., Williams, K., Brain, P. & Rabkin, S. (1997) Report of the Canadian Hypertension Society Consensus Conference:1. Definitions, evaluation and classification of hypertensive disorders in pregnancy. *Canadian Medical Association Journal*: 157:6:715–25.

Henderson v Henderson (1955) 1 BMJ 672.

Herman, N., Choi, K., Affleck, P., Calicott, R., Brackin, R., Singhal, A., Andreasen, A., Gadalla, F. & Fong, J. (1999) Analgesia, pruritus, and ventilation exhibit a dose-response relationship in parturients receiving intrathecal fentanyl during labor. *Anesthesia and Analgesia*:89:378–83.

Herpolsheimer, A. & Schretenthaler, J. (1994) The use of intrapartum intrathecal narcotic analgesia in a community-based hospital. *Obstetrics and Gynaecology*:84:6:931–6.

Hess, P., Pratt, S., Soni, A., Sarna, M. & Oriol, N. (2000) An association between severe labor pain and cesarean delivery. *Anesthetic Analgesia*:90:881–6.

Hibbard, B.M. (1988) *Principles of Obstetrics*. London, Butterworth.

Hibbard, E. & Smithells, R. (1965) Folic acid metabolism and human embryopathy. *Lancet*: 1965;i:1254–6.

Hildebrandt, H.M. (1999) Maternal perception of lactogenesis time: a clinical report. *Journal of Human Lactation*:15:4:317–23.

Hill, W.C. (1995) Risks and complications of tocolysis. *Clinical Obstetrics and Gynecology*: 38:4:725–45.

Hillman, R. (1996) Hematopoietic agents. In: Hardman, J., Limbard, L., Molinoff, P., Ruddon, R. & Goodman Gilman, A. (eds) *Goodman & Gilman's: The Pharmacological Basis of Therapeutics*, 9th edition. New York, McGraw-Hill, 1311–40.

Hildebrandt, H. (1999) Maternal perception of lactogenesis time: a clinical report. *Journal of Human Lactation*:15:4:317–23.

Hindmarsh, P., Geary, M., Rodeck, C., Jackson, M. & Kingdom, J. (2000) Effect of early maternal iron stores on placental weight and structure. *Lancet*:356:719–23.

Hirst, J., Chibbar, R. & Mitchell, B. (1993) Role of oxytocin in the regulation of uterine activity during pregnancy and in the initiation of labor. *Seminars in Reproductive Endocrinology*:11:219–23.

Hoffman, B. & Lefkowitz, R. (1996) Catecholamines, sympathomimetic drugs, and adrenergic receptor antagonists. In: Hardman, J., Limbard, L., Molinof, P., Ruddon, R. & Goodman Gilman, A. (eds) *Goodman & Gilman's: The Pharmacological Basis of Therapeutics*, 9th edition. New York, McGraw-Hill.

Hofmeyr, G. (1995) Prophylactic intravenous preloading before epidural anaesthesia in labour. Oxford, *The Cochrane Pregnancy and Childbirth Database*, Issue 2 Oxford, Update Software. Accessed July 2000.

Hofmeyr, G. & Gulmezoglu, A. (2000) Vaginal misoprostol for cervical ripening and labour induction in late pregnancy. Oxford, *The Cochrane Pregnancy and Childbirth Database*, Issue 2 Oxford, Update Software. Accessed Nov. 2000.

Hofmeyr, G., Gulmezoglu, A. & Alfirevic, Z. (2000) Misoprostol for induction of labour at term. (letter) *British Journal of Obstetrics and Gynaecology*:107:576.

Hofmeyr, G., Nikodem, V., de Jager, M. & Gelbart, B. (1998) A randomised placebo trial of oral misoprostol in the third stage of labour. *British Journal of Obstetrics and Gynaecology*: 105:971–5.

Holdcroft, A., Gibberd, F., Hargrove, R., Hawkins, D. & Dellaportas, C. (1995) Neurological complications associated with pregnancy. *British Journal of Anaesthesia*:75:522–6.

Holgate, S. (1997) The cellular and mediator basis of asthma in relation to natural history. *Lancet*:350:(suppl II):5–9.

Holleboom, C., Merkus, J., van Elfereen, L. & Keirse, M. (1996) Randomised comparison between a loading and incremental dose model for ritodrine administration in preterm labour. *British Journal of Obstetrics and Gynaecology*:103:695–701.

Hollmen, A. (1993) The effects of regional anaesthesia on utero and fetoplacental blood flow. In: Reynolds, F. (ed.) *Effects on the Baby of Maternal Analgesia and Anaesthesia*. London, Saunders, 67–87.

Hopkinson, H. (1995) Treatment of cardiovascular diseases. In: Rubin, P. (ed.) *Prescribing in Pregnancy*, 2nd edition. London, BMJ Group.

Hornby, P. & Abrahams, T. (1996) Pulmonary pharmacology. *Clinical Obstetrics and Gynecology*:39:1:17–35.

Howard, H., Martlew, V., McFadyen, I. & Clarke, C. (1997) Preventing rhesus D haemolytic disease of the newborn by giving anit-D immunoglobulin: are the guidelines being followed adequately? *British Journal of Obstetrics and Gynaecology*:104:37–41.

Howden, C. (1995) Treatment of common minor ailments. In: Rubin, P. (ed.) *Prescribing in Pregnancy*, 2nd edition. London, BMJ Group, 22–8.

Howell, C. & Chalmers, I. (1992) A review of prospectively controlled comparisons of epidural with non-epidural forms of pain relief during labour. *International Journal of Obstetric Anesthesia*:1:93 110.

Howell, C.J. (1994) Systemic narcotics for analgesia in labour. In: *Cochrane Database of Systemic Reviews*:03398. Oxford, Update Software, disk issue 1.

Howell, C.J. (1995a) Epidural vs non-epidural analgesia in labour. *Cochrane Pregnancy and Childbirth Database*, Issue 2. Oxford, Update Software. Accessed July 2000.

Howell, C.J. (1995b) Epidural top-ups on maternal request vs scheduled top-ups. *Cochrane Pregnancy and Childbirth Database*, Issue 2. Oxford, Update Software.

Howell, C.J. (1995c) Prophylactic blood patch for dural puncture. *Cochrane Pregnancy and Childbirth Database*, Issue 2. Oxford, Update Software.

Huffman, M. (1994) Agreeing on a keep-vein-open infusion rate. *American Journal of Hospital Pharmacy*:51:2660.

Hughes, S. (1992) Analgesia methods during labour and delivery. *Canadian Journal of Anaesthesia*:39:5:R18–23.

Hunter, K. (1991) *Doctors' Stories*. Princeton, NJ, Princeton University Press.

IASP Subcommittee on Taxonomy (1986) Classification of chronic pain. *Pain Supplement* 3:216–21.

Huxley, R. (2000) Nausea & vomiting in early pregnancy: its role in placental development. *Obstetrics and Gynecology*:95:779–82.

Idama, T. & Lindow, S. (1998) Magnesium sulphate: a review of clinical pharmacology applied to obstetrics. *British Journal of Obstetrics and Gynaecology*:105:260–8.

Imbach, P. & Kuhne, T. (2000) Sequelae of treatment of ITP with anti-D (Rho) immunoglobulin. *Lancet*:356:447–8.

Irestedt, L., Ekblom, A., Olofsson, C., Dahlstrom, A. & Emanuelsson, B. (1998) Pharmacokinetics and clinical effect during continuous epidural infusion with ropivacaine 2.5 mg/ml or bupivacaine 2.5 mg/ml for labour pain relief. *Acta Anaesthesiologica Scandinavia*:42:8:890–6.

Isarangkura, P., Shearer, M.J., Pindit, P., Grueter, J., Sanmanoj, T., Chuansumrit, A., Sasanakul, W., Hanck, A. & Hathirat, P. (1994) Vitamin K (Konakion MM) by oral route in the prevention of the haemorrhagic disease of the newborn and idiopathic vitamin K deficiency in Infants. *International Symposium Vitamin K in Infancy*, 7–8 October 1994, Basel, Switzerland.

J v. Distillers Co (Biochemicals) (1969) 8 C.L. 99.

Jacobson, B., Nyberg, K., Gronbladh, L. et al (1990) Opiate addiction of adult offspring through possible imprinting after obstetric treatment. *BMJ*:301:1067–70.

Jadad, A., Sigouin, C., Mohide, P., Levine, M. & Fuentes, M. (2000) Risk of congenital malformations associated with treatment of asthma during early pregnancy. *Lancet*:355:119.

Jarrett, R. (1997) Should we screen for gestational diabetes? *BMJ*:315:736–7.

Jewell, D. & Young, G. (2000) Interventions for nausea and vomiting in early pregnancy. *Cochrane Database Systematic Review*: Issue 2. Oxford, Update Software. Accessed July 2000.

Jone, P., Johanson, R., Baldwin, K.J., Lilford, R. & Jones, P. (1998) Changing belief in obstetrics: impact of two multicentre randomised controlled trials. *Lancet*:352:1988–9.

Jordan, S. (1997) Teaching pharmacology by case study. *Nurse Education Today*:17:386–93.

Jordan, S. (1998) From classroom theory to clinical practice: evaluating the impact of a postregistration course. *Nurse Education Today*:18:293–302.

Jordan, S. & Hughes, D. (1996) Bioscience knowledge and the health care professions. *Social Science in Health*:2:2:80–92.

Jordan, S. & Tait, M. (1999) Antibiotic therapy. *Nursing Standard*:13:45:49–54.

Jordan, S. & Torrance, C. (1995) Bionursing: explaining falls in elderly people. *Nursing Standard*:9:50:30–2.

Jordan, S. & White, J. (2001) Bronchodilators: implications for nursing practice. *Nursing Standard*:15:45–52.

Jorgensen, J., Romsing, J., Rasmussen, M., Sonnergaard, J.M., Vang, L. & Musaeus, L. (1996) Pain assessment of subcutaneous injections. *Annals of Pharmacotherapy*:30:729–32.

Joshua, A. & King, T. (1997) *Guy's Hospital 1997–8 Nursing Drug Reference*, 4th edition, London, Mosby.

Kan, R. & Hughes, S. (1995) Recent developments in analgesia during labour. *Drugs*:50: 417–22.

Karch, A. (1992) *Handbook of Drugs and the Nursing Process*, 2nd edition. Philadelphia, Lippincott.

Katz, P. & Castell, D. (1998) Gastroesophageal reflux disease during pregnancy. *Gastroenterology Clinics of North America*:27:1:153–67.

Katz, V. & Farmer, R. (1999) Controversies in tocolytic therapy. *Clinical Obstetrics and Gynecology*:42:802–19.

Katz, V., Farmer, R. & Kuller, J. (2000) Pre-eclampsia into eclampsia: toward a new paradigm. *American Journal of Obstetrics*:182:1389–96.

Kawabata, K.M. (1996) Two cases of asthmatic attack caused by spinal anaesthesia. *Masui*:45:1:102–6.

Keenlyside, D. (1992) Every little detail counts; infection control in IV therapy. *Professional Nurse*:5:1:226–32.

Kelsey, J. & Prevost, R. (1994) Drug therapy during labour and delivery. *American Journal of Hospital Pharmacy*:51:2394–402.

Kendell, R., Chambers, J. & Platz, C. (1987) Epidemiology of puerperal psychoisis. *British Journal of Psychiatry*:150:662–73.

Kendell, R., McInneny, K., Juszczak, E. & Bain, M. (2000) Obstetric complications and schizophrenia. *British Journal of Psychiatry*:176:516–22.

Kennedy, S. & Longnecker, D. (1996) History and principles of anaesthesiology. In: Hardman, J., Limbird, L., Molinoff, P., Ruddon, R. & Goodman Gilman, A. (eds) *The Pharmacological Basis of Therapeutics*, 9th edition. New York, McGraw Hill, 917–36.

Khamashta, M. & Mackworth-Young, C. (1997) Antiphospholipid (Hughes') syndrome. *BMJ*: 314:244.

Khan, G., John, I., Chan, T., Wani, S., Hughes, A. & Stirrat, G. (1995) Abu Dhabi third stage trial. *European Journal of Obstetrics and Gynecology*:58:147–51.

Khan, K. & Chien, P. (1997) Seizure prophylaxis in hypertensive pregnancies: a framework for making clinical decisions. *British Journal of Obstetrics and Gynaecology*:104:1173–9.

Kinsler, V., Thornton, S., Ashford, M., Melin, P. & Smith, S. (1996) The effect of the oxytocin antagonists F314 and F792 on the *in vitro* contractility of human myometrium. *British Journal of Obstetrics and Gynaecology*:103:373–5.

Klinger, G. & Koren, G. (2000) Controversies in antenatal corticosteroid treatment. *Canadian Family Physician*:46:1571–3.

Klingman, W.O. (1954) The effect of ion exchange resins in the paroxysmal disorders of the nervous system. *American Journal of Psychiatry*:111:184–95.

Knight, M., Duley, L., Henderson-Smart, D. & King, J. (2000) Antiplatelet agents for preventing and treating pre-eclampsia. *Cochrane Pregnancy and Childbirth Database*, Issue 2. Oxford, Update Software. Accessed July 2000.

Knox, T. & Olans, L. (1996) Liver disease in pregnancy. *The New England Journal of Medicine*:335:8:569–76.

Koren, G., Pastuszak, A. & Ito, S. (1998) Drugs in pregnancy. *New England Journal of Medicine*:338:16:1128–37.

Kramer, M., Coates, A., Michoud, M., Dagenais, S., Moshonas, D. & Davis, G.M. (1995) Maternal asthma and idiopathic preterm labor. *American Journal of Epidemiology*: 142:10:1078–88.

Kuhnert, B. (1993) Human perinatal pharmacology: recent controversies. In: Reynolds, F. (ed.) *Effects on the Baby of Maternal Analgesia and Anaesthesia*. London, Saunders.

Kulb, N. (1990) Oxytocin Induction/augmentation of labor. In: Buckley, K. & Kulb, N. (eds) *High Risk Maternity Nursing Manual*. Baltimore, Williams and Wilkins.

Kuoppala, T. (1988) Alterations in vitamin D metabolites and minerals in diabetic pregnancy. *Gynecologic and Obstetric Investigation*:25:99–105.

Lamont, R. (2000) The pathophysiology of pulmonary oedema with the use of beta-agonists. *British Journal of Obstetrics and Gynaecology*:107:439–44.

Lamont, R., Mason, R. & Adinkra, P. (2001) Advances in the use of antibiotics in the prevention of preterm birth. In: Bonnar, J. (ed.) *Recent Advances in Obstetrics and Gynaecology 21*. Edinburgh, Churehill Livingstone, 35–44.

Lander, C.M., Edwards, V.E., Eadie, M.J. & Tyrer, J.H. (1977) Plasma anticonvulsant concentrations during pregnancy. *Neurology*:27:128–31.

Landsteiner, K. (1900) Blood groups. *Zbl. Bakt.* 27:357.

Lanseiner, K. & Wiener, A.S. (1940) Agglutinable factor in human blood recognised by immune sera for Rhesus blood. *Proceedings of Society of Experimental Biology (NY)*. 43:223.

Larimore, W. & Cline, M. (2000) Keeping normal labor normal. *Primary Care*:27:221–36.

Laskin, C., Bombardier, C., Hannah, M., Mandel, F., Ritchie, J., Farewell, V., Farine, D., Spitzer, K., Fielding, L., Solonnika, C. & Yeung, M. (1997) Prednisone and aspirin in women with autoantibodies and unexplained recurrent fetal loss. *New England Journal of Medicine*: 337:148–53.

Laurence, K.M., James, N., Miller, M., Tennant, G. & Campbell, H. (1981) Double-blind randomised controlled trial of folate treatment before conception to prevent recurrence of neural-tube defects, *BMJ*:282:1509–11.

Lauszus, F., Klebe, J. & Bek, T. (2000) Diabetic retinopathy in pregnancy during tight metabolic control. *Acta Obstetrica Gynecologica*:79:367–70.

Le Coq, G., Ducot, B. & Benhamou, D. (1998) Risk factors of inadequate pain relief during epidural analgesia for labour and delivery. *Canadian Journal of Anaesthesia*:45:8:719–23.

Lee, A. & McManus, P. (1995) Psychiatric and neurological disorders: part 2. *The Pharmaceutical Journal*:254:118–21.

Lee, A. & Schofield, S. (1994a) Common medical problems in pregnancy. *The Pharmaceutical Journal*:253:6797:57–60.

Lee, A. & Schofield, S. (1994b) Drug use in pregnancy. *The Pharmaceutical Journal*: 253:6796:27–30.

Lensing, A., Prandoni, P., Prins, M. & Buller, H. (1999) Deep-vein thrombosis. *Lancet*: 353:479–85.

Lertakyamanee, J., Chinachoti, T., Tritrakarn, T., Muangkasem, J., Somboonnanonda, A. & Kolatat, T. (1999) Comparison of general and regional anaesthesia for Cesarean section. *Journal of the Medical Association of Thailand*:82:672–80.

Letsky, E.A. & Warwick, R. (1994) Haematological problems. In: James, D.K., Steer, P.J., Weiner, C.P. & Gonik, B. (eds) *High Risk Pregnancy. Management Options* Philadelphia, W.B. Saunders.

Levine, R., Hauth, J., Curet, L., Sibai, B., Catalano, P., Morris, C., Dersimonian, R., Esterlitz, J., Raymond, E., Bild, D., Clemens, J. & Cutler, J. (1997) Trial of calcium to prevent pre-eclampsia. *New England Journal of Medicine*:337:69–76.

Levy, J., Montes, F., Szalam, F. & Hillyer, C. (2000) The in vitro effects of antithrombin III on the activated coagulation time in patients on heparin therapy. *Anesthetic Analgesia*:90: 5:1076–9.

Lieberman, E., Lang, J., Richardson, D., Frigoletto, F., Heffner, L. & Cohen, A. (2000) Intrapartum maternal fever and neonatal outcomes. *Pediatrics*:105:1:8–13.

Liljestrand, J. (1999) Reducing perinatal and maternal mortality in the world: the major challenges. *British Journal of Obstetrics and Gynaecology*:106:877–80.

Lilley, L.L., Aucker, R.S. & Albanese, J.A. (1996) *Pharmacology and the Nursing Process*. St. Louis, Mosby.

Lima, F., Khamashta, M., Buchanan, N., Kerslake, S., Hunt, B. & Hughes, G. (1996) A study of sixty pregnancies in patients with the anti-phospholipid syndrome. *Clinical and Experimental Rheumatology*:14:2:131–6.

Lindhoff-Last, E., Willeke, A., Thalhammer, C., Nowak, G. & Bauersachs, R. (2000) Hirudin treatment in a breastfeeding woman. *Lancet*:355:467–8.

Lipkin, G. (1993) Drug therapy in maternal care. In: Spencer, R.T., Nicolls, L., Lipkin, G., Henderson, H. & West, F. (eds) *Clinical Pharmacology and Nursing Management*, 4th edition Philadelphia, Lippincott.

Lipworth, B.J. (1997) Treatment of acute asthma. *Lancet*:350:(suppl II):18–23.

Little, R., Kirkman, E., Driscoll, P., Hanson, J. & Kackway-Jones, K. (1995) Preventable deaths after injury: why are the traditional 'vital' signs poor indicators of blood loss? *Journal of Accident and Emergency Medicine*:12:1–14.

Littlewood, J. & McHugh, N. (1997) *Maternal Distress and Postnatal Depression*, London, Macmillan.

Lockwood, C.J. (1997) Calcium-channel blockers in the management of preterm labour. *Lancet*:350:1339–40.

Loeb, S., Holmes, N.H., Charnow, J., Fandek, N., Johnson, P. & Sloan G. (1993) *Clinical Skillbuilders: Medication Administration and IV Therapy Manual*, 2nd edition., Springhouse, Pennsylvania, Springhouse Corporation.

Loebstein, R., Lalkin, A. & Koren, G. (1997) Pharmacokinetic changes during pregnancy and their clinical relevance. *Clinical Pharmacokinetics*:33:5:328–43.

Loeser, J. & Melzack, R. (1999) Pain: an overview. *Lancet*:353:1607–9.

Long, P. (1995) Rethinking iron sypplementation during pregnancy. *Journal of Nurse-Midwifery*:40:1:36–40.

Loudon, J. (1995) Psychotropic Drugs. In: Rubin, P. (ed.) *Prescribing in Pregnancy*. London, BMJ Publishing Group, 72–84.

Lougher, C. (1999) Medical Information Officer, Organon Laboratories Ltd., Cambridge Science Park, Cambridge CB4 4FL. Personal letter.

Lu, J. & Nightingale, C. (2000) Magnesium sulfate in eclampsia and pre-eclampsia: pharmacokinetic principles. *Clinical Pharmacokinetics*:38:305–15.

Lucas, C. (1992) Antihistaminics. In: Baer, C. & Williams, B. *Clinical Pharmacology and Nursing*, 2nd edition. Springhouse, Pennsylvania, Springhouse Corporation.

Lumbiganon, P., Hofmeyr, J., Gulmezoglu, A., Pinol, A. & Villar, J. (1999) Misoprostol dose-related shivering and pyrexia in the third stage of labour. *British Journal of Obstetrics and Gynaecology*:106:304–8.

Lutomski, D., Bottorff, M. & Sangha, K. (1995) Pharmacokinetic optimisation of the treatment of embolic disorders. *Clinical Pharmacokinetics*:28:1:67–92.

Lyons, G., Columb, M., Hawthorne, L. & Dresner, M. (1997) Extradural pain relief in labour: bupivacaine sparing by extradural fentanyl is dose dependent. *British Journal of Anaesthesia*: 78:493–7.

MacArthur, C., Lewis, M., Knox, E.G. & Crawford, J.S. (1990) Epidural analgesia and long term backache after childbirth. *BMJ*:301:9–12.

MacKay, H.T. & Evans, A. (1995) Gynecology and obstetrics. In: Tierney, L., McPhee, S. & Papadakis, M. (eds) *Current Medical Diagnosis and Treatment*. Norwalk, Appleton and Lange.

Magee, L., Ornstein, M. & Dadelszen, P. (1999) Management of hypertension in pregnancy. *BMJ*:318:1332–6.

Mahmood, K. (2000) Zinc supplementation in pregnancy. Oxford, *The Cochrane Pregnancy and Childbirth Database*, Issue 2 Oxford, Update Software. Accessed Nov 2000.

Mahmood, T., Rayner, A., Smith, N. & Beat, I. (1995) A randomized prospctive trial comparing single dose prostaglandin E2 vaginal gel with forewater amniotomy for induction of labour. *European Journal of Obstetrics and Gynecology and Reproductive Biology*:58:111–17.

Majerus, P., Brozc, G., Milctich, J. & Tollcfscn, D. (1996) Anticoagulant, thrombolytic and antiplatelet drugs. In: Hardman, J., Limbard, L., Molinoff, P., Ruddon, R. & Goodman Gilman, A. (eds) *Goodman & Gilman's: The Pharmacological Basis of Therapeutics*, 9th edition. New York, McGraw-Hill.

Makrides, M. & Crowther, C. (2000) Magnesium supplementation in pregnancy. *Cochrane Pregnancy and Childbirth Database* (issue 2). Oxford, Update Software.

Malone, F.D. & D'Alton, M.E. (1997) Drugs in pregnancy: antiepileptics. *Seminars in Perinatology*:21:2:114–25.

Malseed, R.T., Goldstein, F.J. & Balkon, N. (1995) *Pharmacology: Drug Therapy and Nursing Considerations*, 4th edition. Philadelphia, Lippincott.

Mander, R. (1994) Epidural analgesia 2: research basis. *British Journal of Midwifery*:2:1:12–16.

Marcus, R. & Coulston, A. (1996) Fat-soluble vitamins. In: Hardman, J., Limbard, L., Molinoff, P., Ruddon, R. & Goodman Gilman, A. (eds) *Goodman & Gilman's: The Pharmacological Basis of Therapeutics*, 9th edition. New York, McGraw-Hill.

Marshall, B. & Longnecker, D. (1996) General anaesthetics. In: Hardman, J., Limbird, L., Molinoff, P., Ruddon, R. & Goodman Gilman, A. (eds) *Goodman & Gilman's: The Pharmacological Basis of Therapeutics*, 9th edition. New York, McGraw Hill, 331–48.

Marx, G. & Rabin, J. (1993) Anaesthesia for Caesarean section and neonatal welfare. In: Reynolds, F. (ed.) *Effects on the Baby of Maternal Analgesia and Anaesthesia*. London, Saunders.

Mas, J. & Lamy, C. (1998) Stroke in pregnancy and the puerperium. *Journal of Neurology*: 245:305–13.

Massie, B. (1995) Management of hypertension. In: Tierney, L., McPhee, S. & Papadakis, M. (eds) *Current Medical Diagnosis and Treatment*. Norwalk, Appleton and Lange.

Mather, H., Morgan, D., Pearson, N., Read, K., Shaw, D., Steed, G., Thome, M., Lawrence, C. & Riley, I. (1976) Myocardial infarction: a comparison between home and hospital care for patients, *BMJ*:1976:6015:925–9.

Mathews, F., Yudkin, P. & Neil, A. (1998) Folates in the periconceptual period: are women getting enough? *British Journal of Obstetrics and Gynaecology*:105:954–9.

Mazzotta, P. & Magee, L. (2000) A risk-benefit assessment of pharmacological and nonpharmacological treatments for nausea and vomiting of pregnancy. *Drugs*:59:781–800.

McCarthy, M.F. (1996) Magnesium taurate for the prevention and treatment of pre-eclampsia/eclampsia. *Medical Hypotheses*:47:4:269–72.

McCartney, D. (1995) Constipation. *Update*:May 5:597–8.

McCowan, L., Buist, R., North, R. & Gamble, G. (1996) Perinatal morbidity in chronic hypertension. *British Journal of Obstetrics and Gynaecology*:103:123–9.

McCrae, A.F., Jozwiak, H. & McClure, J.H. (1995) Comparison of ropivacaine and bupivacaine in extradural analgesia for the relief of pain in labour. *British Journal of Anaesthesia*:74:3:261–5.

McDonald, S., Prendeville, W. & Blair, E. (1993) Randomised trial of oxytocin alone versus oxytocin and ergometrine in active management of third stage of labour. *BMJ*:307:1167–71.

McDonald, S., Prendeville, W. & Elbourne, D. (2000) Prophylactic syntometrine versus oxytocin for delivery of the placenta. *Cochrane Pregnancy and Childbirth Database*, Issue 2. Oxford, Update Software. Accessed July 2000.

McElhatton, P., Bateman, D., Evans, C., Pughs, K. & Thomas, S. (1999) Congential anomalies after prenatal ecstasy exposure. *Lancet*:354:1441–2.

McFadden, E.R. (1991) Asthma. In: Wilson, J., Braunwald, E., Isselbacher, K. et al *Harrison's Principles of Internal Medicine*, 12th edition. New York, McGraw Hill.

MCHRC (Maternal and Child Health Research Consortium) (1997) *Confidential Enquiry into Stillbirths and Deaths in Infancy. 4th Annual Report*. London, MCHRC.

MCHRC (Maternal and Child Health Research Consortium) (2000) *Confidential Enquiry into Stillbirths and Deaths in Infancy. 7th Annual Report*. London, MCHRC.

McKenry, L. & Salerno, E. (1995) *Pharmacology in Nursing*, 19th edition. St.Louis, Mosby.

McKenry, L. & Salerno, E. (1998) *Pharmacology in Nursing*, 20th edition. St.Louis, Mosby.

McKinney, P., Jusszczak, E., Findlay, E. & Smith, K. (1998) Case control study of childhood leukaemia and cancer in Scotland. *BMJ*:316:173–7.

McLaughlin, J. & Thompson, D. (1995) Drugs for the treatment of nausea and vertigo. *Prescriber*:6:9:31–8.

McNamara, J.O. (1996) Drugs effective in the therapy of the epilepsies. In: Hardman, J.G., Limbard, L.E., Molinoff, P.B., Ruddon, R.W. & Gilman, A.G. (ed.) *Goodman & Gilman's: The Pharmacological Basis of Therapeutics*, 9th Edition. New York, McGraw-Hill, 461–86.

McNinch, A. & Tripp, J. (1991) Haemorrhagic disease of the newborn in the British Isles; two year prospective study. *BMJ*:303:1105–9.

McNinch, A., Upton, C., Samuels, M., Shearer, M., McCarthy, P., Tripp, J. & L'E Orme, R. (1985) Plasma concentrations after oral and intramuscular vitamin K1 in neonates. *Archives of Disease in Childhood*:60:814–18.

McQuaid, K. (1995) Alimentary tract. In: Tierney, L., McPhee, S. & Papadakis, M. (eds) *Current Medical Diagnosis and Treatment*. Norwalk, Appleton and Lange.

McRae-Bergeron, C., Andrews, C. & Lupe, P. (1998) The effect of epidural analgesia on the second stage of labor. *AANA (American Association of Nurse Anaesthetists Journal*: 66:2:177–82.

Medawar, C. (1992) *Power and Dependence*. London, Social Audit Ltd.

Medawar, C. (1997) The antidepressant web – marketing depression and making medicines work. *International Journal of Risk & Safety in Medicine*:10:2:75–126.

Mehta, K., Kalkwarf, H., Mimouni, F., Khoury, J. & Tsang, R. (1998) Randomized trial of magnesium administration to prevent hypocalcemia in infants of diabetic mothers. *Journal of Perinatalogy*:18:352–6.

Melzack, R. & Wall, P. (1996) *The Challenge of Pain*. London, Penguin.

Milman, N., Bergholt, T., Byg, K., Eriksen, L. & Graudal, N. (1999) Iron status and iron balance during pregnancy. A critical reappraisal of iron supplementation. *Acta Obstetrica Gynecoligica Scandinavia*:78:9:749–57.

Minerbi-Codish, I., Fraser, D., Avnun, L., Glezerman, M. & Heimer, D. (1998) Influence of asthma in pregnancy on labor and the newborn. *Respiration*:65:130–5.

Mitchelson, F. (1992a) Pharmacological agents affecting emesis: a review (Part I). *Drugs*: 43:295–315.

Mitchelson, F. (1992b) Pharmacological agents affecting emesis: a review (Part II). *Drugs*:43:443–63.

Moldin, P.G. & Sundell, G. (1996) Induction of labour: a randomised clinical trial of amniotomy versus amniotomy with oxytocin infusion. *British Journal of Obstetrics and Gynaecology*:103:306–12.

Moncrieff, J. (1995) Lithium revisited. *British Journal of Psychiatry*:167:569–74.

Montoro, M. (1997) Management of hypothyroidism during pregnancy. *Clinical Obstetrics and Gynecology*:40:1:65–80.

Moore, J. (1993) The effects of analgesia and anaesthesia on the maternal stress response. In: Reynolds, F. (ed.) *Effects on the Baby of Maternal Analgesia and Anaesthesia*. London, Saunders, 148–62.

Moore, S., Turnpenny, P., Quinn, A., Glover, S., Lloyd, D., Montgomery, T. & Dean, J. (2000) A clinical study of 57 children with fetal anticonvulsant syndromes. *Journal of Medical Genetics*:37:489–97.

Morisake, H., Yamamoto, S., Morita, Y., Kotake, Y., Ochiai, R. & Takeda, J. (2000) Hypermagnesemia-induced cardiopulmonary arrest. *Journal of Clinical Anesthesia*:12:224–6.

Morrell, M.J. (1992) Hormones and epilepsy through the lifetime. *Epilepsia*:33:S49–S61.

Morrell, M.J. (1996) The new antiepileptic drugs and women: efficacy, reproductive health, pregnancy and fetal outcome. *Epilepsia*:37(Supplement 6):S34–S44.

Mortola, J.F. (1989) The use of psychotropic agents in pregnancy and lactation: *Psychiatric Clinics of North America*:12:53–68.

Mousa, H., McKinley, C. & Thong, J. (2000) Acute postpartum myocardial infarction after ergometrine administration in a woman with familial hypacholsterolaemia. *British Journal of Obstetrics and Gynaecology*:107:939–40.

MRC Vitamin Study Research Group (1991) Prevention of neural tube defects; results of the MRC vitamin study. *Lancet*:338:132–7.

Muir, H., Writer, D., Douglas, J., Weeks, S., Gambling, D. & MacArthur, A. (1997) Double-blind comparison of epidural ropivacaine 0.25% and bupivacaine 0.25% for the relief of childbirth pain. *Canadian Journal of Anaesthesia*:44:599–604.

Muir, M. (1998) Anticonvulsant agents. In: Williams, B. & Baer, C. (eds) *Essentials of Clinical Pharmacology in Nursing*, 3rd edition. Springhouse, Pennsylvania, Springhouse Corporation, 152–70.

Mulder, E., Derks, J. & Visser, G. (1997) Antenatal corticosteroids therapy and fetal behaviour: a randomised study of the effects of betamethasone and dexamethasone. *British Journal of Obstetrics and Gynaecology*:104:1239–47.

Mulinare, J., Cordero, J.F., Erickson, J.D. & Berry, R.J. (1988) Periconceptual use of multivitamins and the occurrence of neural tube defects. *Journal of the American Medical Association*:260:3141–5.

Munn, M., Groome, L., Atterbury, J., Baker, S. & Hoff, C. (1999) Pneumonia as a complication of pregnancy. *Journal of Maternal and Fetal Medicine*:8:151–4.

Mycek, M., Harvey, R. & Champe, P. (1997) *Pharmacology*. Philadelphia, Lippincott-Raven.

Nachum, Z., Ben-Sholomo, B., Weiner, E. & Shalev, E. (1999) Twice daily versus four times daily insulin dose regimes for diabetes in pregnancy: randomised controlled trial. *BMJ*:319:1223–7.

Nagelhout, J. (1992) General anaesthetic agents. In: Baer, C. & Williams, B. (eds) *Clinical Pharmacology and Nursing*, 2nd edition. Springhouse, Pennsylvania, Springhouse Corporation.

Naidu, S., Payne, A.J., Moodley, J., Hoffmann, M. & Gouws, E. (1996) Randomised study assessing the effect of phenytoin and magnesium sulphate on maternal cerebral circulation in eclampsia using transcranial Doppler ultrasound. *British Journal of Obstetrics and Gynaecology*:103:111–16.

Nash v Eli Lilly & Co (1993) 1 W.L.R. 782.

National Blood Transfusion Service Immunoglobulin Working Party (1991) Recommendations for the use of anti-D immunoglobulin. *Prescribers' Journal*:31:137–45.

Neale, R. (1996) Intrapartum stillbirths and deaths in infancy: the first CESDI report. In: Studd, J. (ed.) *Progress in Obstetrics and Gynaecology: volume 12*. Edinburgh, Churchill Livingstone, 193–214.

Nelson-Piercy, C. (1996) Decisions in prescribing for hypertension in pregnancy. *Prescriber*: 7:2:29–36.

Nelson-Piercy, C. (1997) Hazards of heparin: allergy, heparin-induced thrombocytopenia and osteoporosis. *Ballieres Clinical Obstetrics and Gynaecology*:11:3:489–509.

Nelson-Piercy, C., Letsky, E. & de Swiet, M. (1997) Low-molecular-weight heparin for obstetric thromboprophylaxis. *American Journal of Obstetrics and Gynecology*:176:1062–8.

Nelson-Piercy, C. & Moore-Gillon, J. (1995) Treatment of asthma. In: Rubin, P. (ed.) *Prescribing in Pregnancy*, 2nd edition. London, BMJ Group.

Ngai, S., Chan, Y., Lam, S. & Lao, T. (2000) Labour characteristics and uterine activity. *British Journal of Obstetrics and Gynaecology*:107:222–7.

NHS Executive (1998) *Achieving Effective Practice: A Clinical Effectiveness and Research Instruction Pack for Nurses*. Leeds, NHS Executive.

Nichols, L. (1993) Drug reactions and interactions. In: Spencer, R.T., Nichols, L., Lipkin, G., Henderson, H. & West, F. *Clinical Pharmacology and Nursing Management*. Philadelphia, Lippincott.

Nicolson, P. (1998) *Postnatal Depression Psychology, Science and the Transition to Motherhood*, London, Routledge.

Nickells, J., Vaughan, D., Lillywhite, N., Loughnan, B., Hasan, M. & Robinson, P. (2000) Speed of onset of regional analgesia in labour: a comparison of the epidural and spinal routes. *Anaesthesia*:55:1:17–20.

NIH Consensus Development Panel on the Effect of Corticosteroids for Fetal Maturation on Perinatal Outcomes (1995) Effect of corticosteroids for fetal maturation on perinatal outcomes. *JAMA*:273:413–18.

Nisell, H., Lintu, H., Lunell, N., Mollerstrom, G. & Pettersson, E. (1995) Blood pressure and renal function seven years after pregnancy complicated by hypertension. *British J. of Obstetrics and Gynaecology*:102:876–81.

Nishiguchi, T., Saga, K., Suminoto, K., Okada, K. & Terao, T. (1996) Vitamin K prophylaxis to prevent neonatal vitamin K deficient intercranial haemorrage in Shizuka prefecture. *British Journal of Obstetrics and Gynaecology*:103:1078–84.

Nissen, E., Lilja, G., Matthiesen, A., Pansjo-Arvidsson, A., Unvas-Moberg, K. & Widstrom, A. (1995) Effects of maternal pethidine on infants' developing breast feeding. *Acta Paediatrica*:84:2:140–5.

Nissen, E., Widstrom, A., Lilja, G., Matthiesen, A., Unvas-Moberg, K. & Boreus, J. (1997) Effects of routinely given pethidine during labour on infants' developing breastfeeding behaviour. *Acta Paediatrica*:86:2:201–8.

Niven, C. (1992) *Psychological Care for Families; Before During and After Birth*. Oxford, Butterworth Heinemann.

Nkata, M. (1996) Rupture of uterus: a review of 32 cases in a general hospital in Zambia. *BMJ*:312:1204–5.

Nolan, S. & Scoggin, J.A. (1999) Serotonin syndrome: recognition and management. Http:/www.uspharmacist.com

Nordstrom, L., Fogelstam, K., Fridman, G., Larsson, A. & Rydhstroem, H. (1997) Routine oxytocin in the third stage of labour: a placebo controlled randomised trial. *British Journal of Obstetrics and Gynaecology*:104:781–6.

Norris, M., Grieco, W., Borkowski, M., Leighton, B., Arkoosh, V., Huffnagle, H.J. & Huffnagle, S. (1994) Complications of labor analgesia: epidural versus combined spinal epidural techniques. *Anesthesia and Analgesia*:79:529–37.

Nulman, I., Laslo, D. & Koren, G. (1999) Treatment of epilepsy in pregnancy. *Drugs*:57:535–44.

Nulman, I., Rovet, J., Stewart, D., Wolpin, J., Gardner, H., Jochen, G., Kulin, N. & Koren, G. (1997) Neurodevelopment of children exposed in utero to antidepressant drugs. *New England Journal of Medicine*:336:258–62.

Nurses, Midwives and Health Visitors (Midwives Amendment) Rules 1998, London, UKCC.

Nuutila, M. & Kajanoja, P. (1996) Local administration of prostaglandin E2 for cervical ripening and labor induction: the appropriate route and dose. *Acta Ostetrica et Gynecologica Scandinavica*:75:2:135–8.

Oates, J. (1996) Antihypertensive agents and the drug therapy of hypertension. In: Hardman, J., Limbard, L., Molinoff, P., Ruddon, R. & Goodman Gilman, A. (eds) *Goodman & Gilman's: The Pharmacological Basis of Therapeutics*, 9th edition. New York, McGraw-Hill.

Oates, M. (1988) The development of an integrated community service for severe postnatal mental illness. In: Kumar, S. & Brockington, I. (eds) *Motherhood and Mental Illness*. London, Wright, 133–58.

O'Brien, M.D. & Gilmour-White, S. (1993) Epilepsy and pregnancy. *British Medical Journal*:307:492–5.

O'Connor, R.A. (1995) Induction of labour – not how but why? *British Journal of Hospital Medicine*:52:11:559–63.

Ogueh, O., Khastgir, G., Studd, J., Jones, J., Zadeh, J.A. & Johnson, M. (1998) Antenatal corticosteroid therapy and risk of osteoporosis. *British Journal of Obstetrics and Gynaecology*: 106:977–9.

O'Hara, M. & Swain, A. (1996) Rates and risk of postpartum depression: a meta-analysis. *International Review of Psychiatry*:8:37–54.

Okojie, P. & Cook, P. (1999) Update on some aspects of the use of epidural analgesia in labour. *International Journal of Clinical Practice*:53:6:418–20.

Olah, K. & Gee, H. (1996) The active mismanagement of labour. *British Journal of Obstetrics and Gynaecology*:103:8:729–31.

Olofsson, C., Ekblom, A., Ekman-Ordeberg, G., Hjelm, A. & Irestedt, L. (1996) Lack of analgesic effect of systemically administered morphine or pethidine on labour pain. *British Journal of Obstetrics and Gynaecology*:103:968–72.

Olofsson, C., Ekblom, A., Ekman-Ordeberg, G. & Irestedt, L. (1997) Post-partum urinary retention. *European Journal of Obstetrics, Gynaecology and Reproductive Biology*:71:1:31–4.

Olofsson, C., Ekblom, A., Ekman-Ordeberg, G. & Irestedt, L. (1998) Obstetric outcome following epidural analgesia with bupivacaine-adrenaline 0.25% or bupivacaine 0.125% with sufentanil. *Acta Anaesthesiologica Scandinavia*:42:284–92.

Olofsson, C. & Irestedt, L. (1998) Traditional analgesic agents: are parenteral narcotics passé and do inhalational agents still have a place in labour? *Ballieres Clinical Obstetrics and Gynaecology*:12:3:409–21.

Olsen, K. & D'Oria, L. (1992) Uterine motility agents. In: Baer, C. & Williams, B. (eds) *Clinical Pharmacology and Nursing*. Springhouse, Pennsylvania, Springhouse Corporation.

Olsen, S., Secher, N., Tabor, A., Weber, T., Walker, J. & Gluud, C. (2000) Randomised clinical trials of fish oil supplementation in high risk pregnancies. *British Journal of Obstetrics and Gynaecology*:107:382–95.

Orioli, I. & Castilla, E. (2000) Epidemiological assessment of misoprostol teratogenicity. *British Journal of Obstetrics and Gynaecology*:107:519–23.

Osler, M. (1987) A double blind study comparing meptazinol and pethidine for pain relief in labour. *European Journal of Obstetrics, Gynecology and Reproductive Biology*:26:1:15–18.

Ostrow, C.L. & McCoy, C.A. (1998) Hematinic agents. In: Williams, B. & Baer, C. (eds) *Essentials of Clinical Pharmacology in Nursing*. Springhouse, Pennsylvania, Springhouse Corporation, 301–10.

Palmer, A., Waugaman, W., Conklin, K. & Kotelko, D. (1991) Does the administration of oral Bicitra before elective cesarean section afect the incidence of nausea and vomiting in the parturient? *Nurse Anesthetist*:2:3:126–33.

Pangle, B. (2000) Drugs in pregnancy and lactation. In: Herfindal, E. & Gourley, D. (eds) *Textbook of Therapeutics: Drug and Disease Management*, 7th edition. Philadelphia, Lippincott Williams & Wilkins.

Papatsonis, D., Kok, J., van Geijn, H., Bleker, O., Ader, H. & Dekker, G. (2000) Neonatal effects of nifedipine and ritodrine for preterm labor. *Obstetrics and Gynecology*:95:477–81.

Parker, C. (1996) Pre-pregnancy monitoring for women with diabetes. *Professional Care of Mother and Child*:6:5:135–8.

Parker, L., Cole, M., Craft, A. & Hey, E. (1998) Neonatal vitamin K administration and childhood cancer in the North of England: retrospective case-control study. *BMJ*:316:189–93.

Passmore, S., Draper, G., Brownhill, P. & Kroll, M. (1998a) Case-control studies of relation between childhood cancer and neonatal vitamin K administration. *BMJ*:316:178–84.

Passmore, S., Draper, G., Brownhill, P. & Kroll, M. (1998b) Ecological studies of relation between hospital policies on vitamin K administration and subsequent occurrence of childhood cancer. *BMJ*:316:184–9.

Pattee, C., Ballantyne, M. & Milne, B. (1997) Epidural analgesia for labour and delivery: informed consent issues. *Canadian Journal of Anaesthesia*:44:918–23.

Paul, R.H., Koh, K.S. & Berstein, S.G. (1978) Changes in fetal heart rate-uterine contraction patterns associated with eclampsia. *American Journal of Obstetrics and Gynecology*:130:165–9.

Pearson, J. (1993) Pregnancy and complicated diabetes. *British Journal of Hospital Medicine*:49:10:739–42.

Pedley, T.A., Scheuer, M.L. & Walczak, T.S. (1995) Epilepsy In: Rowlands, L.P. (ed.) *Merrits Textbook of Neurology*, 9th edition. New York, Williams and Wilkins, 845–68.

Perry, C. & Leaper, D. (1994) Care of central venous line exit sites. *Journal of Wound Care*:3:6:279–82.

Perry, K., Morrison, J., Rust, O., Sullivan, C., Martin, R. & Naef, R. (1995) Incidence of adverse cardiopulmonary effects with low-dose continuous terbutaline infusion. *American Journal of Obstetrics and Gynecology*:173:1273–7 .

Perucchini, D., Fischer, U., Spinas, G., Huch, R., Huch, A. & Lehmann, R. (1999) Using fasting plasma glucose concentrations to screen for gestational diabetes mellitus: prospective population based study. *BMJ*:319:812–15.

Peschman, P. (1992) Vitamin, mineral and other nutritional agents. In: Baer, C. & Williams, B. (eds) *Clinical Pharmacology and Nursing*, 2nd edition. Springhouse, Pennsylvania, Springhouse Corporation.

Pfaffenrath, V. & Rehm, M. (1998) Migraine in pregnancy: what are the safest treatment options. *Drug Safety*:19:383–8.

Philipsen, T. & Jensen, N. (1990) Maternal opinion about analgesia in labour and delivery. *European Journal of Obstetrics, Gynecology and Reproductive Biology*:34:3:205–10.

Pickstone, M., Auty, B., Jacklin, A., Langfield, B. & Wootton, R. (1994) Intravenous infusion of drugs. *British Journal of Intensive Care*: November:338–44.

Pinkofsky, H. (1997) Psychosis during pregnancy: treatment considerations. *Annals of Clinical Psychiatry*:9:3:175–9.

Pipkin, F.B., De Swiet, M., Duley, L., Lilford, R., Judd, A., Onwude, J., Prentice, C., Redman, C., Roberts, J. & Walker, J. (1996) Where next for prophylaxis against pre-eclampsia? *British J. of Obstetrics and Gynaecology*:103:603–7.

Pitt, B. (1991) Postnatal depression. *Hospital Update*:17:2:133–40.

Plouin, P., Breart, G., Llado, J., Dalle, M., Keller, M., Goujon, H. & Berchel, C. (1990) A randomized comparison of early with conservative use of antihypertensive drugs in the management of pregnancy-induced hypertension. *British Journal of Obstetrics and Gynaecology*:97:134–41.

Po, A.L.W. & Po, G.L.W. (1992) *OTC Medications*. Oxford, Blackwell Scientific.

Pop, V., Baar, A. & Vulsma, T. (1999) Should all pregnant women be screened for hypothyroidism? *Lancet*:354:1224–5.

Potts, J. (1991) Diseases of the parathyroid gland and other hyper- and hypo-calcaemic disorders. In: Wilson, J., Braunwald, E., Isselbacher, K. et al *Harrison's Principles of Internal Medicine*, 12th edition. New York, McGraw Hill, 1902–21.

Prendergast v Sam & Dee Ltd (1989) 1 Med LR 36.

Prendiville, W., Elbourne, D. & McDonald, S. (2000) Active versus expectant management in the third stage of labour. *Cochrane Database Systematic Review*: (issue 2) Oxford, Update Software. Accessed July 2000.

Prescription Only Medicines (Human Use) Amendment Order 2000 (SI 2000/1917).

Prescrire International (1996) Drug-induced hair loss. *Prescrire International*:5:25:377–9.

Pritchard, J., Cunningham, F. & Pritchard, S. (1984) The Parkland Memorial Hospital protocol for treatment of eclampsia: evaluation of 245 cases. *American Journal of Obstetrics and Gynecology*:148:951–63.

Qarmalawi, A., Morsy, A., Fadly, A., Obeid, A. & Hashem, M. (1995) Labetolol vs. methyldopa in the treatment of pregnancy-induced hypertension. *Int. J Gynaecol. Obstet.*:49:2:125–30.

Rai, R., Cohen, H., Dave, M. & Regan, L. (1997) Randomised controlled trial of aspirin and aspirin plus heparin in pregnant women with recurrent miscarriage associated with phospholipid antibodies. *BMJ*:314:253–7.

Rajan, L. (1993) Perceptions of pain and pain relief in labour: the gulf between theory and observation. *Midwifery*:9:3:136–45.

Rajan, L. (1994) The impact of obstetric procedures and analgesia/anaesthesia during labour and delivery on breast feeding. *Midwifery*:10:2:87–103.

Rang, H., Dale, M. & Ritter, M. (1999) *Pharmacology*, 4th edition. Edinburgh, Churchill Livingstone.

Ranta, P., Spalding, M., Kangas-Saarela, T., Jokela, R., Hollmen, A., Jouppila, P. & Jouppila, R. (1995) Maternal expectations and experiences of labour pain. *Acta Anaesthesiologica Scandinavia*:31:1:60–6.

Rascol, O., Hain, T.C., Brefel, C., Benazet, M., Clanet, M. & Montastruc, J. (1995) Antivertigo medications and drug-induced vertigo. *Drugs*:50:777–91.

Rayburn, W.F. & Conover, E.A. (1993) Non-prescription drugs and pregnancy. In: Studd, J. (ed.) *Progress in Obstetrics and Gynaecology: volume 10*. Edinburgh, Churchill Livingstone, 101–11.

RCN (1996) *Nurses' Involvement in the use of Neuroleptic Drugs.* record no. 000 562 London, Royal College of Nursing (RCN).

Redman, C. & Jefferies, M. (1988) Revised definition of pre-eclampsia. *The Lancet*:1988; 8589:809–12.

Reisine, T. & Pasternak, G. (1996) Opioid analgesics and antagonists. In: Hardman, J., Limbard, L., Molinoff, P., Ruddon, R. & Goodman Gilman, A. (eds) *Goodman & Gilman's: The Pharmacological Basis of Therapeutics*, 9th edition. New York, McGraw-Hill, 521–55.

Renfrew, M., Lang, S. & Woolridge, M. (2000) Oxytocin for promoting successful lactation. *Cochrane Pregnancy and Childbirth Database* (issue 2). Oxford, Update Software.

Review Team on the Prescribing, Supply & Administration of Medicines (CROWN) (1998) *Report on the Supply and Administration of Medicines Under Group Protocols*. London, Department of Health.

Reynolds, F. & Crowhurst, J. (1997) Opioids in labour – no analgesic effect. *Lancet*:349:4–5.

Reynolds, F. (1993a) Pain relief in labour. *British Journal of Obstetrics and Gynaecology*:100:979–83.

Reynolds, F. (1993b) Principles of placental drug transfer. In: Reynolds, F. (ed.) *Effects on the Baby of Maternal Analgesia and Anaesthesia*. London, Saunders, 1–28.

Reynolds, J., Parfitt, K., Parsons, A. & Sweetman, S. (eds) (1996) *Martindale: The Extra Pharmacopoea*, 31st edition. London, Royal Pharmaceutical Society.

Riaz, M., Porat, R., Brodsky, N. & Hurt, H. (1998) The effects of magnesium sulfate treatment on newborns: a prospective controlled study. *Journal of Perinatology*:18:449–54.

Rice, S. (1993) Anaesthesia in pregnancy and the fetus: clinical aspects. In: Reynolds, F. (ed.) *Effects in the Baby of Maternal Analgesia and Anaesthesia*. London, Saunders.

Richardson, M. (2000) Regional anesthesia for obstetrics. *Anesthesiology Clinics of North America*:18:383–406.

Rix, P., Ladehoff, P., Moller, A.M., Tilma, K.A. & Zdravkovic, M. (1996) Cervical ripening and induction of delivery by local administration of prostaglandin E2 gel or vaginal tablets is equally effective. *Acta Ostetrica et Gynecologica Scandinavica*:75:1:45–7.

Roberts, A., Leveno, K., Sidawi, E., Lucas, M. & Kelly, M.A. (1995) Fetal acidaemia associated with regional anesthesia for elective Caesarean delivery. *Obstetrics and Gynecology*:85:1:79–83.

Roberts, J. & Hubel, C. (1999) Is oxidative stress the link in the two-stage model of pre-eclampsia? *Lancet*:354:788–9.

Robertson, R. & Robertson, D. (1996) Drugs used for the treatment of myocardial ischaemia. In: Hardman, J., Limbard, L., Molinoff, P., Ruddon, R. & Goodman Gilman, A. (eds) *Goodman & Gilman's: The Pharmacological Basis of Therapeutics*, 9th edition. New York, McGraw-Hill.

Robson, S.C. (1996) Magnesium sulphate: the time of reckoning. *British Journal of Obstetrics and Gynaecology*:103:99–102.

Robson, S., Lee, D. & Urbaniak, S. (1998) Anti-D immunoglobulin in RhD prophylaxis. *British Journal of Obstetrics and Gynaecology*:105:129–34.

Roche (1995) Konakion *ABPI Data sheet Compendium*. London, Datapharm Publications, 1437–8.

Rodger, M. & King, L. (2000) Drawing up and administering intramuscular injections: a review of the literature. *Journal of Advanced Nursing*:31:3:574–82.

Rogers, C. (1995) *The Women's Guide to Herbal Medicine*. London, BCA.

Rogers, J., Wood, J., McCandish, R., Ayers, S., Truesdale, A. & Elbourne, D. (1998) Active versus expectant management of third stage of labour. *Lancet*:351:693–9.

Rogers, R., Gilson, G., Miller, A., Izquierdo, L., Curet, L. & Qualls, C. (1997) Active Management of labor: does it make a difference? *American Journal of Obstetrics and Gynecology*.177:599–605.

Ross, E. (1996) Pharmacodynamics. In: Hardman, J., Limbard, L., Molinoff, P., Ruddon, R. & Goodman Gilman, A. (eds) *Goodman & Gilman's: The Pharmacological Basis of Therapeutics*, 9th edition. New York, McGraw-Hill.

Ross, S. & Soltes, D. (1995) Heparin and haematoma: does ice make a difference? *Journal of Advanced Nursing*.21:434–9.

Rotchell, Y., Cruickshank, J., Gay, M.P., Griffiths, J., Stewart, A., Farrell, B., Ayers, S., Hennis, A., Grant, A., Duley, L. & Collins, R. (1998) Barbados low dose aspirin study in pregnancy: a randomised trial for the prevention of pre-eclampsia and its complications. *British Journal of Obstetrics and Gynaecology*.105:286–92.

Rothman, K., Moore, L., Singer, M., Nguyen, U., Mannino, S. & Milunsky, A. (1995) Teratogenicity of high vitamin a intake. *New England Journal of Medicine*:333:1369–73.

Rowem, T.F. (1997) Acute gastric aspiration. *Seminars in Perinatology*.21:4:313–19.

Royal College of Psychiatrists (1996) *A Handbook on Perinatal Maternal Mental Health Services*. London, Royal College of Psychiatrists.

Rubin, P. (1995) General Principles. In: Rubin, P. (ed.) *Prescribing in Pregnancy*, 2nd edition. London, BMJ Group.

Rubin, P. (1996) Management of pre-existing disorders in pregnancy: principles of prescribing. *Prescribers' Journal*:36:1:21–7.

Rude, R. & Oldham, S. (1990) Disorders of magnesium metabolism. In: Cohen, R., Lewis, B., Alberti, K. & Denman, A. (eds) *The Metabolic and Molecular Basis of Acquired Disease*. London, Bailliere Tindall.

Ruigomez, A., Rodriguez, G.L., Cattatuzzi, C. & Troncon, M. (1999) Use of cimetidine, omeprazole and ranitidine in pregnant women and pregnancy outcomes. *American Journal of Epidemiology*.150:476–81.

Russell, R., Groves, P., Taub, N., O'Dowd, J. & Reynolds, F. (1993) Assessing long term backache after childbirth. *BMJ*:306:1299–303.

Russell, S. & Doyle, E. (1997) Paediatric anaesthesia. *BMJ*:314:201–3.

Rutishauser, S. (1994) *Physiology and Anatomy*. Edinburgh, Churchill Livingstone.

S.I. (1830) Prescription Only Medicines (Human Use) Order 1997.

Sackett, D., Haynes, R.B., Guyatt, G. & Tugwell, P. (1991) *Clinical Epidemiology: a Basic Science for Clinical Medicine*, 2nd edition. Boston, Little, Brown.

Sadler, L., Davison, T. & McCowan, L. (2000) A randomised controlled trial and meta-analysis of active manaement of labour. *British Journal of Obstetrics and Gynaecology*.107:909–15.

Sadler, L., McCowan, L., White, H., Stewart, A. Bracken, M. & North, R. (2000) Pregnancy outcomes and cardiac complications in women with mechanical, bioprosthetic and homograft valves. *British Journal of Obstetrics and Gynaecology*.107:245–53.

Saeb-Parsy, K., Assomul, R., Khan, F., Saeb-Parsey, K. & Kelly, E. (1999) *Instant Pharmacology*. Chichester, Wiley.

Safari, H., Fassett, M., Souter, I., Alsulyman, O. & Goodwin, T. (1998) The efficacy of methylprednisolone in the treatment of hyperemesis gravidarum. *American Journal of Obstetrics and Gynecology*.179:921–4.

Salama, A., Kiefel, V. & Mueller-Eckhardt, C. (1986) The effect of Ig G anti-Rh$_0$ (D) in adult patients with chronic autoimmune thrombocytopenia. *American Journal of Hematology*. 22:241.

Sanchez-Ramos, L., Kaunitz, A., Gaudier, F. & Delke, I. (1999) Efficacy of maintenance therapy after acute tocolysis. *American Journal of Obstetrics and Gynecology*.181:484–90.

Sandoz (1995) Syntocinon parenteral solution. In: *ABPI Data Sheet Compendium*. London, Datapharm Publications Limited.

Sawle, G. (1995) Epilepsy and anti-convulsant drugs. In: Rubin, P. (ed.) *Prescribing in Pregnancy*, 2nd edition. London, BMJ Group.

Schaefer-Graf, U., Buchanan, T., Xiang, A., Songster, G., Montoro, M. & Kjos, S. (2000) Patterns of congenital anomalies and relationship to initial maternal fasting glucose levels in pregnancies complicated by type 2 and gestational diabetes. *American Journal of Obstetrics & Gynecology*:182:313–20.

Schatz, M. (1999) Asthma and pregnancy. *The Lancet*:353:1202–4.

Schatz, M., Zeiger, R., Harden, K., Hoffman, C.C., Chilingar, L. & Petitti, D. (1997) The safety of asthma and allergy medications during pregnancy. *Journal of Allergy and Clinical Immunology*:100:3:301–6.

Scholz, J., Steinfath, M. & Schulz, M. (1996) Clinical pharmacokinetics of alfentanil, fentanyl and sufentanil. *Clinical Pharmacokinetics*:31:275–92.

Schou, M. & Vestergaard, P. (1996) Lithium treatment problems and precautions. In Burrows, G., Norman, T. & Davies, B. (eds) *Antidepressants*. Amsterdam, Elsevier.

Schwartz, L. (1998) Infertility and pregnancy in epileptic women. *Lancet*:352:1952–3.

Serafin, W. (1996) Drugs used in the treatment of asthma. In: Hardman, J., Limbard, L., Molinoff, P., Ruddon, R. & Goodman Gilman, A. (eds) *Goodman & Gilman's: The Pharmacological Basis of Therapeutics*, 9th edition. New York, McGraw-Hill.

Shafik, A. (1993) Constipation: pathogenesis and management. *Drugs*:45:4:528–40.

Shah, D. & Reed, G. (1996) Parameters associated with adverse perinatal outcome in hypertensive pregnancies. *J. Human Hypertension*:10:8:511–15.

Sharma, P., Day, J. & Webster, S. (1995) Dangerous side-effect of neuroleptic therapy. *Hospital Update*:21:8:374–6.

Shatrugna, V., Raman, L., Kailash, U., Balakrishna, N. & Rao, K. (1999) Effect of dose and formulation on iron tolerance in pregnancy. *National Medical Journal of India*:12:1:18–20.

Sheenan, A., Cooke, V., Lloyd-Jones, F., Morgan, B. & de Swiet, M. (1995) Blood pressure changes during labour and whilst ambulating with combined spinal epidural analgesia. *British Journal of Obstetrics and Gynaecology*:102:192–7.

Sheikh, A. & Tunstall, M. (1986) Comparative study of meptazinol and pethidine for the relief of pain in labour. *British Journal of Obstetrics and Gynaecology*:93:264–9.

Sheiner, E., Shoham, I., Sheiner, E., Press, F., Ram, R., Mazor, M. & Katz, M. (2000) A comparison between the effectiveness of epidural analgesia and parenteral pethidine during labor. *Archives of Gynecology and Obstetrics*:263:3:95–8.

Shuster, J. (1995) Double diuresis? Drug fever and Jarisch-Herxheimer reaction. *Hospital Pharmacy*:30:12:1123–4.

Shyken, J. & Petrie, R. (1995) Oxytocin to induce labor. *Clinical Obstetrics and Gynecology*: 38:2:232–45.

Sibai, B. (1996) Treatment of hypertension in pregnant women. *The New England Journal of Medicine*:335:257–65.

Sibai, B. (1998) Prevention of preeclampsia: a big disappointment. *American Journal of Obstetrics and Gynecology*:179:1275–8.

Silverstone, T. & Romans, S. (1996) Long term treatment of bipolar disorder. *Drugs*:51:367–82.

Silverton, L. (1993) *The Art and Science of Midwifery*. London, Prentice Hall.

Simmons, D. (1997) Persistently poor pregnancy outcomes in women with insulin dependent diabetes. *BMJ*:315:263–4.

Simpkin, P. (1989) Non-pharmacological methods of pain relief during labour. In Chalmers, I., Enkin, M. & Kierse, M.J.N.C. (eds) *Effective Care in Pregnancy and Childbirth*. Oxford, Oxford Medical, 893–912.

Smith, A. (1997) Prescribing iron. *Prescribers' Journal*:37:2:82–7.

Smith, G., Kingdom, J., Penning, D. & Matthews, S. (2000) Antenatal corticosteroids: is more better? *Lancet*:355:251–2.

Smith, G. & McEwan, H. (1997) Use of magnesium sulphate in Scottish obstetric units. *British Journal of Obstetrics and Gynaecology*:104:115–16.

Smith, G.N. & Piercy, W.N. (1995) Methyldopa toxicity in pregnancy: a case report. *Am J. Obstet Gynecol.*:172:1 pt.1:222–4.

Smith, P., Anthony, J. & Johanson, R. (2000) Nifedipine in pregnancy. *British Journal of Obstetrics and Gynaecology*:107:299–307.

Smith v Brighton & Lewes Hospital Management Committee (1958).

Smithells, R.W., Shepherd, S., Schorah, C. et al (1980) Possible prevention of neural-tube defects by periconceptual vitamin supplementation. *Lancet*:1980;8164:339–40.

Soares, J., Dornhorstt, A. & Beard, R. (1997) The case for screening for gestational diabetes. *BMJ*:315:737–9.

Solvay Healthcare Limited (1995) Yutopar® *ABPI Data Sheet Compendium*. London, Datapharm Publications Limited.

Solves, P., Altes, A., Ginovart, G., Demestre, J. & Fontcuberta, J. (1997) Late haemorrhagic disease of the newborn as a cause of intracerebral bleeding. *Annals of Haematology*:75:65–6.

Soriano, D., Dulitzki, M., Schiff, E., Barkai, G., Mashiach, S. & Seidman, D. (1996) A prospective cohort study of oxytocin plus ergometrine compared with oxytocin alone for prevention of postpartum haemorrhage. *British J. of Obstetrics and Gynaecology*:103:1068–73.

Spencer, J. (1995) The management of term labour. *Archives of Disease in Childhood*:72:F55–61.

Spencer, R. (1993) Agents affecting the upper gastrointestinal tract. In: Spencer, R., Nichols, L., Lipkin, G., Henderson, H. & West, F. (eds) *Clinical Pharmacology and Nursing Management*, 4th edition. Philadelphia, Lippincott.

Spencer, R. et al (1993) *Clinical Pharmacology and Nursing Management*, 4th edition. Philadelphia Lippincott Co.

Spencer, R.T. (1993a) Interactions between food and medications. In Spencer, R.T., Nicolls, L., Lipkin, G., Henderson, H. & West, F. (eds) *Clinical Pharmacology and Nursing Management* Philadelphia, Lippincott, 109–23.

Spencer, R.T. (1993b) Agents affecting the lower gastro-intestinal tract. In: Spencer, R.T., Nichols, L., Lipkin, G., Henderson, H. & West, F. *Clinical Pharmacology and Nursing Management*. Philadelphia, Lippincott.

Springhouse Corporation (1999) *Medication Teaching Aids*. Springhouse, Pennsylvania.

Stables, D. (1999) *Physiology in Childbearing*. London, Bailliere Tindall.

Standing Medical Advisory Committee (1976a) *Haemolytic Disease of the Newborn*. London, Department of Health and Social Security.

Standing Medical Advisory Committee (1976b) (1982) *Memorandum on Haemolytic Disease of the Newborn: Addenden 1981* London, Department of Health and Social Security.

Steel, J. & Johnstone, F. (1996) Guidelines for the management of insulin-dependent diabetes mellitus. *Drugs*:52:60–70.

Steer, P. & Flint, C. (1999a) Physiology and management of normal labour. *BMJ*:318:793–6.

Steer, P. & Flint, C. (1999b) Preterm labour and premature rupture of membranes. *BMJ*:318:1059–62.

Steer, P. (1995) Recent Advances: Obstetrics. *BMJ*:311:1209–12.

Steer, P. (1999) Management of preterm labour. Author's reply. *BMJ*:319:257.

Stern, K., Goodmand, H. & Berger, M. (1961) Experimental immunization of haemo-antigens in man. *Journal of Immunology*:87:189–98.

Stewart, D., Klompenhouwer, J., Kendell, R. & van Hulst, A. (1991) Prophylactic lithium in puerperal psychosis the experience of three centres. *British Journal of Psychiatry*:158:393–7.

Stienstra, R., Jonker, T., Bourdrez, P., Kuijpers, J., van Kleef, J.W. & Lundberg, U. (1995) Ropivacaine 0.25% versus bupivacaine 0.25% for continuous epidural analgesia in labor: a double-blind comparison. *Obstetric Anesthesia*:80:285–9.

Stock, M. (1992) Pituitary agents. In: Baer, C. & Williams, B. (eds) *Clinical Pharmacology and Nursing*, 2nd edition. Springhouse, Pennsylvania, Springhouse Corporation.

Stockley, I. (1999) *Drug Interactions*, 5th edition. Oxford Blackwell Science.

Suri, R.A., Altshuler, L., Burt, V.K. & Hendrick, V.C. (1998) Managing psychiatric medications in the breast-feeding woman. *Medscape Women's Health*, 3[1]: 1 Medscape inc. at http://womenshealth.medscape.com/M

Swartjes, J.M. & Van Geijn, H.P. (1998) Pregnancy and epilepsy. *European Journal of Obstetrics, Gynecology and Reproductive Biology*:79:1:3–11.

Swonger, A. & Matejski, M. (1991) *Nursing Pharmacology*, 2nd edition. Philadelphia, Lippincott.

Szal, S., Croughan-Minihane, M. & Kilpatrick, S. (1999) Effect of magnesium prophylaxis and pre-eclampsia on the duration of labor. *American Journal of Obstetrics and Gynecology*. 180:1475–9.

T (A Minor) v Luton & Dunstable Hospital NHS Trust (Unreported, 23 November 1998).

Tan, B. & Hannah, M. (2000) Prostaglandins versus oxytocin for prelabour rupture of membranes at or near term. *Cochrane Database Systematic Review*: (issue 2) Oxford, Update Software. Accessed July 2000.

Tan, L. & Tay, S. (1999) Two dosing regimens for preinduction cervical priming with intravaginal dinoprostone pessary: a randomised clinical trial. *British Journal of Obstetrics and Gynaecology*:106:907–12.

Tay, D., Yeo, S., Chan, S. & Thomas, E. (1994) Continuous spinal analgesia. *Singapore Medical Journal*:35:1:44–6.

Taylor, G. & Cohen, B. (1985) Ergonovine-induced coronary artery spasm and myocardial infarction after normal delivery. *Obstetrics & Gynecology*:66:6:821–2.

Taylor, R. & Taylor, M. (1988) Misuse of oxytocin in labour. *Lancet*:1988;i:352.

Thapa, P., Whitlock, J., Worrell, K., Gideon, P., Mitchel, E., Roberson, P., Pais, R. & Ray, W. (1998) Prenatal exposure to metronidazole and risk of childhood cancer. *Cancer*:83:1461–8.

Thomas, D., Petitti, D., Goldhaber, M., Swan, S., Rappaport, E. & Hertz-Picciotto, I. (1992) Reproductive outcomes in relation to malathion spraying in the San Francisco Bay Area. *Epidemiology*:3:1:32–9.

Thompson, A. & Hillier, V. (1994) A re-evaluation of the effect of pethidine on the length of labour. *Journal of Advanced Nursing*:19:448–56.

Thomson, A., Walker, I. & Greer, I. (1998) Low-molecular weight heparin for immediate management of thromboembolic disease in pregnancy. (letter) *Lancet*:352:1904.

Thornton, J.G. (1996) Active management of labour. *BMJ*:313:378.

Thornton, J.G. (2000) Prophylactic anticonvulsants for pre-eclampsia. *British Journal of Obstetrics and Gynaecology*:107:839–40 .

Thorp, J., Hu, D., Albin, R., McNitt, J., Meyer, B., Cohen, G. & Yeast, J. (1993) The effect of intrapartum epidural analgesia on nulliparous labor: a randomised, controlled, prospective trial. *American Journal of Obstetrics and Gynecology*:169:851–8.

Toglia, M. & Weg, J. (1996) Venous thromboembolism during pregnancy. *New England Journal of Medicine*:335:2:108–14.

Torrance, C. & Jordan, S. (1996) Bionursing: the management of migraine and vomiting. *Nursing Standard*:19:10:40–2.

Tortora, G. & Grabowski, S. (2000) *Principles of Anatomy and Physiology*. New York, Wiley.

Traynor, J., Dooley, S., Seyb, S., Wong, C. & Shadron, A. (2000) Is the management of epidural analgesia associated with an increased risk of cesarean delivery? *American Journal of Obstetrics and Gynecology*:182:1058–62.

Tryba, M. & Kulka, P. (1993) Critical care pharmacotherapy. *Drugs*:45:338–52.

Tsang, R., Chen, I., Friedman, M., Gigger, M., Steichen, J., Koffler, H., Fenton, L., Brown, D., Pramanik, A., Keenan, W., Strub, R. & Joyce, T. (1975) Parathyroid function in infants of diabetic mothers. *Journal de Pediatria*:86:399–404.

Tugwell, C. & Barrett, C. (1995) Do chloramphenicol drops cause blood dyscrasias? *Update*:21:7:98.

Turner, J., Deyo, R., Loeser, J., von Korff, M. & Fordyce, W. (1994) The importance of placebo effects in pain treatment and research. *JAMA*:271:1609–14.

Twycross, R. (1994) *Pain Relief in Advanced Cancer*. Edinburgh, Churchill Livingstone.

United Kingdom Central Council for Nursing, Midwifery and Health Visiting (UKCC) (1992) *Standards for the Administration of Medicines*. London, UKCC.

UKCC (1998) *Midwives Rules and Code of Practice*. London: UKCC.

Ulrich, M., Kristoffersen, K., Rolschau, J., Grinsted, P., Schaumbrug, E. & Foged, N. (1999) The influence of folic acid supplement on the outcome of pregnancies in the county of Funen in Denmark. Part III. Congenital anomalies. An observational study. *European Journal of Obstetrics, Gynecology and Reproductive Biology*:87:2:115–18.

Upjohn (1990a) Hemabate TM sterile solution, carboprost tromethamine. *Drug Reference*. Crawley, Upjohn.

Upjohn (1990b) Prostin E2 tm oral tablets, vaginal tablets, vaginal gel, prepidil gel (dinoprostone). *Drug Reference*. Crawley, Upjohn.

Upjohn (1995) *ABPI Data Sheet Compendium*. London, Datapharm Publications, 1886–90.

Urbaniak, S.J. (1998) Consensus conference on anti-D prophylaxis. *British Journal of Obstetrics and Gynaecology*:105:18.

Valenzuela, G., Ramos, S.L., Romero, R., Silver, H., Koltun, W., Millar, L., Hobbins, J. & Rayburn, W. (2000) Maintenance treatment of preterm labor with the oxytocin antagonist atosiban. *American Journal of Obstetrics and Gynecology*:182:1184–90.

van Dijk, K.G., Dekker, G. & van Geijn, H.P. (1995) Ritodrine and nifedipine as tocolytic agents: a preliminary comparison. *Journal of Perinatal Medicine*:23:5:409–15.

van Dongen, P. & de Groot, A. (1995) History of ergot alkaloids. *European Journal of Gynecology and Reproductive Biology*:60:109–16.

Van Way, C. (1999) *Nutrition Secrets*. Philadelphia, Hanley & Belfus.

Vaughan, N. (1995) Treatment of diabetes. In: Rubin, P. (ed.) *Prescribing in Pregnancy*, 2nd edition. London, BMJ Group, 136–46.

Vesalainen, R., Ekholm, E., Jartii, T., Tahvanainen, K., Kaila, T. & Erkkola, R. (1999) Effects of tocolytic treatment with ritodrine on cardiovascular autonomic regulation. *British Journal of Obstetrics and Gynaecology*:106:238–43.

von Dadelszen, P., Ornstein, M., Bull, S., Logan, A., Koren, G. & Magee, L. (2000) Fall in mean arterial pressure and fetal growth restriction in pregnancy hypertension: a meta-analysis. *Lancet*:355:87–92.

Von Kries, R., Gobel, U., Hachmeister, A., Kaletsch, U. & Michaelis, J. (1996) Vitamin K and childhood cancer: a population based case-control study in Lower Saxony. *BMJ*:313:199–203.

Vutyavanich, T., Wongtra-ngan, S. & Ruangsri, R. (1995) Pyridoxine for nausea and vomiting of pregnancy. *American Journal of Obstetrics and Gynaecology*:173:881–4.

Wagner, M. (1993) Research shows medication of pain is not safe. *MIDIRS Midwifery Digest*:3:3:307–9.

Wald, N.J. & Bower, C. (1995) Folic acid and the prevention of neural tube defects, *BMJ*:310:1019–20 .

Waldenstrom, U. (1999) Experience of labor and birth in 1111 women. *Journal of Psychosomatic Research*:47:471–82.

Walker, J. (1996) Care of the patient with severe pregnancy induced hypertension. *Eur J. Obstet. Gynecol Reprod Biol*:65:1:127–35.

Walker, J. (2000) Severe pre-eclampsia and eclampsia. *Baillieres Best Practice and Research: Clinical Obstetrics and Gynecology*:14:1:57–71.

Walker, N. & O'Brien, B. (1999) The relationship between method of pain management during labor and birth outcomes. *Clinical Nursing Research*:8:119–34.

Walker v South Surrey District Health Authority (1982) CAT, 17 June 1982.

Walkinshaw, S. (2000) Very tight versus tight control for diabetes in pregnancy. *Cochrane Database Systematic Review*: (issue 2) Update Software, Oxford, Accessed July 2000.

Wallace, E., Chapman, J., Stenson, B. & Wright, S. (1997) Antenatal corticosteroid prescribing: setting standards of care. *British Journal of Obstetrics and Gynaecology*:104:1262–6.

Walley, R., Wilson, J., Crane, J., Matthews, K., Sawyer, E. & Hutchens, D. (2000) A double blind placebo controlled randomised trial of misoprostol and oxytocin in the management of the third stage of labour. *British Journal of Obstetrics and Gynaecology*:107:1111–15.

Warkentin, T., Levine, M., Hirsh, J., Horsewood, P., Roberts, R., Tech, M., Gent, M. & Kelton, J. (1995) Heparin-induced thrombocytopenia in patients treated with low-molecular weight heparin or unfractionated heparin. *New England Journal of Medicine*:332:1330–5.

Weiss, G., Klein, S., Shenkman, L., Kataoka, K. & Hollander, C. (1975) Effect of methylergonovine on puerperal prolactin secretion. *Obstetrics and Gynecology*:46:2:209–10.

Welsh Drug Information Centre (1996) Head Lice. *Drug Information Bulletin*. No 2., Cardiff.

Welsh Office (1996) *Helping Practitioners Use the Evidence: A Clinical Effectiveness Initiative for Wales*. Cardiff, Welsh Office.

Wendel, P., Ramin, S., Barnett-Hamm, C., Rowe, T. & Cunningham, F. (1996) Asthma treatment in pregnancy: a randomised controlled study. *American Journal of Obstetrics and Gynecology*:175:150–4.

Werler, M., Hayes, C., Louik, C., Shapiro, S. & Mitchell, A. (1999) Multivitamin supplementation and risk of birth defects. *American Journal of Epidemiology*:150:7:675–82.

West, F. (1993) Toxicology. In: Spencer, R.T., Nichols, L.W., Lipkin, G.B., Henderson, H.S. & West, F. *Clinical Pharmacology and Nursing Management*, Philadelphia, Lippincott.

Whitehouse v Jordan (1981) 1 WLR 246.

Wildsmith, J. (1996) Routes of drug administration: intrathecal and epidural injection, *Prescribers' Journal*:36:2:110–15.

Williams, F.L., Florey, C., Ogston, S., Patel, N., Howie, P. & Tindall, V. (1998) UK Study of intrapartum care for low risk primigravidas: a survey of interventions. *Journal of Epidemiology and Community Health*:52:494–500.

Williams, G. (1991) Hypertensive vascular disease. In: Wilson, J., Braunwald, E., Isselbacher, K., Petersdorf, R., Martin, J., Fauci, A. & Root, R. (eds) (1991) *Harrison's Principles of Internal Medicine*. 12th edition. New York, McGraw-Hill.

Wilson, J. (1994) Preventing infection during iv therapy. *Professional Nurse*:9:3:388–92.

Wisner, K., Gelenberg, A., Leonard, H., Zarin, D. & Frank, E. (1999) Pharmacologic treatment of depression during pregnancy. *JAMA*:282:1264–9.

Witlin, A., Friedman, S. & Sibai, B. (1997) The effect of magnesium sulfate therapy on the duration of labor in women with mild preeclampsia at term: a randomised, double-blind placebo-controlled trial. *American Journal of Obstetrics and Gynecology*:176:623–7.

Wong, C., Walsh, L., Smith, C., Wisniewski, A., Lewis, S., Hubbard, R., Cawte, S., Green, D., Pringle, M. & Tattersfield, A. (2000) Inhaled corticosteroid use and bone mineral density in patients with asthma. *Lancet*:355:1399–403.

Writer, W., Stienstra, R., Eddleston, J., Gatt, S., Griffin, R. & Gutsche, B. (1998) Neonatal outcome and mode of delivery after epidural analgesia for labout with ropivacaine and bupivacaine: a prospective meta-analysis. *British Journal of Anasesthesia*:81:5:713–17.

Xenakis, E.M. & Piper, J.M. Chemotherapeutic induction of labour. A rational approach. *Drugs*:54:61–8.

Yerby, M. (2000) Pharmacological methods of pain relief. In: Yerby, M. & Page, L. (eds) *Pain in Childbearing*. Edinburgh, Bailliere Tindall, 111–30.

Yerby, M. & Page, L. (2000) (eds) *Pain in Childbearing*. Edinburgh, Bailliere Tindall.

Yoshida, K., Smith, B. & Kumar, R. (1999) Psychotropic drugs in mothers' milk: a comprehensive review of assay methods, pharmacokinetics and of safety of breast feeding, *Journal of Psychopharmacology*:13:1:64–80.

Yuen, P., Chan, N., Yim, S. & Chang, A. (1995) A randomised double blind comparison of syntometrine and syntocinon in the management of the third stage of labour. *British Journal of Obstetrics and Gynaecology*:102:377–80.

Zelcer, J., Owers, H. & Paull, D. (1989) A controlled oximetric evaluation of inhalational, opioid and epidural analgesia in labour. *Anaesthesia and Intensive Care*:17:4:418–21.

Zimmerman, S.A., Malinoski, F.J. & Ware, R.E. (1998) Immunologic effects of anti-D (Win Rho-SD) in children with immune thrombocytopenic purpura. *American Journal of Haematology*:57:2:131–8.

Zipursky, A. (1996) Vitamin K at birth. *BMJ*:313:179–80.

Index

Page numbers in *italics* refer to the 'quick reference' lists in Appendix I. Asterisks (*) against page numbers indicate entries in the glossary.